# Soft Tissue Injuries: Diagnosis and Treatment

# Soft Tissue Injuries: Diagnosis and Treatment

*Editors*

**Robert E. Windsor, MD**
Assistant Clinical Professor
Department of Physical Medicine and Rehabilitation
Emory University School of Medicine
Medical Director, Georgia Spine & Sports Physicians, P.C.
Atlanta, Georgia

**Dennis M. Lox, MD**
Medical Director
Florida Spine & Sports Medicine Center
Clearwater, Florida

HANLEY & BELFUS, INC./Philadelphia

HANLEY & BELFUS, INC. / Philadelphia

Publisher:      HANLEY & BELFUS, INC.
                Medical Publishers
                210 South 13th Street
                Philadelphia, PA 19107
                (215) 546-7293; 800-962-1892
                FAX (215) 790-9330
                Website: http://www.hanleyandbelfus.com

**Library of Congress Cataloging-in-Publication Data**

Soft tissue injuries: diagnosis and treatment / Robert E. Windsor.
  Dennis Lox.
      p.  cm.
  Includes bibliographical references and index.
  ISBN 1-56053-212-2 (alk. paper)
  1. Soft tissue injuries.   I. Windsor, Robert E., 1961–
II. Lox, Dennis, 1959-     .
    [DNLM: 1. Soft Tissue Injuries—diagnosis.  2. Soft Tissue
Injuries—therapy.   3. Pain—therapy.    WO 700 S681 1997]
RD93 . S64  1997
617 . 1—dc21
DNLM/DLC                                          97-13858
for Library of Congress                               CIP

**Soft Tissue Injuries: Diagnosis and Treatment**          ISBN 1-56053-212-2

© 1998 by Hanley & Belfus, Inc. All rights reserved. No part of this book may be reproduced, reused, republished, or transmitted in any form, or stored in a data base or retrieval system, without written permission of the publisher.

Last digit is the print number:   9   8   7   6   5   4   3   2   1

*Dedication*

This book is dedicated to my loving wife Sue and my children, Blake, "B.J.," Tyler, Austin, and Justin. Without their support and encouragement, this book would not have become a reality.—REW

I wish to dedicate this book to my family and friends who encouraged me to proceed. It has become for me a symbol of hard work, honor, and integrity—qualities I find in them.—DML

# Contents

# Contributors

**David B. Adams, PhD**
Private practice, Atlanta Medical Psychology, Atlanta, Georgia

**Stephen A. Andrade, MD**
Private practice, Oklahoma City, Oklahoma

**Richard Paul Bonfiglio, MD**
Assistant Professor, Department of Physical Medicine and Rehabilitation, Jefferson Medical College of Thomas Jefferson University, Philadelphia, Pennsylvania

**Christopher R. Brown, DDS, MPS**
Director, Facial Pain Clinic, Decatur County Memorial Hospital, Greensburg, Indiana

**Roger Kenneth Cady, MD**
Director, Headache Care Center, Columbia Hospital North and Columbia Hospital South; Lester E. Cox Medical Centers, Springfield, Missouri

**Krystal W. Chambers, MD**
Fellow, Georgia Spine & Sports Physicians, P.C., Atlanta, Georgia

**Andrew J. Cole, MD**
Clinical Assistant Professor, Department of Physical Medicine & Rehabilitation, Department of Physical Therapy, University of Texas Southwestern Medical Center, Dallas, Texas; Medical Director, Spine Center, Overlake Hospital Medical Center, Bellevue; Puget Sound Sports and Spine Physicians, Seattle, Washington

**L. Anita Cone, MD**
Georgia Spine & Sports Physicians, P.C., Atlanta, Georgia

**David C. Craddock, JD, LLM**
In-house Counsel, Georgia Spine & Sports Physicians, P.C., Atlanta, Georgia

**Susan J. Dreyer, MD**
Assistant Professor of Physical Medicine and Rehabilitation, and Orthopaedic Surgery, The Emory Spine Center, Emory University School of Medicine, Atlanta, Georgia

**Paul Dreyfuss, MD**
Clinical Associate Professor, Department of Rehabilitation Medicine, University of Texas Health Science Center, San Antonio; East Texas Medical Center and Mother Frances Hospitals, and Spine Specialists, P.A., Tyler, Texas

**Frank J.E. Falco, MD**
Clinical Assistant Professor, Department of Physical Medicine and Rehabilitation, Temple University School of Medicine, Philadelphia, Pennsylvania; Comprehensive Spine & Sports Medicine, P.A., Wilmington, Delaware

**Kathleen Usher Farmer, PsyD**
Adjunct Faculty, Forest Institute of Professional Psychology, and Administrator, Headache Care Center, Springfield, Missouri

**Andrew A. Fischer, MD, PhD**
Associate Clinical Professor, Department of Rehabilitation Medicine, Mount Sinai School of Medicine (CUNY), New York; Chief, Rehabilitation Medicine, Veterans Affairs Medical Center, Bronx, New York

**Lawrence W. Frank, MD**
Illinois Spine & Sports Care Centers, Ltd., Bloomingdale, Illinois

**Gary Goldberg, MD**
Co-director, Electrodiagnostic Center, Moss Rehabilitation Hospital; Associate Professor, Department of Physical Medicine and Rehabilitation, Temple University School of Medicine, Philadelphia, Pennsylvania

**Stanley A. Herring, MD**
Puget Sound Sports and Spine Physicians, Seattle; Clinical Associate Professor, Departments of Rehabilitation Medicine and Orthopaedics, University of Washington School of Medicine, Seattle, Washington; Team Physician, Seattle Seahawks

**Francis P. Lagattuta, MD**
Assistant Clinical Professor, Department of Physical Medicine and Rehabilitation, Loyola University Medical Center, Maywood, Illinois

**Jonathan P. Lester, MD**
Georgia Spine & Sports Physicians, P.C., Atlanta, Georgia

**Dennis M. Lox, MD**
Medical Director, Florida Spine & Sports Medicine Center, Clearwater, Florida

**Terry L. Nicola, MD**
Assistant Professor, Director of Sports Medicine Rehabilitation, Department of Rehabilitation Medicine and Restorative Sciences, University of Illinois College of Medicine, Chicago, Illinois; Associate Team Physician, University of Illinois Flames

**Steve Opersteny, MD, PT**
Associate Professor, Department of Surgery, Texas A&M University College of Medicine, College Station, Texas

**Terry C. Sawchuk, MD**
Intermountain Spine Institute, Salt Lake City, Utah

**Curtis W. Slipman, MD**
Director, Penn Spine Center; Assistant Professor, Department of Rehabilitation Medicine, University of Pennsylvania Medical Center, Philadelphia, Pennsylvania

**Steven A. Stratton, PhD, PT, ATC**
Clinical and Associate Professor, Departments of Physical Medicine and Rehabilitation and Physical Therapy, University of Texas Health Science Center at San Antonio, San Antonio, Texas

**Ronald VanDernoord, MD**
Fellow, Georgia Spine & Sports Physicians, P.C., Atlanta, Georgia

**Lori B. Wasserburger, MD**
Private practice, Sports & Spine Associates, Austin, Texas

**Michael Weinik, DO**
Assistant Professor and Assistant Chairman, Department of Physical Medicine and Rehabilitation, Temple University School of Medicine and Temple University Hospital, Philadelphia, Pennsylvania

**Steven L. Wiesner, MD**
Chief, Occupational Health, Kaiser Permanente Medical Center, Oakland, California

**Robert S. Windsor, MD**
Assistant Clinical Professor, Department of Physical Medicine and Rehabilitation, Emory University; President, Georgia Spine & Sports Physicians, P.C., Marietta, Calhoun, Norcross, Forest Park, and Decatur, Georgia

# Preface

Musculoskeletal pain affects all people at some point in their lives. Most of us will visit a physician for advice or treatment for this pain. Most musculoskeletal injuries are confined to the musculoligamentous system. Soft tissue injuries often are more disabling and take longer to heal than a bony injury. Despite this fact, the phrase "soft tissue injury" is occasionally used to minimize the extent of an injury.

The current medical model generally imposes a multidisciplinary approach to musculoskeletal injuries. A very important but all too often ignored component of this treatment is rehabilitation. In addition, rehabilitation is often relegated to the terminal phases of treatment. Indeed, rehabilitation should rightly begin right after an injury occurs. By proactively applying rehabilitation techniques to an injury as soon as it occurs, the disability phase of an injury may be minimized and the overall function of the injured individual may be maintained.

This book seeks to outline many of the major injury processes of the limbs and spine in a clear, readable manner. In addition, it attempts to outline the rehabilitation process in general and as it applies to each injury. This book also delves into the interplay between soft tissue injuries and the legal system as it relates to workers' compensation, personal injury, impairment, and disability.

Robert E. Windsor, MD
Dennis M. Lox, MD

# 1

# Pathophysiology of Soft Tissue Injuries

RICHARD BONFIGLIO, MD
L. ANITA CONE, MD
FRANCIS P. LAGATTUTA, MD

Musculoskeletal soft tissue injury may involve muscle, tendon, ligament, bursa, fascia, adipose tissue, meniscus, intervertebral disc, joint capsule, or cartilage. These connective tissues are the most common sites of nociceptive pain stimuli and functional impairment of patients with musculoskeletal injuries. Such injuries are common among athletes, both professional and amateur, and work-related musculoskeletal injuries are responsible for many emergency department and office visits.[47,62]

Soft tissue injury causes the release of multiple substances that promote an inflammatory response, including histamine, bradykinin, serotonin, prostaglandin, proteolytic enzymes, and lymphokines. In addition, tissue damage may cause bleeding and platelet aggregation, which increases the inflammatory response. The inflammatory response results in localized vasodilatation, increased capillary permeability, clotting of interstitial fluid, and migration of leukocytes. The resulting edema and interstitial accumulation of proteins may lead to further morbidity. Macrophages remove damaged tissue but may further injure viable tissue. The inflammatory process generally leads to activation of fibroblasts and ingrowth of fibrous tissues, which in turn lead to healing.

The natural healing process may be affected by nutritional status, other underlying medical conditions, and the ability to avoid further untoward conditions. Scar tissue often forms during the healing process and is especially significant when range of motion is limited, as with adhesive capsulitis, or when nerves are involved, as with perineural fibrosis. Antiinflammatory medications may reduce secondary tissue trauma by decreasing the inflammatory response. This occurs through multiple effects, including reduced release of prostaglandin, decreased capillary permeability, decreased migration of white blood cells, and reduced vasodilatation.

This chapter presents an overview of the basic physiology and pathophysiology as well as the healing process of soft tissue injuries.

## BASIC MECHANISMS OF INJURY

The soft tissues of any body area can be injured on the job, during sports, or during other activities, but certain people appear more prone to develop injuries to specific areas because of the forces and biomechanics involved. For example, shoulder injuries are common among baseball pitchers, football quarterbacks, and swimmers. Secretaries frequently have repetitive strain injuries involving wrist structures. Runners and football players frequently have knee injuries, and ballerinas most often injure the feet and ankles. Heavy manual laborers most often develop lower back problems. Such injuries are often associated with a specific event, but other factors may predispose some people to injury.[63]

The initiating mechanism of soft tissue injuries may be blunt trauma or impact to the soft tissues. In addition, dynamic overload, overuse, and repetitive or cumulative trauma also may cause soft tissue injuries. Muscle imbalance and rapid growth may increase the extent of injury. Contributing factors often include deconditioning, inflexibility, poor body mechanics and posture, and fatigue.[58]

Blunt trauma or impact injuries are often involved in contact sports such as football, hockey, and lacrosse. Frequent injuries include hip pointers, shoulder dislocations, and knee or ankle ligament sprains. Improper body mechanics, such as blocking or falling improperly with poor body protection, may predispose a player to such injuries or increase the amount of tissue trauma. Inflexibility resulting from decreased length of muscle fibers and tendinous connections also may increase the likelihood of tissue trauma by contributing to muscle imbalance and poor joint protection. Deconditioning increases the likelihood of injury by leading to weakened or poorly conditioned musculature, improper form, poor body mechanics, and poor posture. Fatigue also predisposes to injury or increases the amount of tissue injury.[47,62,63,74]

Dynamic overload injury often occurs with industrial, weightlifting, and wrestling activities. Overstressing of soft tissues leads to muscle strain, ligament sprain, or tendon strain or rupture. Improper body mechanics, deconditioning, inflexibility, and fatigue are common predisposing factors.[74]

Overuse injury results from repetitive activity that leads to cumulative microtrauma. Cumulative microtrauma may cause tendon strains and partial or complete tears; it is common in work-related injuries and among endurance athletes. Muscle imbalance often leads to inflexibility and may cause joint instability. Improper technique or body mechanics and fatigue are predisposing factors. When the shoulder is involved, instability may result in anterior, posterior, or inferior glenohumeral subluxation or dislocation. Rapid growth often leads to inflexibility and muscle imbalance, which may result in injury.[47,62,63,74]

## TISSUE RESPONSE TO INJURY

Acute injuries heal in three phases: phase one, which is a vascular response involving hemostasis; phase two, which involves tissue reconstruction; and phase three, which includes remodeling and functional restoration.[94,95]

Phase one, which is termed the reaction phase, occurs within days of the injury. Bleeding results from vascular and collagen rupture, which causes platelet aggregation and the release of cell-mediating factors. Platelet activation factors initiate the clotting system and a fibrin clot forms, which contains fibrinectin and hyaluronic acid. Microvascular damage results in vasoconstriction followed by vasodilation.[89,94] Vasoactive mediators increase vascular permeability and local blood flow, causing edema. In addition, chemotactic factors activate the complement system, which produces anaphylatoxin and chemotaxis.[4,38] Bradykinin stimulates the release of histamine from mast cells and basophils and the synthesis of prostaglandin, which cause further vasodilation, edema, and inflammation. Fibrinectin and collagen cross-linking initially result in wound strengthening. Inflammation continues, with activation of polymorphonucleocytes that produce arachidonic acid metabolites and proteases. These substances increase prostaglandin, leukotrienes, and thromboxanes.[4,28,42,43,68,78,92]

Phase two, which lasts up to 6–8 weeks, involves tissue reconstruction through repair and regeneration. Macrophages release proteolytic enzymes and growth factors that activate fibroblasts and wound repair.[62,93] Type III collagen fibers are laid down initially and are followed by type I collagen fibrils, which contribute to tissue tensile strength via cross-linkages.[5,38] Angiogenesis (vascular proliferation) leads to the formation of granulation tissue.[29]

Phase three, which generally lasts for months, results in tissue maturation and functional restoration. Synthesis and number of cells decrease, whereas deposition of extracellular matrix increases. Scar tissue, a mixed form of collagen, develops.

Chronic, cumulative microtrauma is associated with a degenerative and hypoxic region that results in tissue hyperplasia and angiogenesis.[42,47,99] Microvascular thrombosis and collagen fiber repair and degeneration lead to microtears and chronic inflammatory granulation tissue or scar tissue and fibrous adhesions.[50,69] Reinjury is common, especially if forces leading to additional microtrauma recur. Training errors (e.g., improper body mechanics or technique), inadequate equipment, inflexibility, muscular imbalance, fatigue, deconditioning, structural abnormalities (e.g., leg length discrepancy and hyperpronation) are predisposing factors.

The range of motion of a joint is influenced by tendons, ligaments, fascial sheaths, and the joint capsule, all of which are composed of organized connective tissues. Effective treatment enhances the healing process of soft tissue injuries, including regeneration and repair with minimal scarring. Such healing results in the full return of range of motion, strength, and pain-free function.[50,54] Ineffective treatment may result in a chronic process that includes formation of scar tissue, adhesions, and pain. These factors cause decreases in range of motion, strength, and function and are associated with an increased incidence of reinjury. Musculotendinous tightness may lead to joint contractures.

## SPECIFIC SOFT TISSUE INJURIES

### Muscle

#### Anatomy

The primary function of skeletal muscles is movement of the bony skeleton, which is accomplished by shortening of muscles. The amount of shortening (contractions) is determined by the size and orientation of muscle. The basic structure is the muscle fiber,[49,57,98] which connects via a tendon to bone. It then crosses one or more joints and ends in another tendon, which is also connected to bone. The individual muscle fiber is enclosed by the endomyosin, and groups of fibers in endomyosin form fascicles. The perimysium surrounds the fascicles. The epimysium surrounds the fascicles and constitutes the fascia. The fascia is a connective tissue that is more resistant to stretch than muscle fibers and determines the amount of stretch before failure of the muscle.[14,57]

Skeletal muscle is controlled by an efferent nerve that enters at the motor point. The single alpha motoneuron and its muscle fibers constitute a motor unit.[39]

There are two types of muscle fibers. Type 1 or slow oxidative fibers are characterized by a smaller motor unit and slower contraction and relaxation times. They have increased resistance to fatigue. Type IIA fibers, called fast oxidative glycolytic motor fibers, are intermediate in size; they have faster contraction and relaxation times and intermediate resistance to fatigue. Type IIB, or the faster glycolytic fibers, are most susceptible to fatigue; they have the lowest aerobic capacity and the highest aerobic capacity.[14,49,52]

Motor units are recruited into action by the central nervous system according to size. The smaller type I fibers are recruited first, followed by type IIA and, finally, type IIB fibers.

## Physiology

Skeletal muscles contract isotonically, isometrically, eccentrically, or isokineti-cally.[44,79] They respond to exercise training by increasing strength and endurance through central nervous system recruitment and by increasing the average size of muscle fibers.[57]

Exercised muscles histologically have higher myoglobin content, more efficient mitochondrial energy systems, and more functional capillaries per muscle fiber. High-intensity, low-repetition exercise increases muscle strength and results in the greatest increase in fiber size, whereas low-intensity, high-repetition exercise improves the endurance of type I fibers.[52,60,94]

Muscle injuries may be categorized as contusions, strains, avulsions, and exercise-induced injury and soreness. Muscle contusions may be mild, moderate, or severe. Contusions are common among athletes engaged in contact sports and may include intermuscular or intramuscular hematomas. Muscular contusions result in damage and partial disruption of the muscle fibers.[90] Frequently capillary rupture and infiltrate bleeding result in intramuscular hematomas. Ecchymosis is seen externally, followed by edema internally and an intense inflammatory reaction.[53,61] After a direct blow to a muscle, damage may occur near muscle fascial sheaths and cause blood to tract down with gravity, especially with an intermuscular hematoma.[9,47,13,78] Therefore, visible sub-cutaneous ecchymosis from a muscle hematoma may be significantly distal to the actual contusion and damage. Unless the contusion is massive or severe enough to cause muscle fiber loss, recovery and functional return are rapid.

Impact to muscle may cause intramuscular damage that results in bleeding within the muscle tissue and an intramuscular hematoma. The inflammatory response is usu-ally increased, with longer recovery time and slower return of function. A com-partment syndrome or myositis ossification may result from large intramuscular hematomas.[53,82]

Significant muscular strains involve acute partial tears of the tendinous insertion into the muscle at the distal myotendinous function. They are caused by excessive use (chronic strain) or excessive stress (acute strain). Muscles that cross two joints are more susceptible to strains and contain more type IIA and type IIB fibers (e.g., gastrocne-mius and hamstring muscles).[23,32,35,48,56,91,92]

Muscle strains also may be classified as mild, moderate, or severe. They usually result from sudden contraction, overstretch, or limb deceleration. Inflexibility or insuf-ficient warm-up may be contributing factors. A mild strain is associated with minimal, almost microscopic damage and rapid recovery and return of function.[32] A mild strain involves no significant disruption of the musculotendinous complex. Pathologic changes include a low-grade inflammatory process with swelling, edema , and pain with use of the muscle. A moderate strain involves a partial muscle tear, which usually leads to a larger hematoma and longer recovery time. It is associated with damage to the musculotendinous complex, which weakens the structure. Inflammation, edema, and discomfort are worse than with a mild strain. A severe muscle strain involves a complete muscle tear with a large hematoma and definite functional loss. Any part of the musculotendinous unit may be ruptured. Histologic characteristics include mild hemorrhage and antiinflammatory response,[75,93] with varying degrees of myofiber sepa-ration and disruption along the myotendinous junction. Healing shows muscular fibro-sis at the site of injury.[3,58,88,93] Magnetic resonance imaging (MRI) shows a similar pattern of injury and healing in all patients.[69,71] Complete muscle disruptions may re-quire surgical repair for reapproximation. Poor reapproximation in a partial or com-plete muscle tear results in increased fibrous scar tissue and decreased function. A muscle tear is more severe and problematic when it involves the musculotendinous junction instead of the muscle belly, because healing is usually less effective and less

**TABLE 1.**
Important P's with Compartment Syndrome

| |
|---|
| Pain at rest |
| Pulselessness |
| Pain out of proportion to muscle stretch |
| Pain out of proportion to palpation |
| Paresthesias in distribution of involved area |
| Pressure that is tense and escalates with palpation |

From Warwick R, Williams PL: Gray's Anatomy, 36th ed. Edinburgh, Churchill Livingstone, 1980, with permission.

complete. Severe muscle tears may lead to a compartment syndrome (Table 1). Early diagnosis is important to prevent more severe secondary injury.[78]

An avulsion usually results from an intense force or dynamic overload transmitted to a bone–thick tendon interphase. Stress fractures, rapid growth, and overdeveloped muscle strength coupled with skeletal immaturity or osteoporosis may predispose to avulsion injury by causing mechanical weakness. Common locations of avulsions are the sartorius muscle at the anterior superior iliac spine, the hamstrings at the ischial tuberosity, and the rectus femoris at the anterior inferior iliac spine.

The pathophysiology of exercise-induced muscle injury or delayed-onset muscle soreness is not fully understood, but it may be associated with an acute inflammatory response. The amount of stress applied to the musculotendinous complex exceeds its ability to elongate without disrupting structural integrity.[2,10] Performance of an unaccustomed activity, viral infection, or excessive eccentric work may predispose to such injury. Symptoms, which are usually present within 24–48 hours after exercise, include excessive muscle tenderness to palpation, swelling, and joint stiffness with loss of function. On a microscopic level, macrophage and fibroblast cellular infiltrates are increased, along with lysosomal activity. In severe cases, compartment syndrome may develop—or even rhabdomyolysis, with elevated serum levels of creatinine kinase, myoglobin, and lactic dehydrogenase.[9,57,99]

## Tendon

Tendons are dense, regularly arranged collagenous structures that connect bone to muscle. They are composed of collagen (85%) and ground substance (15%). Tendons are capable of resisting large, tensile stresses and transmit forces from muscle to bone.[33]

### Structure

A tendon is composed primarily of densely packed collagen fibers arranged parallel to their longitudinal axis. The collagen fibers run the entire length of the structure. Tropocollagen fibers form microfibers. The microfibers in turn form fibers that are mixed with fibroblasts to form a fascicle. Fascicles are surrounded by fascicular membranes, which form the tendon.[36] The epitenon, which surrounds the tendon, is continuous with its inner surface, the endotenon. The endotenon binds collagen fibers, lymph, blood vessels, and nerves. Some tendons are surrounded by a loose, smaller tissue called the paratenon. The paratenon functions as an elastic sheath, permitting free movement of the tendon against the surrounding tissue. The epitenon and paratenon form the peritenon. Tenosynovium refers to replacement of the paratenon with a true synovial sheath or bursa, which consists of two layers lined by synovial cells and allows a greater blood supply to the tendons.[91] The forearm flexors are an example.

The perimysium becomes continuous with the endotenon at the musculotendinous junction; at the tendon–bone interface, collagen fibers enter bone as shaping fibers, and the endotenon becomes continuous with the periosteum.[33] Because of the parallel arrangement of longitudinal tissue, tendons provide effective resistance to tension loading and weak resistance against shear and compression forces.[2,11,25,96]

As tendons age, their tensile strength decreases. Loss of tensile strength is correlated with decreases in both insoluble collagen and total collagen.[91] Exercise training increases the tensile strength of tendons.[86,90,96] Immobilization decreases tensile strength and increases collagen turnover.[6,92] Corticosteroids inhibit the biosynthesis of collagen, thus weakening tendons.[76,90,94] Nonsteroidal antiinflammatory drugs increase tensile strength, with an increase in both total collagen and insoluble collagen.[95] This phenomenon is attributed to an increase in cross-linkage.[26,93]

Tendon injuries may involve microscopic fiber tears associated with inflammation and located at the bony insertion site (enthesopathy or enthesitis). Such injuries may be associated with rapid growth, as in early Osgood-Schlatter disease. Inflammation of the tendinous sheath (peritenon), which is referred to as peritenonitis (tenosynovitis), is often caused by repetitive, cumulative trauma due to overuse. Repetitive microtrauma, such as microtears, results in inflammation about the sheath.[27,74] Localized edema, pain, increased warmth, and tenderness are the clinical symptoms that lead to decreased function. Repetitive microinjuries involving the tendon are referred to as tendinosis or tendinitis.[27,94] Intratendinous inflammation results from vascular and interstitial damage and leads to intratendinous collagen fiber degeneration, necrosis, and/or calcification. This injury may be asymptomatic in the acute stages. A palpable nodule associated with tenderness and edema may be present.[5,28] Chronic histologic changes may include intratendinous collagen fiber degeneration and disorientation, necrosis, and partial or complete tendon fiber tear. Tendinitis is staged clinically as grades I–V:

Grade I      Pain only after activity; no interference with performance.
Grade II     Minimal pain with or during activity; does not interfere with performance.
Grade III    Pain interferes with activity but disappears between activities.
Grade IV     Pain is more constant and does not disappear between activities; severely limits activities[60,95]
Grade V      Pain interferes with all activities, even activities of daily living.

### Biomechanics of Tendon Healing after Surgery

The three phases of tendon healing are defined by the tensile strength of the repaired tendon:

Phase I is characterized by a rapid decrease in tensile strength as a result of wound edema. This phase lasts 5 days. Histologic repair is called exudation and fibrous union.

Phase II involves an increase in tensile strength up to the 16th day. Histologic repair is called fibroplasia.

Phase III is characterized by further increase in tensile strength from day 19 until normal strength is regained. Histologic repair is called maturation, organization, and differentiation.

Mason and Allen encourage mobilization after 3 weeks of immobilization.[80,95]

## Ligament

Skeletal ligaments are similar to tendons and joint capsules in that they consist primarily of highly-oriented, highly-packed collagen fibers that give flexibility and high tensile strength. Ligaments differ from tendons in that they have a much lower length-to-width ratio. Unlike tendons, ligaments connect bone to bone and are layered sheets or lamellae rather than cords of collagen fibers.[21,22]

Ligaments stabilize synovial and nonsynovial joints by guiding normal joint motion and preventing abnormal joint motion. They also provide proprioceptive feedback and initiate protective reflexes.[12,22]

Bundles of collagen fibers form the bulk of ligament substance. Some ligaments, including the interior cruciate ligament, consist of more than one band of fibrils. As the joint moves through its range of motion, different bands of fibrils become taut. This process allows more flexibility.[13,22,30,41,99] Occasionally blood vessels penetrate the ligament substance, forming small-diameter, longitudinal vascular channels parallel to the collagen fibril bands. Nerve fiber is next to the vascular structures.

Ligaments insert into the bone directly and indirectly. In direct insertion (e.g., femoral insertion of the medial collateral ligament of the knee), the ligament inserts directly into the cortex of the bone. The ligament fibers usually pass at right angles to the bone.[19,20,33,75] Indirect insertions (e.g., tibial insertion of the medial collateral ligament of the knee) are less common than direct insertions. The indirect insertion covers more bone surface area and passes obliquely along the bone surface rather than directly into the bone.[19,20,33,65,71,97]

Ligaments consist of four classes of molecules that constitute 40% of the wet weight of most ligaments: collagens (90%), elastin (5%), proteoglycans (17%), and noncollagenous proteins (<1%).[7,17,18,20–22,41,64,65,87,96,100]

Ligament strains disrupt the matrix, damage blood vessels, and injure or kill cells.[21,98] A ligamentous injury or sprain is classified by grades of degrees from 1 to 3. A grade 1 or first-degree ligament sprain involves mild, microscopic stretching or tearing of ligament fibers and results in minimal structural loss with little or no bruising and swelling. Localized tenderness is present. The joint is stable with normal motion and often no obvious injury. Functional loss is minimal (at most a few days), with early return to activity with or without protective bracing via taping or orthotics.[5,42]

A grade 2 or second-degree ligament sprain involves moderate tearing of ligamentous collagen fibers and therefore significant structural loss and weakening. Examination reveals obvious swelling, bruising and loss of motion associated with marked tenderness. Joint hemarthrosis and effusion also may be present. The joint may or may not be stable, but it has a firm endpoint. Functional loss is significant and may require up to 6 weeks for return to activity. Protective bracing is usually necessary and may shorten the time to return of normal activities. Protective measures are necessary to reduce the risk of further injury, especially since these injuries tend to recur.

A grade 3 or third-degree ligament sprain involves severe loss of structural integrity and complete ligament tear with marked bruising, swelling, hemarthrosis, abnormal joint motion, and tenderness. The joint is unstable with a soft endpoint. Management includes prolonged protective bracing, and surgery is often indicated. Functional loss is severe and the return to normal activity takes a minimum of 6–8 weeks. Functional instability may be permanent, especially with insufficient treatment.[5,27,28,38,42]

## Ligament Repair

Repair of damaged ligaments by cell proliferation and synthesis of a new matrix depends on the migration of fibroblasts into the injured area.[21] At 2-3 days after injury the fibroblasts synthesize a new matrix consisting of a higher concentration of water, glycosaminoglycans, and type III collagen.[21] At 3–4 days vascular buds grow into the area under repair. As with tendons, there is little tensile strength.

After 3 weeks, type I collagen replaces type III collagen. The glycomonoglycans and water decrease, along with inflamed cells. The fibrils increase in size and begin to form tightly packed bundles, and the density of the fibroblasts decreases. Matrix organization increases[19,20,29,60] as fibrils align along lines of stress and blood vessels decrease. Elastin decreases as tensile strength increases.[30,31,40,73]

Variables that influence ligament healing include: type, size, and amount of loading applied to repair tissue. Injuries to capsular and extracapsular ligaments stimulate repair. Injuries to intracapsular ligaments, such as the anterior cruciate ligament, fail to stimulate repair because of limited vascular ingrowth, lack of fibroblast migration, and other factors. Treatments that approximate the ends of the tear have a much higher success rate with less scar tissue. Early controlled loading promotes healing, but excessive loading may disrupt healing.[4,8,12,21,34,44,77,78,80, 95,98]

## REFERENCES

1. Abbor BC, Aubert XM: Changes of energy in a muscle during very slow stretches. Proc R Soc Lond (Biol) 139:104–117, 1951.
2. Abraham WM: Factors in delayed muscle soreness. Med Sci Sports Exerc 9:11–20, 1977
3. Almekinders LC, Garrett, WE, Seaber AV: Pathophysiologic response to muscle tears in stretching injuries. Presented at the Orthopedic Research Society , Atlanta, 1984
4. Almekinders LC, Gilbert TA: Healing of experimental muscle strains and the effects of nonsteroidal anti-inflammatory medications. Am J Sports Med 14:303, 1986.
5. Almekinders LC, Banes AJ, Ballinger CA: Inflammatory response of fibroblasts to repetitive motion. Trans Orthop Res Soc 17:678, 1992.
6. Amadio PC: Tendon and ligament. In Cohen IK, Diegelman RF, Lindblad WJ, (eds): Wound Healing: Biochemical and Clinical Aspects. Philadelphia, W.B. Saunders, 1992, p 384.
7. Amiel D., Woo SL-Y, Harwood FL, Akeson WH: The effect of immobilization on collagen turnover in connective tissue: A biochemical-biomechanical correlation. Acta Orthop Scand 53:325–332, 1982.
8. Amiel D., Frank C., Harwood F, et al: Tendons and ligaments: A morphological and biochemical comparison. J Orthop Res 1:257–265, 1984.
9. Andriacchi T, Sabiston P. DeHaven K, et al: Ligament: Injury and repair. In Woo SL-Y, Buckwalter JD (eds): Injury and Repair of the Musculoskeletal Soft Tissues. Park Ridge, IL, American Academy of Orthopaedic Surgeons, 1988.
10. Armstrong RB: Mechanisms of exercise-induced delayed onset muscular soreness: A brief review. Med Sci Sports Exerc 16:529–538, 1984.
11. Assmussen E: Observations on experimental muscular soreness. Acta Rhuem Scand 2:109–116, 1956.
12. Bach BR, Warren RF, Wickiewicz TL: Triceps rupture: A case report and literature review. Am J Sports Med 15:285–289, 1987.
13. Barrack RL, Skinner HB: The sensory function of knee ligaments. In Daniel D, Akeson WH, O'Connor DD (eds): Knee Ligaments: Structure, Function, Injury, and Repair. New York, Raven Press, 1990.
14. Best TM, Garrett WE: Muscle and tendon. In Delee JC (ed): Orthopedic Sports Medicine. Philadelphia, W.B. Saunders, 1994, pp 1–45.
15. Best TM, Glisson RR, Seaber AV, Garrett WE: The response of muscle-tendon units of varying architecture to cyclic passive stretching. Presented at the 35th Annual Meeting of the Orthopaedic Research Society, Las Vegas, February 6–9, 1989.
16. Brewers BJ: Mechanism of injury to the musculotendinous unit. Instructional Course Lectures, vol 17. Park Ridge , IL, American Academy of Orthopaedic Surgeons, 1960, pp 354–358.
17. Bray DF, Frank CB, Bray RC: Cytochemical evidence for a proteoglycan-associated filamentous network in ligament extracellular matrix. J Orthop Res 8:1–12, 1990.
18. Buckwalter JA: Cartilage. In Delbecco R (ed): Encyclopedia of Human Biology. San Diego, Academic Press, 1990.
19. Buckwalter JA, Cooper RR: Bone structure and function. Instructional Course Lectures, vol 36. Park Ridge, IL, American Academy of Orthopaedic Surgeons, 1987, pp 27–48.
20. Buckwalter JA, Cooper RR: The cells and matrices of skeletal connective tissues. In Albirgt JA, Brand RA (eds): The Scientific Basis of Orthopaedics. Norwalk, CT, Appleton & Lange, 1987.
21. Buckwalter JA, Cruess R: Healing of musculoskeletal tissues. In Rockwood CA, Green DP (eds): Fractures. Philadelphia, J.B. Lippincott,1991.
22. Buckwalter JA, Woo SLY: Basic science of soft tissue. In Orthopedic Sports Medicine: Principles and Practice. Philadelphia, W.B. Saunders, 1994, pp 46–59.
23. Burkett LN: Causative factors in hamstring strains. Med Sci Sports Exerc 2:39–42, 1970.
24. Burks, RT: Gross anatomy. In Daniel D. Akeson WH, O'Connor J (eds): Knee Ligaments: Structure, Function, Injury, and Repair. New York, Raven Press, 1990.
25. Cailliet R: Soft Tissue Pain and Disability, 2nd ed. Philadelphia, F.A. Davis, 1988.
26. Carlstedt CA, Madsen K, Wredmar T: The influence of indomethacin on tendon healing. A biomechanical and biochemical study. Arch Orthop Trauma Surg105(6):332–336, 1986.

27. Clancy WG: Tendon trauma and overuse injuries. In Leadbetter WB, Buckwalter JA, Gordon SL (eds): Sports-Induced Inflammation: Clinical and Basic Science Concepts. Park Ridge, IL, American Academy of Orthopaedic Surgeons, 1990, p 609.
28. Clark JM, Harryman DT: Tendons, ligaments, and capsule of the rotator cuff: Gross and microscopic anatomy. J Bone Joint Surg 74A:713–725, 1992.
29. Clark R, Henson P (eds): The Molecular and Cellular Biology of Wound Repair. New York, Plenum Press, 1988.
30. Clayton ML, Miles JS, Abdulla M: Experimental investigations of ligamentous healing. Clin Orthop Rel Res 61:146–153, 1968.
31. Clayton ML, Weir GJ: Experimental investigations of ligamentous healing. Am J Surg 98:373–378, 1959.
32. Coole WG: The analysis of hamstring strains and their rehabilitation. J Orthop Sport Phys Ther 9:77, 1987.
33. Cooper RR, Misol S: Tendon and ligament insertion: A light and electron microscopic study. J Bone Joing Surg 52A:1–21, 1970.
34. Dalton JB, Seaber AV, Gasrrett WE: Biomechanics of passively stretched muscles: Viscoelasticity versus reflex effects. Surg Forum 40:516–518 1989.
35. Ekstrand, J, Gillquist J: The frequency of muscle tightness and injuries in soccer players. Am J Sports Med 10:75–78, 1982.
36. Edwards DAW: The blood supply and lymphatic drainage of the tendons. J Anat (London) 80:147, 1946.
37. Elftman H: Biomechanics of muscle. J Bone Joint Surg 48A:363, 1966.
38. Eyre DR: The collagens of musculoskeletal soft tissues. In Leadbetter WB, Buckwalter JA, Gordon SA, (eds): Sports-Induced Inflammation: Clinical and Basic Science Concepts. Park Ridge, IL, American Academy of Orthopaedic Surgeons, 1990, p 161.
39. Feinstein B, Lindegard B, Nyman E, Wohlfart G: Morphologic studies of motor units in normal human muscles. Acta Anat 23:127–142,1955.
40. Frank C, Schachar N, Dittrich D: Natural history of healing in the repaired medial collateral ligament. J Orthop Res 1:179–188, 1983.
41. Frank C, Woo S,, Andriacchi T, et al: Normal ligament: Structure, function, and composition. In Woo SL-Y, Buckwalter JA (eds): Injury and Repair of the Musculoskeletal Soft Tissues. Park Ridge, IL, American Academy of Orthopaedic Surgeons, 1988.
42. Frank C, Amiel D, et al: Normal ligament porperties and ligament healing. Clin Orthop 196:15–25, 1985.
43. Frank CB, Hart DA: Cellular response to loading. In Leadbetter WB, Buckwalter JA, Gordon SL (eds): Sports-Induced Inflammation: Clinical and Basic Science Concepts. Park Ridge, IL, American Academy of Orthopaedic Surgeons, 1990.
44. Fronek J, Frank C, Amiel D, et al: The effects of intermittent passive motion (IMP) in the healing of medial collateral ligament. Trans Orthop Res Soc 8:31, 1983.
45. Garrett WE, Alkeminders LC, Seaber AV: Biomechanics of muscle tears in stretching injuries. Trans Orthop Res Soc 9:384, 1987.
46. Gelberman R, Goldgerg V, et al: Tendon. In Woo SL-Y, Buckwalter JA (eds): Injury and Repair of the Musculoskeletal Soft Tissues. Park Ridge, IL, American Academy of Orthopaedic Surgeons, 1988, p 5.
47. Gollnick PD, Matoba H: The muscle fiber composition of skeletal muscle as a predictor of athletic success. Am J Sports Med 12:212–217, 1984.
48. Hardingham TE: Proteoglycans: Their structure, interactions and molecular organization in cartilage. Biochem Soc Trans 9:489–497, 1981.
49. Garrett WE, Best TM: Anatomy and physiology and mechanics of skeletal medicine. In Simon SR (ed): AAOS Orthopedic Basic Science. Chicago, AAOS Press, 1994, pp 89–125.
50. Herring SA, Nilson KL: Introduction to overuse injuries. Clin Sports Med 6:225–239, 1987.
51. Hill AV: The heat of shortening and the dynamic constants of muscle. Proc R Soc Lond (Biol) 126:136–195, 1938.
52. Hill AV: Chemical change and mechanical response in stimulated muscle. Proc R Soc Lond (Biol) 141:314–320, 1953b.
53. Hait-Boswic JA, Stone JJ: Heterotopic bone formation secondary to trauma (myositis ossifications truamatica). J Trauma 10:405–411, 1970.
54. Heisler TM, Weber J, Sullivan G, et al: Prophylaxsis and management of hamstring muscle injuries in intercollegiate football players. Am J Sports Med 12:368–370,1984.
55. Henneman E, Olsen CB: Relations between structure and functions in the design of skeletal muscle. J Neurophysiol 28:581–598, 1965.
56. Jackson DW, Feagin JA: Quadricep contusions in young athletes. J Bone Joint Surg 55A:95–105, 1973.
57. Knockel JP: Rhabdomyolysis and myoglobinuria. Annu Rev Med 33:435–443, 1982.
58. Kibler WB, Chandler TJ, Stracener ES: Musculoskeletal adaptations and injury due to overtraining. Exerc Sports Sci Rev 20:99, 1992.

59. Laros GS, Tipton CM, Cooper RR: Influence of physical activity on ligament insertion in the knees of dogs. J Bone Joint Surg 53A:275–286, 1971.
60. Lee HB: Avulsion and rupture of the tendo calcaneus after injection of hydrocortisone. BMJ 2:395, 1957.
61. Long M, Frank C, Schachar N, et al: The effects of motion on normal and healing ligaments. Trans Orthop Res Soc 7:43, 1982.
62. Madden JW, Arem AJ: Wound healing: Biologic and clinical features. In Sabiston DC (ed): Textbook of Surgery, 14th ed. Philadelphia, W.B. Saunders, 1991, p 167.
63. Martinez-Hernandez A: Repair, degeneration, and fibrosis. In Rubin E, Faber J (eds): Pathology. Philadelphia, J.B. Lippincott, 1988, pp 68–95.
64. Mason ML, Allen HS: The rate of healing of tendons: An experimental study of tensile strength. Ann Surg 113:424–459, 1974.
65. Matyas JR, Brodie D, Anderson M, Frank CB: The developmental morphology of a "periosteal" ligament insertion: Growth and maturation of the tibial insertion of the rabbit medial collateral ligament. J Orthop Res 8:412–424, 1990.
65a. Micheli LJ, Fehlandt AF: Overuse injuries to tendons and apophyses in children and adolescents. Clin Sports Med 11:713–726, 1992.
66. Mello MS, Godo C, Vidal BC, Abujadi JM: Changes in macromolecular orientation on collagen fibers during the process of tendon repair in the rat. Ann Histochem 20:145–152, 1975.
67. Moelleken BRW: Growth factors in wound healing. In Esterhai JL, Gristina AG, Poss R (eds): Musculoskeletal Infection. Park Ridge, IL, American Academy of Orthopaedic Surgeons, 1992, p 311.
68. Muir H: Proteoglycans as organizers of the extracellular matrix. Biochem Soc Trans 11:613–622, 1983.
69. Nikolaou PK, Macdonald BL, Glisson RR: Biomechanical and histological evaluation of muscle after controlled strain injury. Am J Sports Med 15:9–14, 1987.
70. Nimni ME, Bavetta LA: Collagen synthesis and turnover in the growing rat under the influence of methylprednisolone. Proc Soc Exp Biol Med 117:618–623, 1964.
71. Noyes FR: Functional properties of knee ligaments and alterations induced by immobilization. Clin Orthop 123:210–242, 1977.
72. Ohkawa S: Effects of orthodontic forces and anti-inflammatory drugs on the mechanical strength of the periodontium in the rat mandibular first molar. Am J Orthod 81:498–502, 1982.
73. Oxlund H: Changes in connective tissues during corticotropin and corticosteroid treatment. Doctoral dissertation, Institute of Anatomy, University of Aarchus, Aarchus, Denmark, 1983.
74. Paget J: Healing of injuries in various tissue. Lect Surg Pathol 1:262–274, 1853.
75. Poole AR, Webber C, Pidoux I, et al: Localization of a dermatan sulfate proteoglycan (DS-PGII) in cartilage and the presence of an immunologically related species in other tissues. J Histochem Cytochem 34:619–625, 1986.
76. Prockop DJ, Kivirikko KI, Tiderman L, et al: The biosyntheis of collagen and its disorders. N Engl J Med 301:13, 1979.
77. Ralph D: Rhabdomyolysis and acute renal failure. J Am Coll Emerg Phys 7:103–106, 1978.
78. Robbins SL, Cotran RS: Pathologic Basis of Disease, 3rd ed. Philadelphia, W.B. Saunders, 1984.
79. Rosenberg L, Choi HU, Neame PJ, et al: Proteoglycans of soft connective tissue. In Leadbetter WB, Buckwalter JA, Gordon SL (eds): Sports-Induced Inflammation: Basic Science and Clinical Concepts. Park Ridge, IL, American Academy of Orthopaedic Surgeons, 1990.
80. Rotwell AG: Quadraceps hematoma: A prospective clinical study. Clin Orthop 171:97–103, 1982.
81. Rowland LP, Penn AS: Myoglobinuria. Med Clin North Am 56:1233–1261, 1972.
82. Ryan AJ: Quadriceps strain, rupture, and charleyhorse. Med Sci 1:106–111, 1969.
83. Schatzker J, Branemark PI: Intravital observation on the microvascular anatomy and microcirculation of the tendon. Acta Orthop Scand 26(Suppl):1–23, 1969.
84. Schaub MC, Watterson JG: Control of the contractile process in muscle. Trends Pharmacol Sci 2(10):279–282, 1981.
85. Schwane JA, Johnson SR, Vandenakker CB, Armstrong RB: Delayed-onset muscular soreness and plasma CPK and LDK activities after downhill running. Med Sci Sports Exerc 15:51–56, 1983.
86. Simon SR, Riggins RS, Wright CR, Fox ML (eds): Orthopedic Sciences. Chicago, American Academy of Orthopaedic Surgeons, 1986, pp 26–33.
87. Smith LL: Acute inflammation: The underlying mechanism in delayed onset muscle soreness. Med Sci Sports Exerc 123:542–554, 1991.
88. Teitz CC (ed): Scientific Foundation of Sports Medicine. Toronto, B.C. Decker, 1989, p 299.
89. Tipton CM, James SL, Mergner W, Tcheng T-K: Influence of exercise on strength of medial collateral ligaments of dogs. Am J Physiol 218:894–901, 1970.
90. Tipton CM, Schild RJ, Tomanek RJ: Influence of physical activity on the strength of knee ligaments in rats. Am J Physiol 212:783–787, 1967.
91. Travell JG, Simons DG: Myofascial Pain and Dysfunction: The Trigger Point Manual. Baltimore, Williams & Wilkins, 1983.

92. Vailas AC,, Tipton CM, Matthes RD, Gart M: Physical activity and its influence on the repair process of medial collateral ligaments. Connect Tissue Res 9:25–31, 1981.
93. Viidik A: Simultaneous mechanical and light microscopic studies of collagen fibers. Z Anat Entwickl-Ges. 136:204–212, 1972.
94. Viidik A: The effects of training on the tensile strength of isolated rabbit tendons. Scand J Plastic Reconstr Surg 1:141–147, 1967.
95. Vogel HC: Influence of maturation and age on mechanical and biochemical parameters of connective tissue of various organs in the rat. Conect Tissue Res 6:161–166, 1978.
96. Wahl SM, Wahl LM: Inflammation. In Cohen JK, Diegglemann RF, Lindblad WY (eds): Wound Healing. Philadelphia, W.B. Saunders, 1992, p 40.
97. Warwick R, WIlliams PL: Gray's Anatomy, 36th ed. Edinburgh, Churchill Livingstone, 1980.
98. Woo SL-Y, Buckwalter JA (eds): Injury and Repair of the Musculoskeletal Soft Tissues. Park Ridge, IL, American Academy of Orthopaedic Surgeons, 1988.
99. Woo, SL-Y, Ritter MA, Amiel D, et al: The biomechanical and biochemical properties of swine tendons. Long-term effects of exercise on the digital extensions. Connect Tissue Res 7:177–183, 1980.
100. Woo S, Maynard J, Butler D, et al: Ligament, tendon, and joint capsule insertions into bone. In Woo SL-Y, Buckwalter JA (eds): Injury and Repair of the Musculoskeletal Soft Tissues. Park Ridge, IL, American Academy of Orthopaedic Surgeons, 1988.
101. Woo SL-Y, Horibe S, Ohland KJ, Amiel D: The response of ligaments to injury: Healing of the collateral ligaments. In Daniel D, Akeson WH, O'Connor J (eds): Knee Ligaments: Structure, Function, Injury, and Repair. New York, Raven Press, 1990.

# 2

# Cervical Soft Tissue Injuries

FRANK J. E. FALCO, MD
FRANCIS P. LAGATTUTA, MD
JONATHAN P. LESTER, MD
STANLEY A. HERRING, MD

The first known record of cervical spine disorders was found in the papyrus written over 5000 years ago by the physician Imhoptep of the Third Egyptian Dynasty, who described cervical sprains and dislocations.[59] Hippocrates recognized that vertebral injuries to the cervical spine resulted in paralysis and developed the concept of cervical traction to treat such disorders. The Greek physician Paul of Aeginia (625–690 AD) was the first to perform cervical laminectomy.[2] Galen, the physician to the Roman Emperor Marcus Aurelius, performed cervical surgery on gladiators and recorded spinal cord function at different cervical root levels.[67,137] Alban Smith performed the first successful cervical laminectomy in the United States in 1829.[127] The term *whiplash* was first introduced in 1928 by Crowe to describe a mechanism of soft tissue injury to the cervical spine.[36]

Soft tissue injuries of the cervical spine are commonly encountered by health care providers in many outpatient musculoskeletal settings. The advent of motorized vehicles and industrialization has led to the greater incidence of soft tissue injuries in metropolitan areas and western societies. Identifying the site of the injury through a comprehensive evaluation, using a thorough history and physical examination along with diagnostic testing, allows specific treatment and better outcomes. A multidisciplinary approach is the best avenue for successful relief of symptoms and functional restoration.

## EPIDEMIOLOGY

Neck and shoulder pain are common complaints in industrialized societies. One of every three individuals can recall an incident of neck pain at least once in their lifetime.[84] The prevalence of neck or shoulder pain with or without arm pain in the general population is approximately 10–20%, with a slightly higher predilection for women.[84,94]

Cervical whiplash injuries leading to neck pain are commonly associated with motor vehicle accidents, especially with rear-end collisions. Deans et al. reported that 62% of patients evaluated in an emergency department after a motor vehicle accident initially complained of neck pain.[39] They also found that 42% continued to have intermittent neck pain after 1 year, with 6% experiencing continuous pain. In another long-term study with a mean follow-up of 10 years, chronic neck symptoms were found in 28% of patients with whiplash.[50] Twelve percent complained of severe neck pain.[50]

In the workplace, 51–80% of laborers recall an episode of neck and arm pain.[68-70] The frequency of neck complaints increases with age, stress, material handling, and above-shoulder-level activity.[66,68–70] Chronic neck pain has a statistically significant correlation with previous neck, back, or shoulder injury; work-related mental distress; and physical stress.[94] Chronic neck pain is rare in people with a high education level, white collar workers, and housewives.[94] There is no association between chronic neck pain and smoking.[94]

## ANATOMY AND PAIN GENERATORS

The cervical spine is a unique part of the axial skeleton. The neck is the most mobile portion of the spine and serves four major functions: (1) it supports and provides stability for the head; (2) it enables the head to move in all planes of motion; (3) it protects the structures that pass through it, specifically the spinal cord, nerve roots, and the vertebral artery; and (4) it allows attachment of numerous muscles and ligaments.

### Osseous Structures

The cervical column is made up of seven vertebrae, which are divided into an upper (C1–C2) and lower (C3–C7) region (Fig. 1). There are distinct anatomic and functional differences between the two regions.

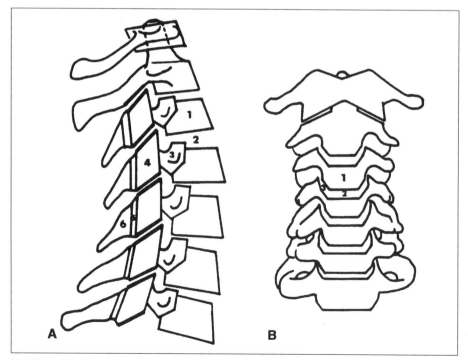

**FIGURE 1.**
A, Lateral view of the cervical spine. 1 = vertebral body, 2 = disc, 3 = nerve root canal, 4 = lateral mass, 5 = lamina, 6 = spinous process. B, Anterior view of the cervical spine. 1 = vertebral body, 2 = disc, 3 = neurocentral joint. (From MacNab I, McCulloch J: Neck Ache and Shoulder Pain. Baltimore, Williams & Wilkins, 1994, with permission.)

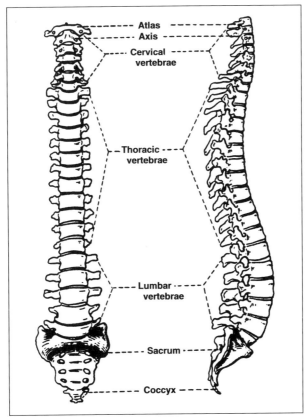

**FIGURE 2.**
Anterior and lateral views of the entire human spine. (From
Hollinshead WH: Textbook of Anatomy, 3rd ed. New York, Harper
& Row, 1974, with permission.)

The atlas (C1) and axis (C2) are considerably different from other cervical vertebrae and the remaining spinal column (Fig. 2). The atlas is a ringlike structure without a
vertebral body. Two lateral masses of the atlas that articulate with the occipital condyles
above allow flexion and extension of the head. The axis has a vertebral body, bifid spinous process, and an upward-projecting odontoid process that represents the congeni-
tally fused atlas body. The odontoid articulates with the anterior arch of the atlas,
making axial rotation of the head possible.

The vertebrae of the lower cervical region are similar in shape and function (Fig. 3).
The C3–C7 vertebrae have small bodies and bifid spinous processes from C3–C6. The
seventh cervical vertebra has the longest spinous process, which is easily palpable in
most people. The spinous processes, transverse processes, and lamina serve as areas for
muscle attachments. All cervical spine motion in the lower region is coupled so that
rotation is associated with lateral bending and vice versa.

The lower cervical zygapophyseal joints have a 45° orientation in the frontal
plane, which contrasts with the 60° and 90° orientation of the facet joints in the thoracic
and lumbar spine, respectively. Unique articulations, called uncovertebral, Luschka, or
neurocentral joints, are present in the lower cervical region (Fig. 4). These pseudojoints
arise from the posterolateral margins of the vertebral bodies and lie anterior to the exiting

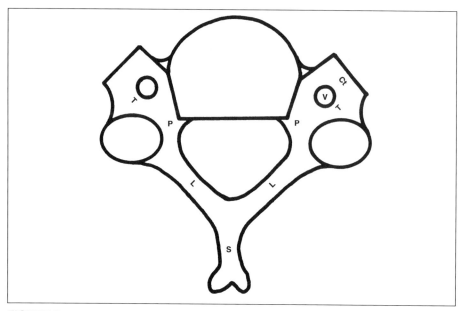

**FIGURE 3.**
Axial schematic of cervical vertebra. P = pedicle, T = transverse process, L = lamina, S = spinous process, ct = costotransverse bar, v = vertebral foramen. (From MacNab I, McCulloch J: Neck Ache and Shoulder Pain. Baltimore, Williams & Wilkins, 1994, with permission.)

nerve roots. They are not present at birth but develop by the end of the first decade. Many believe that they are not true joints because they do not possess synovium and are thought to develop from degenerative clefts or fibrous tissue resorption within the supraposterolateral margins.[62,106,109]

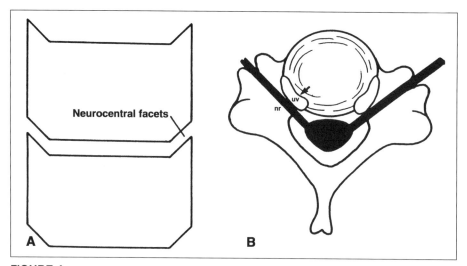

**FIGURE 4.**
Schematic of Luschka's (uncovertebral) joints. *A,* Coronal view of Luschka's (neurocentral joints). *B,* Proximity of the uncovertebral joints (uv) to the cervical nerve roots (nr). (From MacNab I, McCulloch J: Neck Ache and Shoulder Pain. Baltimore, Williams & Wilkins, 1994, with permission.)

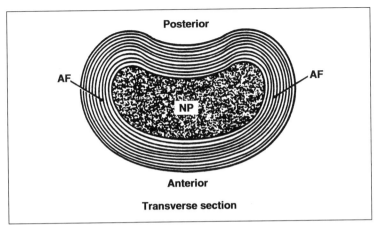

**Posterior**

AF

AF

NP

**Anterior**

**Transverse section**

**FIGURE 5.**
The structural components of the intervertebral disc. NP = nucleus pulposus;
AF = anulus fibrosus. (From Bogduk N, Twomey LT: Clinical Anatomy of the
Lumbar Spine, 2nd ed. New York, Churchill Livingstone, 1991, with permission.)

## Soft Tissue Structures

The intervertebral disc is made up of the eccentrically located nucleus pulposus
and the surrounding anulus fibrosus (Fig. 5). Discs are located throughout the cervical
spine except between the C1 and C2 vertebrae. The ligaments and joint capsules are the
only structures to resist excessive motion between the atlas and axis. The intervertebral
discs below C2 provide shock absorption, accommodate movement, and separate the
vertebral bodies, maximizing the size of the intervertebral foramen.

Several ligaments found at each vertebral level provide strength and stability to the
cervical spine (Fig. 6). The transverse, alar, and accessory atlantoaxial ligaments help to
maintain the integrity of the odontoid and C1 articulation. The anterior (ALL) and posterior longitudinal ligaments (PLL) run along the anterior and posterior surfaces of the
vertebrae and discs, respectively. They provide stability during flexion and extension. The
PLL also reinforces the posterior anulus. The facet capsule, supraspinous, and interspinous ligaments and ligamentum flavum provide flexion stability. The ligamentum nuchae
spans from the occiput to the C7 spinous process and adds support to the posterior neck.

The neck muscles support and provide movement for the cervical spine and head.
The musculature can be divided functionally into the anterior flexor and posterior extensor muscle groups. The anteriorly placed scalene and sternocleidomastoid muscles
are the important flexors and additional rotators of the neck and head. The posterior
muscles are arranged with the longer groups superficial and the shorter groups closest
to the vertebral column. For example, the iliocostalis and longissimus muscles span
many vertebral levels and are superficial, whereas the deeply located, short cervical rotators pass from only one vertebrae to the next. These muscles produce extension of the
spine and head by contracting bilaterally or rotation by acting ipsilaterally.[28]

Some of the extrinsic shoulder muscles, such as the trapezius, rhomboid, levator
scapulae, and latissimus dorsi muscles, have attachments to the cervical spine. Injury to
these structures may lead to neck pain because of this anatomic relationship.[82]

## Neural Structures

The spinal cord originates at the foramen magnum and extends to approximately
the L2 vertebral level. The spinal cord is about 10 mm in size, and the vertebral canal
averages 17 mm in sagittal diameter.[25,108] The spinal canal is the widest at C3–C5 and

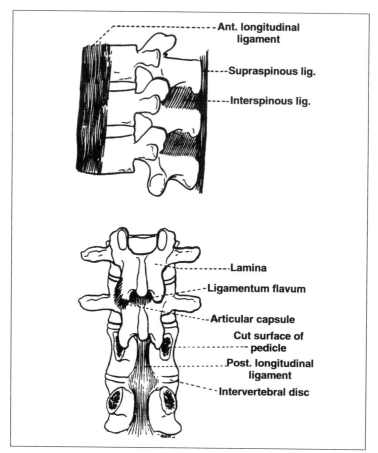

**FIGURE 6.**
Ligaments of the spinal column. (From Hollinshead WH: Textbook of Anatomy, 3rd ed. New York, Harper & Row, 1974, with permission.)

rapidly decreases in size to a small circular lumen throughout the thoracic area. In the cervical region, the transverse diameter of the spinal canal is almost twice that of the anteroposterior diameter. Therefore, the spinal cord has ample room to expand laterally but considerably less room in the anteroposterior direction.

Spinal nerves are formed by ventral (motor) and dorsal (sensory) roots within the neuroforamen (Fig. 7). The cervical nerves contain both motor and sensory fibers. The first cervical nerve emerges from the vertebral canal at the atlantooccipital junction, and the eighth nerve exits between the seventh cervical and first thoracic vertebrae. As the cervical spinal nerves exit through the foramen, they divide into anterior and posterior rami. The anterior rami supply the prevertebral and paravertebral muscles and form the brachial plexus, which innervates the upper limbs. The posterior rami divide into muscular, cutaneous, and articular branches innervating posterior neck structures, including the postvertebral muscles.[28]

The cervical intervertebral discs receive innervation to the outer one-third of the anulus (Fig. 8).[24] The disc receives branches laterally from the vertebral nerve, which accompanies and innervates the vertebral artery. The vertebral nerve is derived predominantly from the sympathetic system but also may carry somatic afferents

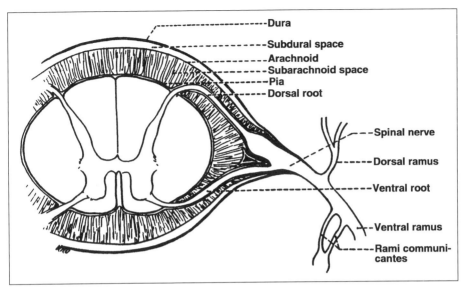

**FIGURE 7.**
Formation of spinal nerves from the spinal cord. (From Hollinshead WH: Textbook of Anatomy, 3rd ed. New York, Harper & Row, 1974, with permission.)

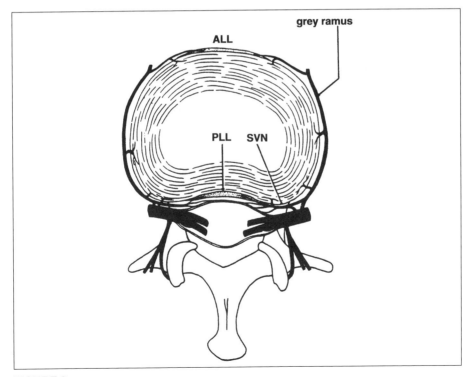

**FIGURE 8.**
Nerve supply of the cervical intervertebral disc. PLL = posterior longitudinal ligament; ALL = anterior longitudinal ligament; SVN = sinovertebral nerve. (From Bogduk N, Twomey LT: Clinical Anatomy of the Lumbar Spine, 2nd ed. New York, Churchill Livingstone, 1991, with permission.)

because of its many connections with the ventral rami. Posterolateral innervation is provided by the sinuvertebral nerve, also known as the recurrent nerve of Luschka, at the level of the disc. The sinuvertebral nerve is formed by branches from somatic and autonomic nerve roots. The sinuvertebral nerve also supplies the disc-one segment cephalad and innervates the posterior longitudinal ligament, pedicle, posterior vertebral periosteum, epidural veins, and dorsal dura mater. Anterolateral cervical disc innervation is suspected but has not been definitively demonstrated.

The cervical zygapophyseal joints are innervated by the medial (articular) branches from the posterior cervical rami. The C3–C4 to C6–C7 joints are supplied by the medial branches that run above and below the joints (Fig. 9).[18,31,86] The medial branch of the C3 dorsal ramus, the third occipital nerve, innervates the ipsilateral C2–C3 joint.[17,31,86] The atlantooccipital and atlantoaxial joints are supplied by the C1 and C2 ventral rami, respectively.[17,31,86]

### Pain Generators

Many structures in the neck are potential pain generators. Pain also can be referred to the neck from other sources, such as the upper limbs. Any structure that receives innervation is a potential pain generator.

Injury or compromise of the cervical spinal nerves may cause radicular pain as well as weakness and sensory loss. Radicular symptoms include pain referred into the

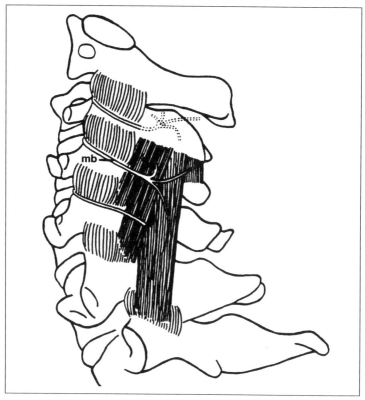

**FIGURE 9.**
Innervation of the cervical zygapophyseal joints. mb = medial branch. (From Bogduk N: The clinical anatomy of the cervical dorsal rami. Spine 7:319–330, 1982, with permission.)

shoulder or other distal structures, sensory loss, paresthesias, and weakness.[26,45,46,133] Specific peripheral nerve injuries in the neck region also may occur. For example, an injury to the occipital nerve may lead to occipital neuralgia, which often results in occipital headaches.[17,83,107]

The cervical vertebrae also may be nociceptive sources, as seen with vertebral body compression fractures from trauma or metabolic abnormalities. Cervical zygapophyseal joint injury secondary to traumatic fracture or osteoporosis with microscopic fractures may lead to pain.[15,18,20,23,92,123,125]

Pain may originate solely from the intervertebral disc without evidence of herniation if there is disruption of the outer anular fibers.[19,24,33,142] Painful disc derangement may develop with acute trauma or chronic repetitive injury. Disc disruption may lead to neck or arm pain.[33]

Cervical muscles and ligaments are also potential sources of pain. The musculature may generate pain when injured from direct trauma or the relatively common traumatic flexion–extension injuries (whiplash).[45,46,71] The highly innervated ligaments may be stretched or even torn during flexion–extension injuries, also resulting in pain.[40,130,132,141]

## CERVICAL SOFT TISSUE INJURIES

### Sprains and Strains

Sprain and strain injuries to cervical spine structures are the most commonly encountered cervical disorders. A sprain is a traumatic overstretching or tearing of ligaments or tendons encompassing a joint. A strain is an injury to muscle or ligamentous structures. Whiplash injuries are the most frequent cause of cervical sprains and strains, with over 1 million cases in the United States every year.[43] This condition is more common in western societies and metropolitan areas with greater concentrations of automobiles. Although the classic mechanism of injury has long been described as a hyperextension insult to the cervical spine from a rear-end motor vehicle collision, soft tissue injuries from whiplash may occur from flexion, extension, lateral, rotational, distraction, and compression forces or any combination thereof.[9,16,93] The incidence is higher in women and in people 30–50 years old.[129] Approximately one- to two-thirds of patients develop neck pain within 24 hours of injury.[39,124] Approximately 60% of whiplash injuries resolve within the first several months with no residual symptoms. About 30–40% improve but continue to be intermittently symptomatic after the first year, and roughly 10% have continuous symptoms.[39,50,104,139] Litigation, psychologic factors, and personality traits may or may not have an effect on treatment outcome.[6,55,96,112]

### Pathophysiology

Whiplash injuries are most often caused by rear-end collisions, and the biomechanics of this injury mechanism has been studied more extensively than the biomechanics of any other injury. The rear-end impact leads to an immediate acceleration of the vehicle and an acceleration of the trunk and shoulders that is delayed by one-tenth of a second after impact from the movement of the car seat. The head and neck are forced into passive extension as the shoulders move anteriorly. The head and neck then move into flexion after the extension moment is overcome by the forward acceleration. Any head rotation at the time of impact leads to further rotation, which places more stress on the zygapophyseal joint capsules, discs, ligaments, and muscles as they are subjected to greater stretch. Extremely elevated G-forces (Fig. 10) cause acceleration and deceleration injuries to ligaments, facet joints, and muscle.[9,33,40,123,124] A 20-mph rear-end collision may result in a level 12 G-force to the head during extension.[125]

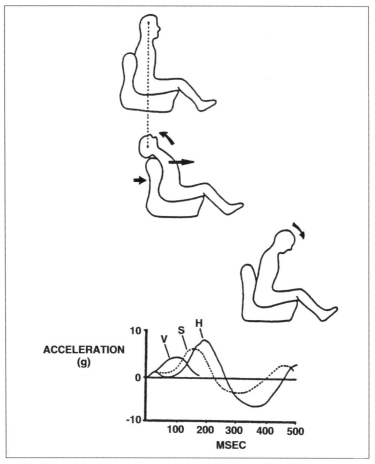

**FIGURE 10.**
Idealized graph showing acceleration curves of the head, shoulders, and vehicle following a rear-end impact at 5 miles per hour. Note that peak acceleration of the head is considerably greater than that of the car, followed by significant deceleration. (From Barnsley L, Lord S, Bogduk N: Pathophysiology of whiplash. Spine State Art Rev 7:330, 1993, with permission.)

The extent of soft tissue damage from whiplash injuries of the cervical spine may be quite severe. Studies in primates have revealed by gross histology tearing of sterno-cleidomastoid and longus colli muscles; retropharyngeal and intraesophageal hematomas; tearing of the cervical sympathetic chain, anterior longitudinal ligament, and facet joint capsules; and internal disc disruption.[92,93] Brain injury, spinal cord damage, and vertebral artery rupture also have been reported in primate models.[136,143] Disruption of the anterior and posterior longitudinal ligaments, ligamentum flavum, and intervertebral disc as well as large disc herniations have been documented by magnetic resonance imaging (MRI) in patients who developed myelopathy after cervical spine hyperextension injuries.[61,74] Osseous abnormalities such as vertebral body compression and fractures of the facet, pedicle, laminae, and transverse process have been described in the literature.[1,73,95]

Neck pain also may occur after lateral or frontal accidents but are less common. There is a lower likelihood of an isolated soft tissue injury from these types of collisions because the shoulder or chest stops the head before the normal physiologic range of cervical spine motion is exceeded. Significant sequelae of hyperflexion injuries are typically associated with concomitant axial compression, leading to fracture, dislocation, and instability as in diving accidents or head-on collisions.[65]

The zygapophyseal joints have been recognized as a frequent cause of neck pain, headaches, and referred symptoms in hyperextension injuries.[9,10,16,19,83,91,93] Studies using fluoroscopically guided diagnostic injections have implicated the facet joint as the source of neck pain in 50–60% of patients with whiplash and as the source of headache in one-third.[10,91] The cervical facet joint has been implicated as a cause for chronic neck pain in as many as 70% of sufferers.[8] Regardless of the cause for chronic cervical zygapophyseal joint pain, the C2–C3 and C5-C6 facet joints have been found to be the most common symptom-producing joints.[8,10,91]

Cervical prevertebral, paravertebral, and postvertebral muscles may develop trigger points—localized bands of tight, well-defined, and painful fibers. They may develop from acute trauma, strain, or, more commonly, repetitive overuse. Frequent overhead reaching and lifting or chronic posturing are typical mechanisms of repetitive overuse. Trigger points may produce referred sclerotomal pain to the head, shoulder, scapula, or upper extremity.[135] In some instances, trigger points are secondary to segmental dysfunction of the intervertebral disc or facet joint.

Others contend that chronic myofascial neck pain is secondary to partial avulsions of musculotendinous and ligamentous attachments to the suboccipital region as well as to the spinous and transverse processes.[113] This mechanism is thought to lead to hemorrhage, inflammation, and fibrotic deposition. Excessive fibrosis, underdeveloped calcification, and immature nerve sprouting follow, resulting in chronic pain.

Nerve root injuries also may occur with radicular features, presumably from a stretch injury or focal hemorrhages.[32,76] The C2 dorsal root ganglia are vulnerable to injury between the axis and atlas vertebral arches during hyperextension, which may lead to occipital neuralgia. In rare instances, an injury to the descending portion of the cranial V nerve sensory nucleus results in facial sensory disturbances. Additional bulbar symptoms, such as blurry vision, dizziness, tinnitus, and Horner syndrome, may result from injuries to other cranial nerves. Temporomandibular joint injuries also may occur with hyperextension whiplash injuries.[113]

Headaches arising after whiplash injuries were originally thought to result from injury to the C2 dorsal ganglia. Compelling evidence in recent literature strongly implicates the atlantooccipital, atlantoaxial, and C2-C3 facet joints as the source for most occipital headaches in whiplash injuries.[8–10,41,91] Injection of these joints or the nerves that innervate them has led to headache relief.[8–10,22,41,91]

An unusual constellation of symptoms known as the Barré-Lieou syndrome has been associated with hyperextension injuries of the cervical spine.[12] The syndrome consists of headaches, tinnitus, aphonia or hoarseness, vertigo, ocular pain, blurry vision, intermittent dysesthesias in the distal upper extremities, and modified auditory perception. The syndrome is thought to result from an injury to the vertebral artery, cervical sympathetic chain, or central nervous system.

## Diagnosis

The history usually includes neck pain, referred symptoms into the upper extremity or torso, and headaches. The patient typically complains of neck fatigue, stiffness and pain associated with movement. Pain patterns should be evaluated carefully to differentiate sclerotomal from radicular features (Fig. 11).[23,42,71,81] As described earlier, associated symptoms include dizziness, lightheadedness, difficulty with concentration and memory, unusual skin sensations over the face, blurred vision, difficulty in hearing, tinnitus, hoarseness, and other complaints from cranial nerve injuries.[7,23,26,39,47,64,107,110,111,132,133]

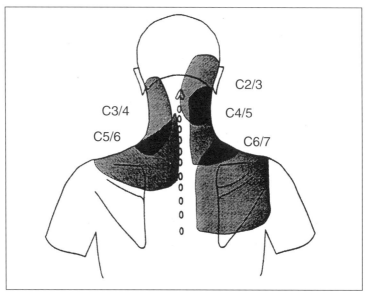

**FIGURE 11.**
Pain referral from C2–C3 through C6–C7 facet joints. (From Barnsley L, Lord S, Wallis BJ, Bogduk N: The prevalence of chronic cervical zygapophyseal joint pain after whiplash. Spine 20:20–26, 1995, with permission.)

The physical examination shows decreased range of motion in the neck with poor quality of movement. Spurling's and Lhermitte's signs are typically negative. Patients frequently show tenderness to palpation in both anterior and posterior soft tissue structures of the neck. Facet joint tenderness on palpation is common from injuries to the joints, ligaments, or capsules.[75] Structural defects may occur with dysfunction of cervical facet movement. The neurologic examination is usually normal, although radicular signs are occasionally present early after injury and usually resolve within the first 2 weeks. In most cases, sensory abnormalities are of sclerotomal rather than dermatomal origin.

Plain neck films may show loss of the normal cervical lordotic curvature. MRI and computed tomography (CT) scans are typically normal but may reveal disc herniations, ligamentous injury, and hemorrhage in severe hyperextension injuries and fracture or dislocation in traumatic hyperflexion injuries.[38] Bone scans may be considered for further evaluation of fracture. Electrodiagnostic studies help to rule out radiculopathy in patients with continued pain and unusual referred limb sensations.

### Treatment

Initial care involves the use of nonsteroidal antiinflammatory drugs (NSAIDs) and analgesics to control pain. Tricyclic antidepressant medications also may be used to decrease pain and decrease sleep disturbances. There is usually no need for muscle relaxants with sufficient use of analgesics and physical modalities.

Physical therapy modalities include mobilization, which may be effective after acute injury.[27,44,58,63] Cervical instability in patients of all ages and vertebral insufficiency in the elderly need to be ruled out before performing mobilization. There is a small risk for stroke with high-velocity movements.[30,101] Massage is of benefit in increasing circulation, decreasing pain, and facilitating exercises that are the mainstay of treatment. Ultrasound and electrical stimulation are also beneficial, as is postural reeducation.[87] Orthotic devices should not be used continuously for more than 72 hours because they can delay healing and lead to soft tissue tightening—unless instability is a major clinical concern.[99,100,111]

Spinal manipulation and mobilization are used to restore normal range of motion and to decrease pain. Although there is no clear explanation of how manipulation works, some believe that adjustments to zygapophyseal joints improve afferent signals from mechanoreceptors to the peripheral and central nervous systems.[44] The normalization of afferent impulses results in better muscle tone, decreased muscle guarding, and more effective local tissue metabolism. These physiologic modifications led to improved range of motion and pain reduction. Spinal manipulation has been shown to have beneficial short-term results in acutely injured patients.[27,44,58,63] No evidence suggests that manipulation provides long-term benefits, improves chronic conditions, or alters the natural course of the disorder.[103]

Proper movement patterns need to be reestablished within the cervical segments. Poor posture may lead to rounding of the shoulders, dorsal thoracic kyphosis, forward head thrusting from the lower cervical spine, and extension of the upper cervical spine.[28,29] Poor neck posture may cause microtrauma to the cervical facets, disc, ligaments, and muscles,[28,29] resulting in bony hypertrophy, ligamentous laxity, and breakdown of the disc and facet articulations. Correct segmental movement depends on balancing the head, cervical spine, and thoracic spine. This provides optimal mechanical balance within all three structures and is achieved through increased cervical flexibility and proprioception. Flexibility is achieved with mobilization and repetitive self-stretching techniques. Proprioception is improved with instruction from the therapist or physician and visual feedback from a mirror. The stabilization exercises in Table 1 allow the muscles to self-correct the neck into proper position and posture, resulting in decreased pain and trauma to the joints.[80,119,130]

Myofascial trigger points may be treated with passive stretching after spraying the overlying skin with a vapocoolant such as ethyl chloride. Theoretically, the superficial coolant inhibits pain and spinal stretch reflexes, allowing more effective stretching with the goal of obtaining normal resting muscle length and restoring range of motion.[135] Trigger points also may be treated with dry needling, with or without use of an anesthetic injection. The needling attempts to break up fibrotic scar that has formed in the damaged soft tissue and to interrupt the trigger point mechanism.[135] The use of an injectable anesthetic adds to the mechanical disruption of scar, blocks the pain from dry needling, and may help to limit associated muscle spasm. The myofascial area can be sprayed with a vapocoolant after trigger point injection if residual pain remains. Specific therapy, such as aggressive stretching and massage as well as other exercises, should follow the anesthetic injection and dry needling to maximize results. Steroids and soft tissue techniques, such as shiatsu or Rolfing, probably have no place in trigger point therapy.

Prolotherapy is an option to treat trigger points of a different kind. Trigger points are thought to occur not only within muscles but also in ligaments and joint capsules.[57,67,77] Tendon and ligamentous attachments to bone have been described as pain generator sites that may lead to chronic symptoms when stretched or weakened by injury.[57,67,77] Prolotherapy is the injection of proliferant solutions at the attachment site of ligaments and tendons to periosteum. The proliferants are thought to induce new tissue formation at the injection sites, leading to ligament and tendon strengthening as well as joint stability and reducing pain by eliminating chronic nociception from formally weakened periosteal attachments.[79,88,105]

There is a high incidence of facet joint pain in patients with chronic neck pain and headaches.[4,19] Such patients can be identified with facet joint nerve blocks. Although intraarticular steroid injections have been shown not to provide significant relief,[11] rhizotomy of the facet joint nerves in properly identified patients may provide longer

**TABLE 1.**
Cervicothoracic Stabilization Exercises

| | Cervicothoracic Stabilization Levels | | |
|---|---|---|---|
| | I<br>Basic | II<br>Intermediate | III<br>Advanced |
| Direct<br>Cervical stabilization<br>Exercises | Cervical active range<br>of motion<br>Cervical isometrics | Cervical gravity<br><br>Resisted isometrics | Cervical active<br><br>Range gravity resisted |
| Indirect<br>Cervical Stabilization<br>Exercises | | | |
| Supine, head<br>supported | Theraband chest press<br>Bilateral arm raise<br>Supported dying bug | Unsupported dying bug | Chest flyes<br>Bench press<br>Incline dumbbell press |
| Sit | Reciprocal arm raise<br>Unilateral arm raise<br>Bilateral arm raise<br>Seated row<br>Latissimus pulldown | Swiss ball reciprocal<br>Arm raises<br>Chest press | Swiss ball bilateral<br>Shoulder shrugs<br>Supraspinatus raises |
| Stand | Theraband reciprocal<br>Chest press<br>Theraband straight<br>Arm latissimus<br>Pulldown<br>Theraband:<br>  Chest press<br>  Latissimus pulldown<br>Standing rowing<br>Crossovers<br>Tricep press | Standing rowing<br>Bicep pulldown | Upright row<br>Shoulder shrugs<br>Supraspinatus raises |
| Flexed hip-hinge<br>position | 0–30°<br>Reciprocal arm raise<br>Unilateral arm raise<br>Bilateral arm raise<br>Interscapular flyes | 30–60°<br>Incline prone flyes<br>Reciprocal deltoid<br>  raise<br>Cable crossovers | 60–90°<br>Bilateral anterior<br>Deltoid raises<br>Interscapular flyes |
| Prone | Reciprocal arm raise<br>Unilateral arm raise<br>Bilateral arm raise | Quadruped<br>Head unsupported<br>Swiss ball bilateral<br>Anterior deltoid raises<br>Swiss ball prone<br>Rowing<br>Swiss ball prone flyes | Head supported<br>Prone flyes<br>Latissimus flyes |
| Supine, head<br>unsupported | Not advised for level I | Partial sit-ups<br>Arm raises | Swiss ball chest flyes<br>Swiss ball reciprocal |

Reprinted from Sweeney T, Prentice C, Saal JA, et al: Cervicothoracic muscular stabilizing technique. Phys Med Rehabil State Art Rev 4:335–360, 1990, with permission.

relief of symptoms[3,21,89,90,126] and an opportunity for aggressive rehabilitation of patients who do not respond to more conservative measures. Some suggest that radiofrequency cauterization at the sites of musculotendinous and tendinous insertions also offers long-term relief.[113]

## Radiculopathy

Cervical radiculopathy is a relatively common consequence of mechanical compression of a nerve root due to a herniated nucleus pulposus or degenerative changes of the cervical spine. A radiculopathy is any sensory, motor, or reflex abnormality secondary to nerve root injury. Although no data about the true incidence or prevalence of cervical radiculopathy are available, 51% of adults in one study experienced neck and arm pain at some time in their life.[69] Job activities, smoking, and abnormal anatomy are factors that predispose to the development of cervical radiculopathy.[5,13,37]

### Pathophysiology

Cervical radiculopathy may be secondary to mechanical compression or an inflammatory process.[121] In an acute disc herniation, the pain is induced by chemical inflammation from proteoglycans of the nucleus pulposus and/or from compression of the nerve root.[48,49,95,97] Disc herniations typically occur through weakening of the posterolateral anulus from repetitive stress and only rarely result from a single traumatic incident.[53]

Degenerative changes may occur within the spinal canal, lateral recess, and foramen. Lateral recess or foraminal stenosis often develops from degenerative changes to the joints of Luschka and facet joints, leading to radiculopathy in the presence of nerve root compression.

Radiculopathy also may result from a localized intense inflammatory reaction alone without mechanical nerve root compression. This chemical radiculitis is thought to result from exposure to inflammogenic material from the disc to the epidural space, which promotes an increase in inflammatory mediators.[51,52,98,120,131,139] This increase leads to nerve root inflammation, which in turn may lead to radicular symptoms and eventually injury.

### Diagnosis

Radicular pain may be described as deep, dull, and achy, or sharp, burning, and electric in quality, depending on whether there is primarily motor or dorsal root involvement.[45,46] The pain associated with radiculopathy generally follows a radicular pattern in the shoulder, arm, and hand.[118,121] The most common site of cervical radicular pain is the interscapular region, although pain also may radiate to the occiput, shoulder, or arm. Neck pain is not necessarily associated with radiculopathy and frequently is absent. Patients with radiculopathy may have upper limb numbness or weakness with or without pain.

The radicular patient typically displays decreased cervical range of motion. Pain is usually worse with extension and rotation and improves with neck flexion. There can be decreased sensation to pain, light touch, or vibration. Upper limb weakness may be present with significant motor root compromise but must be differentiated from pain-related weakness. Increased lower extremity reflexes or other upper motor neuron signs suggest the possibility of a myelopathy and require aggressive work-up.

Plain films help to evaluate the disc space, vertebral body height, neuroforamen, and relative anterior-posterior diameter of the spinal canal.[134] Electrodiagnostic studies are helpful to evaluate radiculopathy or to exclude peripheral or focal neuropathy. MRI allows indepth anatomic evaluation of soft tissue structures, including the intervertebral discs, spinal cord, thecal sac, and nerve roots as well as osseous structures such as the foramen and facet joints. CT scanning allows better evaluation than MRI of osseous structures. CT-myelography is usually the imaging test of choice to document spinal and foraminal stenosis. MRI alone is not as sensitive and may give false-positive and false-negative results.[14,102,116,117]

Clinical correlation must be used to interpret the results of diagnostic testing—in particular, imaging studies that evaluate anatomy. Herniated cervical discs are found in 10% of asymptomatic people under 40 years of age and in 5% of people older than 40 years by MRI.[14] Therefore, the presence of a cervical disc herniation on an imaging study does not necessarily indicate a clinical disorder.

Treatment

Initially the patient may be placed on NSAIDs for pain control. An oral steroid taper provides a powerful antiinflammatory effect and may be used to treat a radiculopathy that does not initially respond to NSAIDs. There is little to no risk in developing avascular necrosis from a single use of short-term oral steroids.[72] Steroids should not be given concomitantly with NSAIDs or aspirin products to avoid gastric and other potential side effects. Muscle relaxants can be used as adjuncts to analgesics. Narcotics are used sparingly and for short periods.

Physical modalities may be used initially for acute pain control and later on an as-needed basis. Cervical traction may be beneficial in reducing radicular symptoms by decreasing intradiscal pressure and increasing neuroforaminal size.[34] Cervical spine range of motion is actively and passively performed to help restore normal function. As the acute episode subsides, the patient is advanced from a passive program to an active stretching and flexibility routine for the cervical spine.

Strengthening and stabilization are the next important parts of the rehabilitation process. Cervicothoracic stabilization is a rehabilitation program designed to limit pain, maximize function, and prevent further injury. Stabilization includes cervical spine flexibility, posture reeducation, and strengthening. The exercises used for stabilization proceed from simple to more advanced routines (see Table 1). Various isometric and isotonic resistance exercises are used to train the cervicothoracic muscles. Elastic bands, weight machines, and free weights are used in a progressive manner. The patient is instructed to maintain a neutral spine position at all times during stabilization exercises. Advanced exercises challenge the patient to maintain this position during dynamic activities. An engram that is achieved through repetition enables the patient to stabilize the cervical spine automatically.

Prevention of recurrent episodes through education is important. The patient should go through a neck school program during treatment and be independently involved in a home program at the time of discharge from rehabilitation.

Patients who progress slowly sometimes require the use of selective spinal injection procedures. Cervical epidurals and selective nerve root blocks in patients with radiculopathy provide diagnostic and therapeutic benefits. An epidural block may give enough relief to allow an aggressive rehabilitation program.

Patients with cervical radiculopathy and neurologic loss from cervical disc herniation may be successfully treated nonoperatively. In one study, patients suffering from a cervical radiculopathy secondary to disc herniation, the majority of which had disc extrusions, were treated conservatively with 1-year follow-up.[122] Fourteen of the patients presented with myotomal weakness, and 6 others had dermatomal sensory loss. Treatment consisted of ice, cervical collar, traction, exercise, antiinflammatory medication, oral steroids, education, and a home program. Patients with severe cervical stenosis or symptomatic myelopathy were not included in the study. Of the 26 consecutive patients enrolled in the study, 24 were treated successfully without surgery; only 2 required surgical intervention.

Patients who fail conservative treatment may benefit from surgery. Patients with neck pain alone and no radicular features typically do not benefit from surgery as much as patients with radiculopathy unless there is associated instability or myelopathic consequences. The best results of cervical disc surgery are in patients with clear-cut radicular signs and symptoms.[54,140,144]

## Internal Disc Disorders

Internal disc disruption (IDD) and degenerative disc disease (DDD) are cervical disorders involving the substance of the disc. Degenerative disc changes are common in the general population and are considered part of the natural aging process of the cervical spine. MRI demonstrates that degenerative discs are present in 25% of asymptomatic persons under 40 and nearly 60% of those over 40.[14] Younger people tend to have herniated discs, whereas older people tend to have degenerative disc changes.

## Pathophysiology

Internal disc disruption (IDD) is a term used to describe pathologic changes of the internal structure of the disc.[35] IDD is characterized as an abnormality of the nucleus pulposus and/or the anulus fibrosus with no external disc deformation. IDD is believed to result from either nuclear degradation related to trauma or isolated anular injury from a combination of cervical flexion and rotation movements. Some have implicated cervical whiplash injuries as a cause of cervical internal disc disruption.[60] The outer anulus of the cervical disc is innervated and may be a source of pain and pain referral.[19,24,142] Discrete circumferential or radial anular fissures involving the outer third of the disc are believed to be responsible for symptomatic internal disc disruption.

Disc degeneration disease (DDD) is thought to be part of the normal aging process. Age-related cervical disc changes are indistinguishable from symptomatic degenerative discs. Degenerative disc changes on radiographic studies are simply a reflection of the natural aging process and do not necessarily indicate a symptomatic process.

The disc begins to degenerate in the second decade of life. Circumferential tears begin in the anulus, particularly in the posterolateral aspects, after recurrent strains. Theoretically, several circumferential tears often consolidate to form radial fissures that eventually progress to radial fissures extending to the nucleus. The disc then becomes completely and diffusely disrupted, with tears passing through the disc. There is also loss of disc height with subsequent anular bulging at the periphery. Proteoglycans and water from nuclear degradation are lost through the fissures. Finally, the disc space becomes thin and is associated with vertebral sclerotic changes and osteophyte formation.

## Diagnosis

Either IDD or DDD may lead to neck and arm pain. Discogenic pain is typically vague and diffuse in an axial distribution. Pain referred from the disc to the arm is usually in a nonradicular pattern. Symptoms may vary according to changes in intradiscal pressure. Activities such as lifting and Valsalva maneuvers, which tend to increase disc pressure, may intensify symptoms, whereas lying supine may provide relief by decreasing intradiscal pressure. Vibration also has a tendency to exacerbate discogenic pain.

The patient with discogenic pain has decreased range of motion and is usually neurologically intact on physical examination. Pain is worse with axial compression and better with distraction. Myofascial tender or trigger points are commonly palpable.

Clinical correlation is advised in interpreting the results of radiograph or imaging studies. Seventy percent of asymptomatic people over 70 years of age have degenerative cervical spine changes in one form or another.[78,85] Twenty-five percent of asymptomatic individuals under the age of 40 and almost 60% over the age of 40 have DDD on MRI.[14]

Cervical discography has remained controversial since its introduction in 1957 by Smith.[128] Discography is used for the evaluation of IDD or DDD to determine whether the cervical disc is responsible for the neck pain. Plain films evaluate the disc space and osseous structures, and MRI or CT scan provides a detailed anatomic evaluation of the intervertebral discs. Only provocative discography can determine whether the disc is painful. Discography is an invasive procedure, not without risk. The major potential complications of cervical discography are spinal cord injury and disc infection. There are no reported cases in the literature of permanent spinal cord injury from direct needle trauma during cervical discography. Cervical discitis due to discography has a reported incidence of 0.1–0.5%.[56,114]

### Treatment

Conservative treatment is generally the same for discogenic pain as for cervical radiculopathy. Most patients with DDD are elderly, and NSAIDs, like any medication, are prescribed with caution. Patients with discogenic pain alone typically do not respond in the long term to epidural procedures but may benefit from short-term relief. In patients with DDD but without radicular symptoms, significant segmental facet pain may result from poor articular mechanics due to the DDD. Such patients may benefit from intraarticular cortisone injections or facet rhizotomy after an appropriate response to facet joint nerve (medial branch) injections. Patients who fail with conservative treatment of IDD or DDD may benefit from surgical fusion.

### CONCLUSION

The cervical spine is a complicated structure that is frequently involved in soft tissue injuries. Successful treatment depends on making the right diagnosis and providing appropriate treatment and prevention through education. Identifying the pain generator is important in establishing the diagnosis and prescribing specific treatment. The use of selective spinal procedures may be helpful in establishing the source of pain and allowing maximal benefit from rehabilitation efforts. An aggressive multidisciplinary approach to treatment often provides the best results.

### REFERENCES

1. Abel MS: Occult traumatic lesions of the cervical vertebrae. Crit Rev Clin Radiol Nucl Med 6:469–553, 1975.
2. Adams F: Paulus Aeginata, vol. 2. London, Sydenham Society, 1816.
3. Anderson KH, Mosdal C, Vaernet K: Percutaneous radiofrequency facet denervation in low-back and extremity pain. Acta Neurochir 87:48–51, 1987.
4. Aprill C, Bogduk N: The prevalence of cervical zygapophyseal joint pain: A first approximation. Spine 17:744–747, 1992.
5. Astrand NE: Medical, psychological, and social factors associated with back abnormalities and self-reported back pain. Br J Ind Med 44:327–336, 1987.
6. Awerbuch NE: Whiplash in Australia: Illness or injury? Med J Aust 157:193–196, 1992.
7. Balla JI: The late whiplash syndrome. Aust NZ J Surg 50:610–614, 1980.
8. Barnsley L, Lord S, Bogduk N: Comparative local anaesthetic blocks in the diagnosis of cervical zygapophysial pain. Pain 55:99–106, 1993.
9. Barnsley L, Lord S, Bogduk N: Pathophysiology of whiplash. Spine State Art Rev 7:330, 1993.
10. Barnsley L, Lord S, Wallis BJ, Bogduk N: The prevalence of chronic cervical zygapophyseal joint pain after whiplash. Spine 20:20–26, 1995.
11. Barnsley L, Lord SM, Wallis BJ: Lack of effect of intraarticular corticosteroids for chronic pain in the cervical zygapophyseal joints. N Engl J Med 330:1047–1050, 1994.
12. Barre JA: Sur un syndrome sympathetique cervicale posterior, et sa cause frequent: l'arthtrite cervicale. Rev Neurol 45:1246, 1926.
13. Bigos SJ, Spengler DM, Martin NA, et al: Back injuries in industry: A retrospective study III: Employee-related factors. Spine 11:252–256, 1986.
14. Boden SD, McCowin PR, Davis DO, et al: Abnormal magnetic-resonance scans of the cervical spine in asymptomatic subjects. J Bone Joint Surg 72A:1178–1184, 1990.
15. Bogduk N: Back pain: Zygapophysial joint blocks and epidural steroids. In Cousins MJ, Bridenbaugh PO (eds): Neural Blockade in Clinical Anesthesia and Pain Management, 2nd ed. Philadelphia, J.B. Lippincott, 1988, pp 935–954.
16. Bogduk N: The anatomy and pathophysiology of whiplash. Clin Biomech 1:92–101, 1986.
17. Bogduk N: The anatomy of the occipital neuralgia. Clin Exp Neurol 17:167–184, 1980.
18. Bogduk N: The clinical anatomy of the cervical dorsal rami. Spine 7:319–330, 1982.
19. Bogduk N, Aprill C: On the nature of neck pain, discography and cervical zygapophysial joint blocks. Pain 54:213–217, 1993.

20. Bogduk N, Aprill C, Dwyer A: Cervical zygapophysial joint pain patterns. II: A clinical evaluation. Spine 15:458–461, 1990.
21. Bogduk N, Long DM: Percutaneous lumbar medial branch neurotomy. A modification of facet denervation. Spine 5:193–201, 1980.
22. Bogduk N, Marsland A: On the concept of third occipital headache. J Neurol Neurosurg Psychiatry 49:775–780, 1986.
23. Bogduk N, Marsland A: The cervical zygapophysial joints as a source of neck pain. Spine 13:610–617, 1988.
24. Bogduk N, Windsor M, Inglis A: The innervation of the cervical intervertebral discs. Spine 13:2–8, 1988.
25. Bohlman HH, Emery SE: The pathophysiology of cervical spondylosis and myelopathy. Spine 13:844, 1988.
26. Braaf MM, Rosner S: Symptomatology and treatment of injuries of the neck. NY J Med 55:237, 1955.
27. Brunarski DJ: Clinical trials of spinal manipulation. J Manip Physiol Ther 7:4, 1984.
28. Cailliet R:˙Neck and Arm Pain, 3rd ed. Philadelphia, F.A. Davis, 1991.
29. Cailliet R: Soft Tissue Pain and Disability, 2nd ed. Philadelphia, F.A. Davis, 1988, pp 123–169.
30. Cantu R, Grodin A: Soft tissue mobilization. In Basmajian JV, Nyberg R (eds): Rational Manual Therapies. Baltimore, Williams & Wilkins, 1993, pp 199–221.
31. Cave AJE: The innervation and morphology of the cervical intertransverse muscles. J Anat 71:497–515, 1927.
32. Clemens HJ, Burow K: Experimental investigation on injury mechanisms of cervical spine and frontal and rear-frontal vehicle impacts. In Proceedings of the Sixteenth STAPP Car Crash Conference. Warrendale, Society of Automotive Engineers, 1972, pp 76–104.
33. Cloward RB: Cervical discography: A contribution to the etiology and mechanism of neck, shoulder, and arm pain. Ann Surg 150:1052, 1959.
34. Colachis S, Strohm B: Cervical traction: Relationship of traction time to varied tractive force with constant angle of pull. Arch Phys Med Rehabil 46:815, 1965.
35. Crock HV: A reappraisal of intervertebral disc lesions. Med J Aust 1:983–989, 1970.
36. Crowe H: Injuries to the cervical spine. Presented at the Annual Meeting of the Western Orthopedic Association, San Francisco, 1928.
37. Damkot DK, Pope MH, Lord J, et al: The relationship between work history, work environment and low-back pain in men. Spine 9:395–399, 1984.
38. Davis SJ, Teresi LM, Bradley WG, et al: Cervical spine hyperextension injuries: MR findings. Radiology 180:245–251, 1991.
39. Deans GT, Magalliard JN, Kerr M: Neck sprain—A major cause of disability following car accidents. Injury 18:10–12, 1987.
40. Deng YC: Anthropomorphic dummy neck modeling and injury considerations. Accid Anal Prev 21:85–100, 1989.
41. Dreyfuss P, Michaelsen M, Fletcher D: Atlanto-occipital and lateral atlanto-axial joint pain patterns. Spine 19:1125–1131, 1994.
42. Dwyer A, Aprill C, Bogduk N: Cervical zygapophyseal joint pain patterns. I: A study in normal volunteers. Spine 15:453–457, 1990.
43. Evans RW: Some observations on whiplash injuries. Neurol Clin 10:975–997, 1992.
44. Farrell JB, Twomey LT: Acute low back pain. Comparison of two conservative treatment approaches. Proceedings of Manipulative Therapists Association of Australia, Perth, Western Australia, 1983, p 162.
45. Feinstein B: Referred pain from paravertebral structures. In Buerger AA, Tobis JS (eds): Approaches to the Validation of Manipulative Therapy. Springfield, IL, Charles C Thomas, 1977, pp 139–174.
46. Feinstein B, Langton JNK, Jameson RM, et al: Experiments on pain referred from deep somatic tissues. J Bone Joint Surg 36A:981–997, 1954.
47. Fisher CM: Whiplash amnesia. Neurology (NY) 32:667–668, 1982.
48. Franson R, Saal J: Human disc phospholipase A2 in inflammatory disease. Spine 17(Suppl 6): S129–S132, 1992.
49. Garfin SR, Rydevik BL, Brown RA: Compressive neuropathy of spinal nerve roots. A mechanical or biological problem? Spine 16:162–165, 1991.
50. Gargan MF, Bannister GC: Long-term prognosis of soft-tissue injuries of the neck. J Bone Joint Surg 72B:901–903, 1990.
51. Gertzbein SD: Degenerative disc disease of the lumbar spine: Immunological implications. Clin Orthop Rel Res 129:68–71, 1977.
52. Gertzbein SD, Tile M, Gross A, Falk R: Autoimmunity in degenerative disc disease of the lumbar spine. Orthop Clin North Am 6:67–73, 1975.
53. Gordon SJ, King YH, Mayer PJ, et al: Mechanism of disc rupture. A preliminary report. Spine 16:450–456, 1991.

54. Gore D, Sepic S: Anterior cervical fusion for degenerated or protruded discs. Spine 9:667, 1984.
55. Gotten N: Survey of one hundred cases of whiplash injury after settlement of litigation. JAMA 162:865–867, 1956.
56. Guyer RD, Collier R, Stith WJ, et al: Discitis after discography. Spine 13:1352–1354, 1988.
57. Hackett GS: Ligament and tendon relaxation treated by prolotherapy, 3rd ed. Springfield, IL, Charles C Thomas, 1956.
58. Hadler NM, Curtis P, Gillings DB, et al: A benefit of spinal manipulation as adjunctive therapy for acute low-back pain: A stratified controlled trial. Spine 12:7, 1987.
59. Hamada G, Rida A: Orthopaedics and orthopaedic diseases in ancient and modern Egypt [letter]. Clin Orthop 89:253, 1972.
60. Hamer J, Gargan MF, Bannister GC: Whiplash injury and surgically treated cervical disc disease. Injury 24:549–550, 1993.
61. Harris JH, Yeakley JW: Hyperextension-dislocation of the cervical spine. Ligament injuries demonstrated by magnetic resonance imaging. J Bone Joint Surg 74B:567–570, 1992.
62. Hayashi K, Yabuki T: Origin of the uncus and of Luschka's joint in the cervical spine. J Bone Joint Surg 67A:788–791, 1985.
63. Hoehler FK, Tobis JS, Buerger AA: Spinal manipulation for low back pain. JAMA 245:1835, 1981.
64. Hohl M: Soft tissue injuries of the neck in automobile accidents: Factors influencing prognosis. J Bone Joint Surg 56A:1675–1681, 1974.
65. Holdsworth F: Fractures, dislocations, and fracture-dislocations of the spine. J Bone Joint Surg 52A:1534–1551, 1970.
66. Holmstrom EB, Lindell J, Mortiz U: Low back and neck/shoulder pain in construction workers: Occupational workload and psychosocial risk factors. Spine 17:672, 1992.
67. Howorth B, Petrie G: Injuries to the Spine. Baltimore, Williams & Wilkins, 1964.
68. Hult L: Cervical, dorsal, and lumbar spinal syndromes. Acta Orthop Scand 17(Suppl):1, 1954.
69. Hult L: Frequency of symptoms for different age groups and professions. In Hirsch C, Zotterman Y (eds): Cervical Pain. New York, Pergamon Press, 1971, pp 17–20.
70. Hult L: The Munkford investigation. Acta Orthop Scand 16(Suppl):1, 1954.
71. Inman VT, Saunders JB: Referred pain from skeletal structures. J Nerv Ment Dis 99:660–667, 1944.
72. Jones JP: Do short-term corticosteroids increase osteonecrosis risk? J Musculoskel Med 13:10, 1996.
73. Jónsson H, Bring G, Rauschning W, et al: Hidden cervical spine injuries in traffic accident victims with skull fractures. J Spin Disord 4:251–263, 1991.
74. Jónsson H, Cesarini K, Sahlstedt B, et al: Findings and outcome in whiplash-type neck distortions. Spine 19:2733–2743, 1994.
75. Jull G, Bogduk N, Marsland A: The accuracy of manual diagnosis for cervical zygapophysial joint pain syndromes. Med J Aust 148:233–236, 1988.
76. Kallieris D, Mattern R, Schmidt G, et al: Kinematic and spinal columnar injuries in active and passive passenger protection: Results of simulated frontal collisions. In Proceedings of the 1984 International Conference on Biomechanics of Impact. Bron, France, IRCOBI, 1984, pp 279–295.
77. Kelegren JH: Observations on referred pain arising from muscle. Clin Sci 3:280–281, 1975.
78. Kellegren JH, Lawrence JS: Osteoarthritis and disk degeneration in an urban population. Ann Rheum Dis 17:388–397, 1958.
79. Klein RG, Dorman TA, Johnson CE: Proliferant injections for low back pain: Histologic changes of injected ligaments and objective measurements of lumbar spine mobility before and after treatment. J Neurol Orthop Med Surg 10:123–126, 1989.
80. Knott M, Voss D: Proprioceptive Neuromuscular Facilitation: Patterns and Techniques. New York, McGraw-Hill, 1956.
81. Kurz LT: The differential diagnosis of cervical radiculopathy. In Herkowitz HN (ed): Seminars in Spinal Surgery. Philadelphia, W.B. Saunders, 1989, pp 194–199.
82. Kvist M, Jarvenen M: Clinical, histochemical and biochemical features in repair of muscle and tendon injuries. Int J Sports Med 3:12–14, 1982.
83. LaBan M: "Whiplash": Its evaluation and treatment. In Saal JA (ed): neck and Back Pain. Phys Med Rehabil State Art Rev 4:293–308, 1990.
84. Lawrence JS: Disc degeneration: Its frequency and relationship to symptoms. Ann Rheum Dis 38:121, 1969.
85. Lawrence JS, Brenner JM, Bier F: Osteoarthrosis: Prevalence in the population and relationship between symptoms and x-ray changes. Ann Rheum Dis 5:1–24, 1966.
86. Lazorthes G, Gaubert J: L'innervation des articulations interapophysiares vertebrales. C R Assoc Anat 43:488–494, 1956.
87. Lehmann J, deLateur BJ: Diathermy and superficial heat and cold therapy. In Kottke EJ, Stillwell GK, Lehmann JF (eds): Krusen's Handbook of Physical Medicine and Rehabilitation. Philadelphia, W.B. Saunders, 1982, pp 275–350.
88. Liu YK, Tipton CM, Mathes RD, et al: An in-situ study of the influence of a sclerosing solution in rabbit medial collateral ligaments and its junction strength. Connect Tissue Res 11:95–102, 1983.

89. Lora J, Long D: So-called facet denervation in the management of intractable back pain. Spine 1:121–126, 1976.
90. Lord S, Barnsley L, Bogduk N: Percutaneous radiofrequency neurotomy in the treatment of cervical zygapophysial joint pain: A caution. Neurosurgery 36:732–739, 1995.
91. Lord S, Barnsley L, Wallis BJ, et al: Chronic cervical zygapophysial joint pain after whiplash. A placebo-controlled prevalence study. Spine 21:1737–1745, 1996.
92. Macnab I: Acceleration injuries of the cervical spine. J Bone Joint Surg 46A:1797–1799, 1964.
93. Macnab I: The "whiplash syndrome." Orthop Clin North Am 2:389–403, 1971.
94. Makela M, Heliovaara M, Sievers D, et al: Prevalence, determinants, and consequences of chronic neck pain in Finland. Am J Epidemiol 134:1356–1367, 1991.
95. Marshall L, Trethewie E, Curtain C: Chemical irritation of nerve root in disc prolapse. Lancet 7824:320, 1973.
96. Mayou R, Bryant B, Duthie R: Psychiatric consequences of road traffic accidents. BMJ 307:1047–1050, 1993.
97. McCarron RF, Wimpee MW, Hudkins PG: The inflammatory effect of nucleus pulposus: A possible element in the pathogenesis of low-back pain. Spine 12:760–764, 1987.
98. McCarron RF, Winjed MW, Hudgins PG, et al: The inflammatory effect of nucleus pulposus: A possible element in the pathogenesis of low back pain. Spine 12:760–764, 1987.
99. McKinney LA: Early mobilization of acute sprain of the neck. BMJ 299:1006–1008, 1989.
100. Mealy K, Brennan H, Fenelon GC: Early mobilization of acute whiplash injury. BMJ 292:1656–1657, 1986.
101. Miller R, Burton R: Stroke following chiropractic manipulation of the spine. JAMA 229:189, 1974.
102. Modic MT, Masaryk TJ, Mulopulos GP, et al: Cervical radiculopathy: Prospective evaluation with surface coil MR imaging: CT with metrizamide and metrizamide myelography. Radiology 161:753–759, 1986.
103. Mortiz U: Evaluation of manipulation and other manual therapy. Criteria for measuring the effect of treatment. Scand J Rehabil Med 11:173, 1979.
104. Norris SH, Watt I: The prognosis of neck injuries resulting from rear-end vehicle collisions. J bone Joint Surg 65B:608–611, 1983.
105. Ongley MJ, Dorman TA, Esk BC, et al: Ligament instability of knees: A new approach to treatment. Man Med 3:152–154, 1988.
106. Orofino C, Sherman MS, Schechter D: Luschka's joint—a degenerative phenomenon. J Bone Joint Surg 42A:853–858, 1964.
107. Pand LQ: The otological aspects of whiplash injuries. Laryngoscope 81:1381–1387, 1971.
108. Park WW: Correlative anatomy of cervical spondylotic myelopathy. Spine 13:831, 1988.
109. Payne EE, Spillane JD: The cervical spine. An anatomico-pathological study of 70 specimens (using a special technique) with particular reference to the problem of cervical spondylosis. Brain 80:571–596, 1957.
110. Pennie B, Agambar L: Patterns of injury and recovery in whiplash. Injury 22:57–59, 1991.
111. Pennie BH, Agambar LJ: Whiplash injuries. Trial of early management. J Bone Joint Surg 72B:277–279, 1990.
112. Radanov BP, Stefano G, Schnidrig A, et al: Role of psychosocial stress in recovery from common whiplash. Lancet 338:712–715, 1991.
113. Rogal OJ, Todorczuk JM, Sumerson LF, et al: New study revolutionizes treatment of pain. Headache Relief 13:2–6, 1995.
114. Roosen K, Bettag W, Fiebach O: Komplikationen der cervikalen diskographie. ROFO 122:520–527, 1975.
115. Roydhouse RH: Torquing of the neck and jaw due to belt restraint in whiplash-type accidents. Lancet 1:1341, 1985.
116. Russell E: Cervical disc disease. Radiology 177:313–325, 1990.
117. Russell E, D'Angelo C, Zimmerman R, et al: Cervical disc herniation: CT demonstration after contrast enhancement. Radiology 152:703–712, 1984.
118. Rydevik B, Brown M, Lundborg G: Pathoanatomy and pathophysiology of nerve root compression. Spine 9:7–15, 1984.
119. Saal JS: Flexibility training. Phys Med Rehabil State Art Rev 1:537–554, 1987.
120. Saal JS, Franson RC, Debrow R, et al: High levels of inflammatory phospholipase $A_2$ activity in lumbar disc herniations. Spine 15:674–678, 1990.
121. Saal JS, Saal JA, Herzog R: The natural history of lumbar intervertebral disk extrusions treated nonoperatively. Spine 15:683–686, 1990.
122. Saal JS, Saal JA, Yurth EF: Nonoperative management of herniated cervical intervertebral disc with radiculopathy. Spine 21:1877–1883, 1996.
123. Schneider LW, Foust DR, Bowman BM, et al: Biomechanical properties of the human neck in lateral flexion. In Proceedings of the 19th STAPP Car Crash Conference. Warrendale, Society of Automotive Engineers, 1975, pp 453–485.

124. Selecki BR: Whiplash. Aust Fam Phys 13:243–247, 1984.

125. Severy DM, Mathewson JH, Bechtol CO: Controlled automobile rear end collisions: An investigation of related engineering and medical phenomena. Can Serv Med J 11:727–759, 1955.

126. Silvers HR: Lumbar percutaneous facet rhizotomy. Spine 15:36–40, 1990.

127. Smith AG: Account of a case in which portions of three dorsal vertebrae were removed for the relief of paralysis from fracture, with partial success. N Am Med Surg J 8:94, 1829.

128. Smith GW, Nichols P: The technic of cervical discography. Radiology 68:718–720, 1957.

129. Su HC, Su RK: Treatment of whiplash injuries with acupuncture. Clin J Pain 4:233, 1988.

130. Sweeney T, Prentice C, Saal JA, et al: Cervicothoracic muscular stabilizing technique. Phys Med Rehabil State Art Rev 4:335–360, 1990.

131. Takahashi H, Suguro T, Okazima Y, et al: Inflammatory cytokines in the herniated disc of the lumbar spine. Spine 21:218–224, 1996

132. Taylor JR, Womey T: Acute injuries to cervical joints. Spine 18:1736–1745, 1993.

133. Teasell RW, McCain G: The clinical spectrum and management of whiplash injuries. In Tollison CD (ed): Painful Cervical Trauma: Diagnosis and Rehabilitation Treatment in Neuromuscular Injuries. Baltimore, Williams & Wilkins, 1992, pp 292–318.

134. Torg JS, Pavlov H, Geneuaro SE, et al: Neuropraxia of the cervical spinal cord with transient quadriplegia. J Bone Joint Surg 68A:1354–1370, 1986.

135. Travell JG, Simmons DG: Myofascial Pain and Dysfunction. The Trigger Point Manual. Baltimore, Williams & Wilkins, 1983.

136. Unterharnscheidt F: Traumatic alterations in the Rhesus monkey undergoing GX-impact accelerations. Neurotraumatology 6:151–167, 1983.

137. Walker EA: A history of neurological surgery. New York, Hafner, 1967.

138. Watkinson A, Gargan MF, Bannister GC: Prognostic factors in soft tissue injuries of the cervical spine. Injury 22:307–309, 1991.

139. Weinstein J, Claverie W, Gibson S: The pain of discography. Spine 13:1344–1348, 1988.

140. White A, Southwick W, Deponte RJ: Relief of pain by anterior cervical spine fusion for spondylosis. J Bone Joint Surg 55A:525, 1973.

141. White AA, Panjabi MM: Biomechanics of the Spine, 2nd ed. Philadelphia, J.B. Lippincott, 1978, pp 229–235.

142. Whitecloud TS, Seago RA: Cervical discogenic syndrome: Results of operative intervention in patients with positive discography. Spine 12:313–316, 1987.

143. Wickstrom JK, Martinez JL, Rodriguez R, et al: Hyperextension and hyperflexion injuries to the head and neck of primates. In Gurdijian ES, Thomas IM (eds): Neckache and Backache. Springfield , IL, Charles C Thomas, 1970, pp 108–117.

144. Williams J, Allen M, Harkess J: Late results of cervical discectomy and interbody fusions: Some factors influencing the results. J Bone Joint Surg 50A:227, 1968.

# 3

# Discopathy

CURTIS W. SLIPMAN, MD
TERRY C. SAWCHUK, MD

## EPIDEMIOLOGY

Back pain results in more lost productivity than any other medical condition.[26,85,88] It is second only to upper respiratory tract complaints as a cause of time lost from work. It is estimated to account for 175.8 million days of restricted activity annually in the United States.[83] At any given time, 2.4 million Americans are disabled by low back pain; 1.2 million of these are chronically disabled.[5] The National Center for Health Statistics reported that 14.3% of new patient visits to physicians each year can be attributed to complaints of low back pain. Each year almost 13 million physician visits are required to care for chronic low back pain.[73]

In most industrialized nations, the overall lifetime prevalence of back pain exceeds 70%.[24] In the United States, the 1-year prevalence rate has been estimated at 15–20%.[23,27] In 1990, 400,000 industrial low back injuries resulted in disability in the United States. A prospective Swedish study of residents aged 20–65 years, conducted over an 18-month interval, reported 7,526 episodes of absence related to low back pain.[20] Of these patients with acute back pain, 57% recovered within 1 week, 90% in 6 weeks, and 95% after 12 weeks. Deyo and Tsui-Wu[27] reported a more protracted course of recovery for low back pain in the United States. Only 33.2% of patients with low back pain reported symptoms of less than 1 month, 33% reported pain for 1–5 months, and 32.7% reported pain for longer than 6 months. During the first 2 years after an acute episode of low back pain, recurrence rates from 60–85% have been reported.[96,98]

When asked, "Have you ever had leg pain in association with back pain?," 40% responded affirmatively.[34] If the questions are refined to determine pain distribution and associated symptoms such as numbness and weakness, this percentage drops significantly. Only 1% of adult respondents in the United States reported symptoms indicative of true sciatica. Translating the frequency of back pain into economic terms emphasizes the magnitude of the problem. Low back injuries account for approximately 22% of compensable workplace injuries but 31% of compensation payments.[34] In the United States, the direct costs of spinal disorders were estimated to exceed $23 billion during 1990.[19] This estimate represented an increase of nearly 47% over Holborock's 1984 estimated costs.[34]

## BASIC AND FUNCTIONAL ANATOMY

The lumbar spine is composed of five vertebrae with an intervertebral disc interposed between adjacent vertebral bodies. A cartilaginous endplate is located between the disc and the adjacent vertebral bodies. The disc itself is composed of a central nucleus pulposus surrounded peripherally by the anulus fibrosus. In normal young adults the nucleus is a semifluid mass of mucoid material (with the consistency more or less of toothpaste).[12] The nucleus pulposus is approximately 70–90% water in a young healthy disc, but this percentage varies and generally decreases with age.[4,37,74,76,84,90] The main constituents within the nucleus include glycosaminoglycans, proteoglycans, and collagen. Type II collagen predominates in the nucleus. Proteoglycans are the largest molecules in the body and possess an enormous capacity to imbibe water to the point of increasing their weight by 250%. This ability to attract and hold water results in predictable morphology. An intact nucleus is considered gel-like. Biomechanically it may display properties of either a solid or liquid substance, depending on transmitted loads and posture.[52]

The anulus fibrosus consists of collagen fibers, which, in contrast to the nucleus, are primarily type I. These fibers are arranged in 10–20 concentric layers, known as lamellae, that surround the nucleus pulposus.[3,95] The orientation of the collagen fibers within each lamella is parallel and angled about 65–70° from vertical.[46,47] The direction of this inclination from vertical alternates with each lamella. This alternation of the direction of fibers in consecutive lamellae is integral to the ability of the disc to resist twisting.[14]

The vertebral endplate is a thin layer of cartilage located between the vertebral body and the intervertebral disc. Although normally composed of both hyaline and fibrocartilage, the endplates are virtually entirely fibrocartilage in older discs. Because the intervertebral disc is the largest avascular structure in the body, it depends on diffusion across the endplate for nutrition and waste removal.

The principal functions of the disc are to allow movement between vertebral bodies and to transmit loads from one vertebral body to the next.[12] When axial loads are transmitted to the spine, the complex, interwined roles of the anulus fibrosus and nucleus pulposus allow pressure dispersal. The nucleus pulposus has the capacity to sustain and transmit pressure. This ability is principally invoked during weight-bearing, when the nucleus pulposus transmits loads and braces the anulus, as described below.[13] The densely packed collagen lamella of the healthy anulus is capable of sustaining an axial load on the basis of its bulk. Application of an axial load to the nucleus pulposus tends to reduce the height of the nucleus. The nucleus attempts to expand radially, thereby exerting pressure on the anulus. Anular resistance efficiently opposes this outward pressure, therefore creating a hoop tension effect. The intervertebral disc is so effective at resisting axial loads that a 40-kg load to a disc causes only 1 mm of vertical compression and only 0.5 mm of radial expansion of the disc.[50]

During movement, the anulus fibrosus acts like a ligament to restrain movements and to stabilize the interbody joint to some degree.[13] Because of their oblique orientation, the anular fibers provide resistance to movement vertically, horizontally, and during pure sliding movements forward, backward, or laterally. Twisting movements are a special consideration. During twisting, only anular fibers inclined in the direction of the movement have their points of attachment separated, thus allowing them to resist the movement. Therefore, at any time the anulus resists twisting movements with only half of its collagen fibers; this accounts for its increased susceptibility to injury from shear stress.

## DISC DEGENERATION

A series of events chronicling the degeneration of the lumbar intervertebral disc has been well described by Kirkaldy-Willis et al.[60] This widely accepted pathophysiologic process has been termed the degenerative cascade.[17] The following discussion highlights sequential changes affecting the entire motion segment during degeneration and how these anatomic changes relate to specific clinical presentations.

The process occurs in three phases. Typically, the phases overlap one another. Changes in the anterior disc, endplate, vertebral body, and posterior spinal columns (facet joints) are intimately related. Readers are referred to Kirkaldy-Willis[17] for a detailed discussion.

## Phase I

Phase I, or the dysfunctional phase, is characterized anatomically by circumferential tears in the outer anulus. These tears may be accompanied by endplate separation or failure, either of which interrupts blood supply to the disc and thus impairs nutritional supply and waste removal. These changes are believed to be secondary to repetitive microtrauma. Tears within the substance of the outer one-third of the anulus may be painful, because this portion of the disc is innervated.[10] Strong experimental evidence suggests that most episodes of low back pain are a consequence of a disc injury rather than a musculotendonous strain or ligamentous sprain.[64,82]

As the degenerative process advances, two structural changes may occur. Circumferential tears may coalesce to form radial tears, and the nucleus pulposus may lose its normal water-imbibing abilities. The second change is a direct result of biochemical changes in aggregating proteoglycans. Several studies suggest that proteoglycan destruction results from an imbalance between matrix metalloproteinase-3 (MMP-3) and tissue inhibitor of metalloproteinase-1 (TIMP-1).[25,56,61,65] These alterations result in diminished water-imbibing capacity, which manifests morphologically as a bulging disc and radiologically as a desiccated disc with diminished disc height. A bulging disc results in focal protrusion, extrusion, or sequestration if a full thickness radial anular tear develops. With these changes, the degenerating disc moves into the second phase.

It is commonly accepted that structural alteration of the facet joint follows discogenic degeneration, but, in fact, this pathologic alteration does not necessarily occur.[17,100] Changes related to the zygapophyseal joints during the dysfunction phase are believed to include synovitis and hypomobility. The facet joint may cause pain during this and all subsequent phases.

## Phase II

Phase II, or the unstable phase, is believed to result from the progressive loss of mechanical integrity of the three-joint complex. Disc-related changes include multiple anular tears, internal disruption, and disc resorption. Disc space height may be lost because of biochemical alteration and destruction of type II proteoglycans, impaired nuclear hydrophilic properties, and disc resorption. Concomitant changes in the zygapophyseal joints include cartilage degeneration, capsular laxity, and subluxation, according to the model of Kirkaldy-Willis. The biomechanical result of these alterations may lead to segmental instability. The clinical syndromes of segmental instability and intranuclear disc disruption syndrome most likely occur during this phase.

## Phase III

The stabilization phase is characterized by further disc resorption, intervertebral disc space narrowing, endplate destruction, disc fibrosis, and osteophyte formation and bridging. Pain emanating from such discs is generally believed to have a lower incidence than pain from discs in phases I and II. During this phase degenerative scoliotic symptoms present.

## NEUROPHYSIOLOGY OF LOW BACK PAIN

Three criteria must be met for a structure to be considered a pain generator: (1) it must have a nerve supply; (2) it must be susceptible to diseases or injuries known to be painful; and (3) it should be capable of causing pain similar to that seen clinically.[12]

The first criterion may be met by an established nociceptive source. Weinstein et al. identified substance P, calcitonin gene-related peptide (CGRP), and vasoactive intestinal polypeptides (VIP)—all of which are important chemicals related to pain perception—in nerves among the outer anular fibers of rat disc.[105,106] Further studies have found substances P, encephalon, dopamine, B-hydroxylase, and choline acetyltransferase immunoreactive nerve fibers among the surgically removed human longitudinal ligaments.[58]

Several studies have proven the presence of nerve fibers in the superficial layers of the anulus fibrosus.[11,15,49,54] A variety of free and complex nerve endings in the outer third of the anulus was demonstrated by Malinsky.[66] Several intrinsic painful disorders may affect lumbar discs, including discitis and internal disc disruption. Discitis often presents with complaints of lower back pain, and internal disc disruption has been shown to be a common cause of chronic low back pain.[91] These conditions satisfy the second criterion.

The third criterion has been evaluated through the performance of invasive imaging. Various investigators have demonstrated provocation of concordant pain with lumbar discography.[18,21,30,33,40,59,99,109] Although pain can be evoked with provocative discography, it has not been conclusively demonstrated that this diagnostic technique actually elicits pain from the disc or that such pain is due to a circumferential tear.[45] Moneta et al. provide the most suggestive evidence linking peripheral anular tears as the nociceptive source during discography.[71] Weinstein et al. have demonstrated that the disc has the capability of producing pain, thus fulfilling the third criterion.[105,106]

## THE ROLE OF INFLAMMATION

The following discussion centers on the current data establishing a causal relationship between inflammation and radicular pain. Back pain without radicular symptoms may be a consequence of a biochemical and/or mechanical process, with the development of the latter entirely dependent on the former.[86] The evidence indicating that inflammation underpins the radicular pain associated with symptomatic lumbar disc herniation continues to mount.[28,43,48,53,57,67–69,77,92–94,104] The notion that, in most instances, lumbar radiculopathy secondary to disc protrusion is not purely the result of a mechanical process is widely accepted. It is believed the inflammatory process sensitizes the dorsal root ganglion (DRG) to all incoming messages. In such a scenario, even minor mechanical stimulation of the DRG may evoke severe pain. Acceptance of this paradigm by spine physicians has led to two interesting position papers concerning treatment of acute radicular pain. The North American Spine Society has recommended epidural space steroid installation in the management of lumbar radicular syndromes.[107] In his presidential address Kraemer implored members of the International Society for the Study of the Lumbar Spine to use epidural perineural injection (selective nerve root block/transforaminal epidural) before surgical intervention.[62] Of note is a recent meta-analysis demonstrating the statistically significant benefit of this therapeutic approach.[44] Basic scientific evidence supporting the inflammatory model can be found in both animal and human research.

An autoimmune response has been suggested.[6–8,16,28,35,36,68,75] After embryologic formation, under normal conditions the nucleus pulposus is not in contact with the systemic circulation. It is postulated that a focal protrusion leads to exposure of nuclear material to the immune system. Because it is detected as a foreign body, an autoimmune response may be mounted.

Bobechko and Hirsch demonstrated the inflammatogenic potential of nuclear material in a rabbit model.[8] Olmarker et al. showed that the epidural application of autologous nucleus pulposus without mechanical compression in pigs may induce pronounced changes in nerve root structure and function.[80] An epidural inflammatory reaction followed application of both nucleus pulposus and fat. Olmarker et al. implanted titanium chambers containing autologous nucleus pulposus and retroperitoneal fat or empty sham chambers subcutaneously into pigs.[78] They observed increased numbers of inflammatory cells in comparison with chosen controls, thereby demonstrating that the nucleus pulposus had marked inflammagenic properties. This study also contained a second experimental model in which suspensions of homologous nucleus pulposus and homologous subcutaneous fat were injected locally into the hamster cheek pouch.[78] The results demonstrated that the nucleus pulposus suspension induced a rapid macromolecular leakage from blood vessels as well as thrombus formation within vessels. In a follow-up study, electronmicroscopic analyses of normal-appearing neural tissue revealed axonal injury and Schwann cell damage.[79] These results demonstrate that nuclear material can cause morphologic damage to neural tissue without a concurrent mechanical process such as compression. The potential for the nucleus pulposus to produce an inflammatory reaction was also demonstrated by McCarron et al., who injected autologous nucleus pulposus suspension epidurally in dogs.[69] Histologic examinations revealed that the nucleus pulposus suspension induced an epidural inflammatory reaction. A similar response was absent in a control group injected with normal saline.

Observations in human studies essentially mirror the results obtained in animal studies. Saal et al.[87] reported the presence of phospholipase A2 (PLA2) in human disc samples surgically removed for the treatment of radiculopathy secondary to lumbar disc disease. PLA2 is an enzyme responsible for the liberation of arachidonic acid from cell membranes at the site of inflammation. It plays a central role in the inflammatory process via regulation of the arachidonic acid cascade and ultimately leads to the production of prostaglandin and leukotrienes.[29,32,97] The activity of intervertebral disc-derived PLA2 was shown to be from 20–10,000 times greater than PLA2 activity derived from any other human source.[87] Franson et al. demonstrated that PLA2 extracted from human lumbar discs has a powerful ability to induce inflammatory activity in vitro.[31] Ozaktay et al. injected PLA2 into the nerve receptive fields of surgically isolated facet joint capsules in rabbits and demonstrated evidence of both neurotoxic and inflammatory effects.[81] The neurotoxic effects included loss of spontaneous nerve discharge after PLA2 injection and lack of response to mechanical stimulation in previously responsive units. Histologically, typical leukocyte infiltration with polymorphonuclear leukocytes, vascular congestion, focal extravasation, and edema provided evidence for the inflammatory effects of PLA2. These reports initiated a widespread effort to expand the understanding of the relationship between painful herniations and inflammation. Grönblad et al. demonstrated the presence of an abundant number of macrophages in human disc herniation specimens removed at the time of surgery.[39] Control discs contained only a few macrophages.[39] They also identified an important inflammatory cytosine, interleukin-beta immunoreactive cells, in herniated disc tissue. Interleukin-1 beta seems to be a significant element in the pathophysiology of rheumatoid arthritis and perhaps in osteoarthritis as well.[38,41,42] Haro et al. obtained similar data about the presence of macrophage.[43] In addition, they demonstrated statistically significant quantities of factor VII, monocyte chemotactic protein-1, and macrophage inflammatory protein-1 positive cells in symptomatic herniations. Doita et al.[28] showed infiltration of mononuclear cells along the margins of extruded discs expressing inflammatory mediators. Takahashi et al. demonstrated the presence of inflammatory cytokines in human tissue adjacent to nerve roots at the level of a symptomatic herniated disc removed at the time of surgery.[94] What, if any, role these inflammogens—interleukin-1α, interleukin-1β, interleukin-6, and tumor necrosis factor—play in the production of pain is yet to be elucidated. One possibility involves their ability to stimulate production of prostaglandin E2, which Takahashi demonstrated in vitro.[94] An interesting component of this study involved the demonstration that production of cytokine and prostaglandin E2 was "dramatically decreased" after the addition of betamethasone.

## INTERNAL DISC DISRUPTION

Internal disc disruption (IDD) is a syndrome that also may be termed incompetent disc disease. This disorder may account for one-third of all chronic low back pain.[91] Alterations in the internal structure and metabolic functions of the disc account for the associated symptoms. IDD may present after significant trauma such as sudden or unexpected lifting or forces transmitted through the disc secondary to high-speed accidents or substantial axial load. Some individuals develop IDD in the absence of an inciting event. For as yet inexplicable reasons, a small number of individuals with insidiously progressing degenerative disc disease develop IDD.

The major clinical characteristic is spinal pain in the form of a deep-seated ache. It typically worsens over several months after onset and is aggravated by activities that increase compressive forces on the spine. An explanation of why such activities cause pain is not yet widely accepted, although several theories have been offered. One proposed chemical mechanism depends on leakage of disc catabolites. These chemicals first create adverse reactions in the regional nerves around the disc and spinal canal. They also may produce constitutional disturbances, possibly mediated through the immune system.[22] Adams et al. proposed an appealing biomechanical model. They suggest that creep leads to concentrated areas of stress within the anulus.[1] Combining this concept with the results of Nachemson's intradiscal pressure studies leads to an explanation of why patients with IDD have predictable symptoms and examination findings.[72] For example, symptoms do not rapidly improve with rest but may be ameliorated by unloading the spine. Partial pain relief is achieved by resting in the lateral decubitus position, changing from unsupported to supported sitting, and assuming the standing rather than sitting position. Aerobic and anaerobic deconditioning, which result from prolonged inactivity, lead to easy fatigability, weight gain, and soft tissue contractures. Some patients experience weight loss as described by Crock,[22] but in our experience weight loss tends to be the exception. Extremity or perineal pain may be described. An insidious history is typical, and peripheral symptoms fluctuate directly with the back pain intensity. Radicular complaints are rarely confused with these sclerotomally referred symptoms. A deep achy pain, a sense of weakness without corroborative objective evidence, and a feeling of heaviness are commonly experienced. Some degree of psychologic disturbance, particularly depression, is common. In patients with IDD, as with any chronic pain disorder, psychologic factors must be critically assessed, particularly when surgical intervention is considered.

Physical examination findings consistent with IDD syndrome—but not found in every case—include provocation of back pain with pelvic rocking, straight leg raise, partial forward flexion in the standing position with the knees extended, pressure application over the intervertebral disc space, and sustained hip flexion. Sustained hip flexion is performed with the patient supine, the cervical spine in neutral or slightly flexed, and both hands clasped on the abdomen. The examiner assists the patient in flexing the hips to approximately 70° by supporting both calcanei. The knees are kept fully extended throughout the test. After telling the patient to maintain the current position, the examiner removes his hands. The patient is questioned about the presence of low back pain. Both legs are then simultaneously lowered to three or four sequentially lower positions so that the lower extremities progress toward a position parallel with the floor. A positive result entails complaints of higher intensity pain provocation at lower angles to the horizontal plane. These provocative maneuvers should not be accompanied by exorbitant demonstrations of perceived pain. Such overt pain behavior should alert the clinician to important psychosocial issues.[63,101–103] Partial pain relief is achieved through the diminishment of axially transmitted forces. While sitting at the edge of the bed, the individual is asked to shift weight to the hands by slightly lifting the buttock off the bed.

Such symptoms and examination findings are generally accepted but have not been proved by scientific study. To date, one study assessing which components of history or physical examination predict the presence of IDD has been completed, and none could be identified.[91]

Imaging studies such as MRI may be helpful in showing changes in the signals generated by the nucleus pulposus and occasionally in the adjacent vertebral bodies. However, studies have shown the same types of MRI changes in life-long asymptomatic individuals.[9,55] An interesting development in the noninvasive radiographic identification of a symptomatic disc was reported by both Aprill[2] and Schellhaus,[89] who suggest that a high-intensity zone lesion observed on MRI may be a marker of a painful disc.

Once a clinical diagnosis of probable IDD has been made, the patient has failed conservative treatment, and an MRI suggests lumbar disc degeneration, a presurgical evaluation should be completed. Psychologic testing, provocative discography, and disco-CT are performed. According to preliminary analyses at the Penn Spine Center, the probability that patients with an unremarkable psychological examination and a single positive disc will achieve a good or excellent result is approximately 80–90%.[92] In contrast, numerous studies have reported a range of 40-89% for various types of fusions for single and/or multiple symptomatic discs.[92]

## CONCLUSION

An onslaught of new research has led to a refined, albeit incomplete, understanding of the causes of low back pain. For decades a purely mechanical construct has been postulated for both axial back pain and radicular pain. This conceptual paradigm evolved from the degenerative cascade model of Kirkaldy-Willis and the observations of Mixter and Barr.[60,70] Although applicable in some instances, these postulates have failed to explain asymptomatic disc herniations[9,51,108] or asymptomatic single or multilevel lumbar spondylosis.[9,55] A biochemical model is quite appealing, because it explains the deficiencies of a purely mechanical basis for low back disorders. Hence stems the current focus of identifying inflammatory mediators and our decision to devote most of this chapter to new developments in the inflammatory model. However, a mechanical model should not be ignored. We underscore this belief with a discussion of a previously and widely doubted diagnosis: internal disc disruption syndrome.

The future for low back care is exciting. As the biochemical model is developed, new medications will be developed to abort and possibly prevent radicular pain. With advancement of the mechanical paradigm, patients who experience primarily mechanical pain will be specifically identified. This identification will allow the selection of homogeneous populations and completion of much-needed outcome studies. Results from these studies will elucidate when and on whom surgery should be performed, who should participate in extended exercise programs, and for whom medical care is unnecessary.

## REFERENCES

1. Adams MA, McMillan DW, Green TP, Dolan P: Sustained loading generates stress concentrations in lumbar intervertebral discs. Spine 21:434–438, 1996.
2. Aprill C, Bogduk N: High-intensity zone: A diagnostic sign of painful lumbar disc on magnetic resonance imaging. Br J Radiol 65:361–369, 1992.
3. Armstrong JR: Lumbar Disc Lesions, 3rd ed. Edinburgh, Churchill-Livingstone, 1965, p 13.

4. Beard HK, Stevens RL: Biochemical changes in the intervertebral disc. In Jayson MIV (ed): The Lumbar Spine and Backache, 2nd ed. London, Pitman, 1980, pp 407–436.
5. Bigos SJ, Battié MC: The impact of spinal disorders in industry. In Frymoyer JW (ed): The Adult Spine. New York, Raven Press, 1991.
6. Bisla RS, Marchisello PJ, Lockshin MD, et al: Autoimmunological basis of disc degeneration. Clin Orthop 123:149–154, 1976.
7. Bobechko WT, Hirsch C. Autoimmune response to nucleus pulposus in the rabbit. J Bone Joint Surg 47B:574, 1965.
8. Bobechko WT, Hirsch C. Autoimmune response to nucleus pulposus in the rabbit. J Bone Joint Surg 47B:574–580, 1965.
9. Boden SD, Davis DO, Dina TS, et al: Abnormal magnetic resonance scans of the lumbar spine in asymptomatic subjects: A prospective investigation. J Bone Joint Surg 72A:403–408, 1990.
10. Bogduk N: The innervation of the human lumbar intervertebral discs. J Anat 132:39–56, 1981.
11. Bogduk N: The innervation of the lumbar spine. Spine 8:286, 1983.
12. Bogduk N, Twomey LT: Clinical Anatomy of the Lumbar Spine, 2nd ed. London, Churchill Livingstone, 1991, p 12.
13. Bogduk N, Twomey LT: Clinical Anatomy of the Lumbar Spine, 2nd ed. London, Churchill Livingstone, 1991, p 25.
14. Bogduk N, Twomey LT: Clinical Anatomy of the Lumbar Spine, 2nd ed. London, Churchill Livingstone, 1991, p 125.
15. Bogduk N, Twomey LT: Clinical Anatomy of the Lumbar Spine, 2nd ed. London, Churchill Livingstone, 1991, p 161.
16. Braun IF, Lin JR, Benjamin MU, Kriecheff II: Compound tomography of the asymptomatic postsurgical lumbar spine: Analysis of the physiologic scar. AJR 139:149–152, 1984.
17. Butler D, Trafimow JH, Andersson GB, et al: Discs degenerate before facets. Spine 15:111–113, 1990.
18. Butt WP: Lumbar discography. J Can Assoc Radiol 14:172, 1964.
19. Cats-Baril WL, Frymoyer JW: The economics of spinal disorders. In Frymoyer JW (ed): The Adult Spine. New York, Raven Press, 1991.
20. Choler U, Larsson R, Nachemson A, Peterson LE: Back Pain. Spri Report 188, 1985 [in Swedish].
21. Colhoun E, McCall IW, Williams L, Cassar Pullicino VN: Provocation discography as a guide to planning operations on the spine. J Bone Joint Surg 70B:267, 1988.
22. Crock HV: Internal disc disruption. In Frymoyer JW (ed): The Adult Spine: Principles and Practice. New York, Raven Press, 1991, p 2015.
23. Cunningham LS, Kelsey JL: Epidemiology of musculoskeletal impairments and associated disability. Am J Public Health 74:574, 1984.
24. Damkot DK, Pope MH, Lord J, Frymoyer JW: The relationship between work history, work environment and low back pain in men. spine 9:395, 1984.
25. Dean DD, Pelletier MJ, Pelletier JP, Howell DS: Evidence for metalloproteinase and metalloproteinase inhibitor imbalance of human osteoarthritic cartilage. J Clin Invest 84:678–685, 1989.
26. Deyo RA, Bass JE: Lifestyle and low back pain. Spine 14:501, 1989.
27. Deyo RA, Tsui-Wu Y-J: Descriptive epidemiology of low back pain and its related medical care in the United States. Spine 12:264–268, 1987.
28. Doita M, Kanatani T, Harada T, Maizuno K: Immunohistologic study of the ruptured intervertebral disc of the lumbar spine. Spine 21:235–241, 1996.
29. Famaey JP: Phospholipases, eicosanoid production and inflammation. Clin Rheumatol 1:84–94, 1982.
30. Feinberg SB: The place of discography in radiology as based on 2,320 cases. AJR 92:1275, 1964.
31. Franson RC, Saal JS, Saal JA: Human disc phospholipase $A_2$ is inflammatory. Spine 17(6S):S129, 1992.
32. Franson RC, Weir DL: Inhibition of a potent phospholipase $A_2$ activity in the synovial fluid of patients with arthritis by nonsteroidal anti-inflammatory agents. Clin Res 31:650A, 1983.
33. Friedman J, Goldner MZ: Discography in evaluation of lumbar disc lesions. Radiology 65:653, 1955.
34. Frymoyer JW: Epidemiology: The magnitude of the problem. In Wiesel SW, et al (eds): The Lumbar Spine, 2nd ed. Philadelphia, W.B. Saunders, 1992.
35. Gertzbein SD: Degenerative disc disease of the lumbar spine: Immunological implications. Clin Orthop Res Res 129:68–71, 1977.
36. Gertzbein SD, Tile M, Gross A, Falk R: Autoimmunology in degenerative disc disease of the lumbar spine. Orthop Clin North Am 6:67–73, 1975.
37. Gower WE, Pedrimi V: Age-related variation in protein polysaccharides from human nucleus pulposus, annulus fibrosus and costal cartilage. J Bone Joint Surg 51A:1154–1162, 1969.
38. Grönblad M, Tolonen J, Virri J, et al: Immunohistochemical characterization of pro-inflammatory cell types in disc herniation tissue. Presented at the Annual Meeting of the International Society for the Study of the Lumbar Spine, Marseilles, France, 1993.

39. Grönblad M, Virri J, Tolonen J, et al: A controlled immunohistochemical study of inflammatory cells in disc herniation tissue. Spine 19:2744–2751, 1994.
40. Grubb SA, Lipscomb HJ, Guilford WB: The relative value of lumbar roentgenograms, metrizamide myelography and discography in the assessment of patients with chronic low back syndrome. Spine 12:282, 1987.
41. Guyton AC: The blood cells. In Function of the Human Body, 3rd ed. Philadelphia, W.B. Saunders, 1965, pp 85–98.
42. Hardy MA: The biology of scar formation. Phys Ther 69:1014–1024, 1989.
43. Haro H, Shinomiya K, Komori H, et al: Unregulated expression of chemokines in herniated nucleus pulposus resorption. Spine 21:1647–1652, 1996.
44. Haselkorn JK, Rapp S, Ciol M, et al: Epidural steroid injections and the management of sciatica: A meta-analysis. Arch Phys Med Rehabil 76:1037, 1995.
45. Heggeness M, Doherty BJ: Discography causes endplate deflection. Spine 18:1050–1053, 1993.
46. Hickey DS, Hukins SWL: X-ray diffraction studies of the arrangement of collagen fibers in human fetal intervertebral disc. J Anat 131:81–90, 1980.
47. Hickey DS, Hukins SWL: Relation between the structure of the annulus fibrosis and the function and failure of the intervertebral spine. Spine 5:100–116, 1980.
48. Hirabayashi S, Kumano K, Tsuiki T, et al: A dorsally displaced free fragment of lumbar disc herniation and its interesting histologic findings. Spine 15:1231–1233, 1990.
49. Hirsch C, Ingelmark BE, Miller M: The anatomical basis for low back pain. Acta Orthop Scand 33:1–17, 1963.
50. Hirsch C, Nachemson A: New observations on mechanical behavior of lumbar discs. Acta Orthop Scand 23:254–283, 1954.
51. Hitselberger W, Witten R: Abnormal myelograms in asymptomatic patients. J Neurosurg 28:204–206, 1968.
52. Iatridis JC, Weidenbaum N, Setton LA, Mow VC: Is the nucleus pulposus a solid or a fluid? Mechanical behaviors of the nucleus pulposus of the human intervertebral disc. Spine 21:1174–1184, 1996.
53. Ito T, Yamada M, Ikuta F, et al: Histologic evidence of absorption of sequestration-type herniated disc. Spine 21:230–234, 1996.
54. Jackson HC, Winkelmann RK, Bickel WH: Nerve endings in the human lumbar spinal column and related structures. J Bone Joint Surg 48A:1272–1281, 1966.
55. Jensen MC, Brant-Zawadzki MN, Obuchowski N, et al: Magnetic resonance imaging of the lumbar spine in people without back pain. N Engl J Med 2:69–73, 1994.
56. Kanemoto M, Hukuda S, Komiya Y, et al: Immunohistochemical study of matrix metalloproteinase-3 and tissue inhibitor metalloproteinase-1 in human intervertebral discs. Spine 21:1–8, 1996.
57. Kang JD, Georgescu HI, McIntyre-Larkin L, et al: Herniated lumbar intervertebral discs spontaneously produce matrix metalloproteinases, nitric oxide, interleukin-6, and prostaglandin $E_2$. Spine 21:271–277, 1996.
58. Kawakami M: Histochemical and immunohistochemical demonstrations of nerve fibers on human perispinal soft tissue. J Wakayama Med Soc 40:621, 1989 [in Japanese].
59. Keck C: Discography: Technique and interpretation. Arch Surg 80:580, 1960.
60. Kirkaldy-Willis WH: The pathology and pathogenesis of low back pain. In Kirkaldy Willis WH (ed): Managing Low Back Pain. New York, Churchill Livingstone, 1988, p 49.
61. Komiya Y: Immunohistochemical localization of tissue inhibitor of metalloproteases (TIMP) and stromelysin in human joint synovium. Jpn J Rheum Joint Surg 11:59–70, 1992.
62. Kraemer J: Presidential Address: National Course and Prognosis of Intervertebral Disc Diseases. Spine 20:635–639, 1995.
63. Kummel BM: Nonorganic signs of significance in low back pain. Spine 21:1077–1081, 1996.
64. Kuslich SD, Ulstrom CL, Michael CJ: The tissue origin of low back pain and sciatica: A report of pain response to tissue stimulation during operations on the lumbar spine using local anesthesia. Orthop Clin North Am 22:181–187, 1993.
65. MacNaul KL, Chartrain N, Lark M, et al: Discoordinate expression of stromelysin, collagenase, and tissue inhibitor of metalloproteinase-1 in rheumatoid human synovial fibroblast: Synergistic effects of inter-leukin-1 and tumor necrosis factor alpha on stromelysin expression. J Biol Chem 265:17238–17245, 1990.
66. Malinsky J: The ontogenetic development of nerve terminations in the intervertebral discs of man. Acta Anat 38:96–113, 1959.
67. Marshall LL, Trethewie ER: Chemical irritation of nerve-root in disc prolapse. Lancet ii:320, 1973.
68. Marshall LL, Trethewie ER, Curtain CC: Chemical radiculitis: A clinical physiological and immunological study. Clin Orthop Rel Res 129:61–67, 1987.
69. McCarron RF, Wimpee MW, Hudkins PG, Laros GS: The inflammatory effect of nucleus pulposus: A possible element in the pathogenesis of low back pain. Spine 12:760–764, 1987.
70. Mixter WJ, Barr JS: Rupture of the intervertebral disc with involvement of the spinal canal. N Engl J Med 211:210–215, 1934.

71. Moneta GB, Videman T, Kaivanto K, et al: Reported pain during lumbar discography as a function of annular ruptures and disc degeneration. Spine 19:1968–1974, 1994.
72. Nachemson A, Morris JM: In vivo measurements of intradiscal pressure: Discometry, a method for the determination of pressure in the lower lumbar discs. J Bone Joint Surg 46A:1077, 1964.
73. National Center for Health Statistics: Prevalence of Selected Impairment, United States—1977. Hyattsville, MD, Department of Health and Human Services Publication, series 10, no. 134, 1984.
74. Naylor A: Intervertebral disc prolapse and degeneration. The biochemical and biophysical approach. Spine 1:108–114, 1976.
75. Naylor A, et al: Enzymic and immunologic activity in the intervertebral disc. Orthop Clin North Am 6:51–58, 1975.
76. Naylor A, Shental R: Biochemical Aspects of Intervertebral Discs in Aging and Disease. In Jayson MIV (ed): The Lumbar Spine and Backache. New York, Grune & Stratton, 1976, pp 317–326.
77. O'Donnell JL, O'Donnell AL: Prostaglandin $E_2$ content in herniated lumbar disc disease. Spine 21:1653–1656, 1996.
78. Olmarker K, Blomquist J, Strömberg J, et al: Inflammatogenic properties of nucleus pulposus. Spine 20:665–669, 1995.
79. Olmarker K, Nordborg C, Larsson K, Rydevik B: Ultrastructural changes in spinal nerve roots induced by autologous nucleus pulposus. Spine 21:411–414, 1996.
80. Olmarker K, Rydevik B, Nordborg C: Autologous nucleus pulposus induces neurophysiologic and histologic changes in porcine cauda equina nerve roots. Spine 18:1425–1432, 1993.
81. Ozaktay AC, et al: Phospholipase A2-induced electrophysiologic and histologic changes in rabbit dorsal lumbar spine tissues. Spine 20:2659–2668, 1995.
82. Palmgren T, Grönblad M, Virri J, et al: Immunohistochemical demonstration of sensory and autonomic nerve terminals in herniated lumbar disc tissue. Spine 21:1301–1306, 1996.
83. Praemer A, Furner S, Rice DP: Musculoskeletal Conditions in the United States. Elk Grove, IL, American Academy of Orthopaedic Surgeons, 1992, pp 23–33.
84. Puschel J: Der wassergehalt normaler und degenerierter swischenwirbelscheiben. Beitr Path Anat 84:123–130, 1930.
85. Rowe ML: Low back pain in industry. A position paper. J Occup Med 11:161, 1969.
86. Saal J: The role of inflammation in lumbar pain. Spine 20:1821–1827, 1995.
87. Saal JS, Franson RC, Dobrow R, et al: High levels of inflammatory phospholipase $A_2$ activity in lumbar disc herniations. Spine 15:674–678, 1990.
88. Salkever DS: Morbidity Costs: National Estimates and Economic Determinants. NCHSR Research Summary Series, October 1985, Department of Health and Human Services Publication No. 86-3393, 1986.
89. Schellhas KP, Pollei SR, Gundry CR, Heithoff KB: Lumbar disc high-intensity zone. Spine 21:79–86, 1996.
90. Schmorl G, Junghanns H: The Human Spine in Health and Disease, 2nd American ed. New York, Grune & Stratton, 1971, p 18.
91. Schwarzer AC, Aprill CN, Derby R, et al: The prevalence and clinical features of internal disc disruption in patients with chronic low back pain. Spine 20:1878–1883, 1995.
92. Slipman CW: Discography. In Gonzalez E (ed): Acute Low Back Pain: Assessment and Management. Demos Vermande, [in press].
93. Smyth MJ, Wright V: Sciatica and the intervertebral disc: An experimental study. J Bone Joint Surg 40A:1401–1418, 1958.
94. Takahashi H, Suguro T, Okazima Y, et al: Inflammatory cytokines in the herniated disc of the lumbar spine. Spine 21:218–224, 1996.
95. Taylor JR: The development and adult structure of lumbar intervertebral discs. J Man Med 5:43–47, 1990.
96. Troup JDG, Martin JW, Lloyd DCEF: Back pain in industry: A prospective survey. Spine 6:61–69, 1981.
97. Vadas P, Stefanski E, Pruzanski W: Influence of plasma proteins on activity of pro-inflammatory enzyme phospholipase. Inflammation 10:183–193, 1986.
98. Valkenburg HA, Haanen HCM: The epidemiology of low back pain. In White AA III, Gordon SL (eds): American Academy of Orthopaedic Surgeons Symposium on Idiopathic Low Back Pain. St. Louis, Mosby, 1982.
99. Vanharanta H, Sachs BL, Spivey MA, et al: The relationship of pain provocation to lumbar disc deterioration as seen by CT/discography. Spine 12:295–298, 1987.
100. Vernon-Roberts B, Pirie CJ: Degenerative changes in the intervertebral discs and their sequelae. Rheumatol Rehabil 16:13–22, 1977.
101. Waddell G, Bircher M, Finlayson D, Main CJ: Symptoms and signs: Physical disease or illness behavior. BMJ 289:739–741, 1984.
102. Waddell G, McCulloch JA, Kummel E, Verner RM: Nonorganic physical signs in low back pain. Spine 5:117–125, 1980.

103. Walsh TR, Weinstein JN, Spratt KF, et al: Lumbar discography in normal subjects: A controlled prospective study. J Bone Joint Surg 72A:1081–1088, 1990.
104. Wehling P, Bandra G, Evans CH, Schulitz KP: Synovial cytokines impair the function of the sciatic nerve in rats: A possible element in the pathophysiology of radicular syndromes. Orthop Trans 14:338–339, 1990.
105. Weinstein J, Claverie W, Gibson S: The pain of discography. Spine 13:1344, 1988.
106. Weinstein J: Mechanisms of spinal pain: The dorsal root ganglion and its role as a mediator of low back pain. Spine 11:999, 1986.
107. Weinstein S, Herring SA, Derby R: Contemporary concepts in spine care: Epidural steroid injections. Spine 20:1842–1846, 1995.
108. Wiesel SW, Tsourmas N, Feffer HL, et al: A study of computer assisted tomography. Part I: The incidence of positive CAT scans in an asymptomatic group of patients. Spine 9:549–551, 1984.
109. Wilson DH, MacCarty WC: Discography: Its role in the diagnosis of lumbar disc protrusion. J Neurosurg 31:520, 1969.

# 4

# Zygapophyseal (Facet) Joint Pain: A Functional Approach

ANDREW J. COLE, MD
SUSAN J. DREYER, MD
PAUL DREYFUSS, MD
STEVEN A. STRATTON, Phd, PT, ATC

An anatomically accurate and functionally complete diagnosis of pain originating from the spine and its supporting tissues may improve treatment outcome. After excluding nonspinal causes of back and neck pain, the clinician's challenge is to distinguish whether the intervertebral disc, spinal nerve roots, joints, ligaments, or muscles are responsible for the patient's subjective pain experience. The posterolateral, paired facet joints of the spine are more precisely termed zygapophyseal joints (z-joints). These joints have been implicated as a source of low back pain since 1911.[82]

Both axial and extremity pain may be caused by z-joint pathology.[4,22,57,61,75,92,126,128,172] The z-joint is considered to be a source of discomfort if precise instillation of local anesthetic into the joint or around its nerve supply eliminates all or part of a patient's pain (Fig. 1). Elimination of nociception from a joint with local anesthetic blockade determines whether the anesthetized joint is a source of pain. A recent saline-controlled study of patients with chronic low back pain noted that 40% reported 50% or greater relief of pain with intraarticular z-joint blocks and no relief with placebo injection.[153] Another study designed to eliminate false-positive responses used physiologic pain relief after two separate blocks with different local anesthetics. This study showed that 15% of patients with chronic low back pain who were referred to tertiary spine centers had isolated lumbar z-joint pain.[149] The prevalence of lumbar z-joint pain based on single diagnostic blocks ranges from 7.7–75%.[32–34,42,66,88,109,116,119,128,130,131,140,142] Practice referral patterns, interpretation of imaging results, physical examination selection criteria, and potential placebo responses may be responsible for the wide variation in z-joint pain prevalence. The studies with larger sample groups and fewer inclusion criteria account for lower prevalence rates.[95,96,130,140] The prevalence of isolated cervical z-joint–mediated pain in patients with chronic neck pain is at least 25%.[4,10,17] The prevalence of cervical z-joint pain may approach 64% in patients with neck and nonradicular referred pain if combined cervical discogenic and z-joint pain are included.[17] No studies on prevalence of thoracic z-joint pain are available.

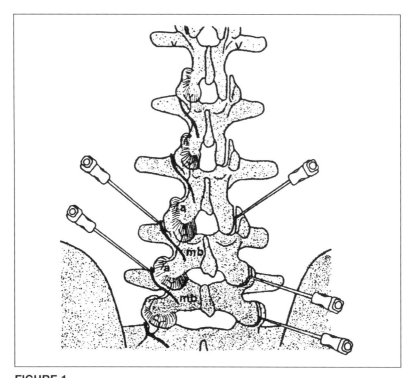

**FIGURE 1.**
Posterior view of the lumbar spine demonstrating location of the medial branches
*(mb)* of the dorsal rami that innervate the lumbar z-joints *(a)*. Needle positions for the
L3 and L4 medial branch blocks are shown on the left half of the diagram and would
be used to anesthetize the L4–L5 z-joint. The right half of the diagram demonstrates
L3–L4, L4–L5, and L5–S1 intraarticular z-joint injection position. (From Bogduk N:
Back pain: Zygapophysial blocks and epidural steroids. In Cousins MJ, Bridenbaugh
PO (eds): Neural Blockade in Clinical Anesthesia and Management of Pain, 2nd ed.
Philadelphia, J.B. Lippincott, 1989, p 937, with permission.)

Injections to diagnose and control pain originating from the z-joints should be
used only as an adjunct to aggressive, conservative spine care and not in isolation.
Conservative care may include oral medication, modalities, traction, instruction in body
mechanics, manual physical therapy, flexibility training, strength training, and aerobic
conditioning. No randomized, prospective studies assess the efficacy of noninjection or
noninvasive conservative care in a population selected for pure z-joint pain as demonstrated by physiologic pain relief with diagnostic intra-articular and/or medial branch
nerve blocks in any spinal segment.

Important diagnostic information is gained from fluoroscopically guided, contrast-enhanced z-joint injections.[4,15,22,41,56,93,168] The therapeutic benefit of z-joint injections remains controversial.[11,15,32–34,42,43,48,51,56,59,65,66,95,96,98,109,117,119,121,128,130,142,143,169] Some
argue that short-term pain relief from the local anesthetic or corticosteroid may facilitate a rehabilitation program and result in decreased pain and improved function.
Others have demonstrated no lasting benefit, for the vast majority of patients, from
z-joint injections used in therapeutic isolation compared with inert injections.[11,32] This
chapter reviews the literature regarding the anatomy, biomechanics, pathophysiology,
diagnosis, and treatment of z-joint pain and dysfunction. Detailed discussion regarding
z-joint injection procedures can be found on pp. 269–271.

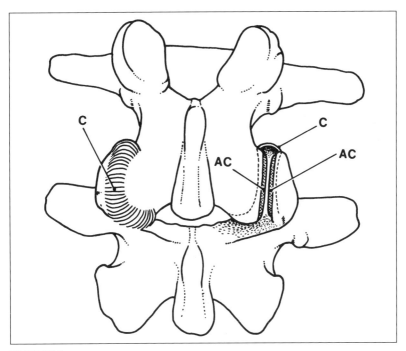

**FIGURE 2.**
Posterior view of the L3–L4 lumbar z-joint. The capsule *(c)* is intact on the left but removed on the right to demonstrate the joint anatomy: articular cartilage *(ac)* separated by the joint space, superior capsule *(c)*, and posterior capsular attachment sites (dotted lines). (From Bogduk N, Twomey LT: Clinical Anatomy of the Lumbar Spine, 2nd ed. London, Churchill Livingstone, 1991, p 27, with permission.)

## ANATOMY

A z-joint is a true synovial joint with a joint space, hyaline cartilage, synovial membrane, and fibrous capsule (Fig. 2). Z-joints have the potential to mediate pain. Cadaver studies have demonstrated that they are innervated by medial branch nerve nociceptive fibers originating from adjacent dorsal rami (see Fig. 1).[15,16,23,24,41,157,176,177]

### Lumbar Anatomy

The lumbar z-joints are paired synovial joints that vary between a "C" and "J" shape.[22,115] The filling volume of each lumbar z-joint has been found to be approximately 1–2 cc.[80] The plane of each lumbar z-joint progresses from the sagittal plane to approximately 45° coronally from L1–L2 to L5–S1. The most inferior joints may approach a coronal orientation. Two subcapsular recesses are created by the 1-mm thick fibrous capsule of the lumbar z-joint that attaches about 2 mm from the articular margins.[39,179] Although their existence is controversial, fibroadipose meniscoids are reported to project into the joint and may protect exposed cartilaginous articular surfaces during movement (Fig. 3).[18,23] The joint capsule resists flexion forces and counteracts a posterior sliding motion during extension.[39] Substantial sensory innervation, including nociceptive nerve fibers, is found in the z-joint capsule.[7,76,77] In degenerative z-joints, subchondral bone nerve fibers containing the pain mediator substance P have been isolated.[12] Autonomic nerve fibers have been found in z-joint capsules.[7] In addition, mechanoreceptors have been demonstrated in rabbit z-joints.[8] Finally, z-joint synovial

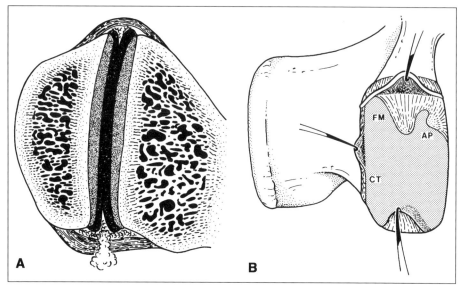

**FIGURE 3.**
*A,* Coronal view of a lumbar z-joint demonstrating the joint's superior and inferior fibroadipose meniscoids. *B,* Lateral view of a lumbar z-joint with the superior articular process removed to show the joint's anatomy. The capsule is retracted with small hooks in the diagram. The fibromeniscoid *(FM)*, adipose tissue pad *(AP)*, and connective tissue *(CT)* rim of the joint are labeled. (From Bogduk N, Twomey LT: Clinical Anatomy of the Lumbar Spine, 2nd ed. London, Churchill Livingstone, 1991, p 33, with permission.)

nociceptors have been identified in some studies,[76,77] whereas other researchers believe that these synovial nerves regulate blood flow.[86,105]

### Cervical Anatomy

True z-joints in the cervical spine are found from C2–C3 to C7–T1. The atlantooccipital and atlantoaxial joints are not true z-joints.[21,49,52,53] From C2–C3 distally, the z-joint superior articular processes from the vertebral level below are oriented posteriorly and superiorly at 45° from the horizontal plane. These superior articular processes form the inferior portion of the cervical z-joint. In a reciprocal manner, the inferior articular processes from the vertebral level above are oriented anteriorly and inferiorly at 45° from the horizontal plane. The angle of z-joint inclination becomes more vertical at the lower cervical z-joints.[60] Cervical z-joint articular surfaces are relatively flat and have only minimal concavity or convexity.

Each cervical z-joint from C3–C4 to C7–T1 is innervated by the medial branches of the dorsal rami from the level above and below that joint.[16] The third occipital nerve, which is the superficial medial branch of the C3 dorsal ramus, innervates the C2–C3 z-joint. The third occipital nerve then continues around the lower lateral and dorsal surface of the C2–C3 joint, embedded in the connective tissue that invests the joint capsule.[16,21]

The volume of a cervical z-joint is usually 1 cc or less.[4,15,61] Like its lumbar spine counterpart, each cervical z-joint is lined with hyaline cartilage and may contain a meniscus.[22,181] The fibrous joint capsule forms superior and inferior capsular recesses. Mechanoreceptors and nociceptors richly innervate each cervical z-joint capsule.[176] The internal margin of the joint capsule is covered by the ligamentum flavum.[13]

## Thoracic Anatomy:

The thoracic z-joints are also paired diarthrodial joints. They probably are innervated by the medial branches of the dorsal rami.[24] The articular surface of each joint is oriented 60° from the horizontal plane and rotated 20° laterally. The medial margin of the joint is positioned more posteriorly.[60,147] The upper thoracic joints are usually more vertically inclined. The lower thoracic z-joints become more sagittally oriented (similar to the orientation of the more proximal lumbar z-joints).[162] Thoracic z-joint capsules are reinforced anteriorly by the ligamentum flavum and posteriorly by the posterior spinal ligaments.[162]

## BIOMECHANICS

Spinal z-joints help to direct segmental motion and share loads with the anterior elements. In the lumbar spine, axial rotation is limited by the sagittal orientation of the z-joints, and translation is limited by the z-joints' coronal orientation.[23] Lumbar end-range forward flexion is achieved by translation of the inferior articular process along the superior articular process. Translation of 5–7 mm occurs during forward flexion.[115] Lumbar spondylosis and hyperlordosis increase lumbar z-joint load sharing.[2,180] Maximal lumbar z-joint intraarticular pressure occurs during extension.[58] The inferior facet may glide beyond the superior facet and contact inferior laminae when the lumbar spine is extended past its normal range of motion.[180] Stretch of the lumbar z-joint capsule also may occur if the joint is overloaded.[180] The capsular ligaments of z-joints protect the posterior anulus of the disc from excessive torsion and flexion stress.[2,23]

As a result of their alignment, cervical z-joints are characterized by greater segmental weight-bearing and less torsional resistance than their lumbar spine counterparts.[24] The C2–C3 joint lies between the upper cervical spine, which primarily accommodates rotation, and the lower cervical spine, which primarily accommodates flexion and extension.[122,135] Therefore, it is considered a transitional joint from both biomechanic and anatomic perspectives.

The thoracic region is the most stable region of the spinal column with the least amount of spinal axis z-joint motion.[169] Thoracic z-joints are reported to bear between 0% and 33% of the axial load, depending on posture.[162]

## Z-JOINT PATHOPHYSIOLOGY

The z-joint as a source of pain has been well established anatomically,[15,16,23] histologically[7,12,76,77] and clinically.[4,20,22,56,57,92,126,128,172] However, the precise cause of most z-joint pain remains unknown.

Common causes of z-joint pain include trauma and degeneration. Microtrauma, such as small articular fractures of the lumbar and cervical z-joints, is not readily apparent on routine radiographs but may be detected with stereoradiography and multidirectional tomography.[156,174] Lumbar z-joint fractures, capsular tears, articular cartilage splits, and articular cartilage hemorrhage have been documented in post-mortem studies of trauma victims who had normal radiographs.[161] The relationship between pain and such pathologic findings was not assessed. A different, open study of 11 patients did not find a correlation between cervical z-joint arthropathy and previous trauma.[93]

Osteoarthritis may be related to z-joint pain. Radiographic changes of z-joint osteoarthritis are strongly correlated with age but not with spinal pain. The incidence of z-joint arthropathy is equal in both symptomatic and asymptomatic patients.[110,123] Some researchers report that degenerative joints are more likely to be symptomatic than nondegenerative joints.[33,116] Other studies have shown that the degenerative joint changes demonstrated with computed tomography (CT) are not always painful.[88,142,171] In addition, lumbar z-joints may be painful, even if they appear normal on both plain radiographs and single-photon emission computed tomography (SPECT) scans.[34,41,63,109,119,131,142,146,152]

Meniscoid entrapment and extrapment,[19] synovial impingement,[19,23,41] chondromalacia facetae,[63] capsular and synovial inflammation,[15,23] and mechanical injury to the joint capsule[7] also have been considered as possible causes of z-joint pain. Occasionally, the z-joints are affected by systemic inflammatory arthritides such as rheumatoid arthritis or ankylosing spondylitis.[9,97] Other rare conditions, such as villonodular synovitis, synovial cysts, and infection, have been reported to cause z-joint pain.[29,89,145]

In summary, it appears that spinal z-joints may become painful for various reasons. Diagnostic, fluoroscopically guided, contrast-enhanced z-joint anesthetic injections may relieve spine and extremity pain, whether or not arthritic changes are present in the z-joint. Fluoroscopically guided, contrast-enhanced injections help identify painful z-joint(s), but they do not differentiate the underlying pathology.

## CLINICAL PICTURE

No noninvasive pathognomonic findings distinguish z-joint-mediated pain from other sources of spine pain.[22,41,95,96,142] The diagnosis of z-joint pain is one of exclusion and confirmation by analgesic injections. However, physicians must still apply their clinical judgment and knowledge of a patient's previous response to treatment to determine whether a z-joint may be a source of pain.[47,48] Potentially important but not diagnostic clinical findings include (1) site of maximal segmental or direct articular tenderness, (2) concordant pain on provocative segmental testing, (3) "articular restriction" and local soft tissue changes such as increased muscle tone,[85] and (4) pain in recognized z-joint referral zones.[36,57,61,126,128] Studies show that certain levels appear to be more commonly involved, including C2–C3, C5–C6, L4–L5, and L5–S1.[22,34,109,131,148,151] No similar data exist for the thoracic spine.

### Signs and Symptoms

The clinical presentation of z-joint–mediated pain appears to overlap considerably with the presentation of spine pain due to other causes. Although patients with z-joint pain are neurologically intact, they may demonstrate pain-inhibited weakness, subjective nondermatomal extremity sensory loss, and other distal sensory complaints.[66,128,148]

The largest study of provocative tests for z-joint pain involved 390 patients who underwent single, fluoroscopically guided, diagnostic lumbar z-joint injections. The authors concluded that none of the 127 potentially predictive variables that they studied absolutely correlated with pain relief upon z-joint injection. However, older age, history of low back pain, absence of leg pain, absence of exacerbation by cough, normal gait, absence of muscle spasm, and maximal pain on extension after forward flexion correlated significantly with postinjection relief.[96]

A more recent study explored potential clinical indicators of z-joint pain in a population with definite lumbar z-joint discomfort. To be included in the analysis, patients were required to achieve physiologic responses to two separate, fluoroscopically guided blocks. If pain relief was not obtained with both injections and if the longer-duration anesthetic did not correlate with a longer period of analgesia, the patients were not believed to have true z-joint pain and were excluded as potential false-positive responders. Despite the tightly controlled population, no correlation was noted between pain relief after lumbar z-joint injection and presenting pain in the groin, buttock, thigh, calf, or foot. No correlation was found between injection-elicited pain relief and pain provocation produced via passive rotation combined with extension. Patients with pain below the knee were equally distributed among responders and nonresponders. Of note, no patients with central back pain responded to diagnostic blocks of the z-joints.[149]

Similar findings were noted in another study of 40 patients receiving single, fluoroscopically controlled lumbar intraarticular z-joint blocks. Specifically, pain on lumbar extension, hip hyperextension, standing, or walking was diminished after the block, although pain with these provocative maneuvers was not specific to responders. Of the 90 maneuvers and symptoms compared among 40 patients (22 responders [55%] and 18 nonresponders [45%]), the preinjection responders were usually older, free of pain exacerbated by coughing, able to obtain relief when recumbent, free of pain exacerbated by forward flexion or return to the erect position after forward flexion, and without increased discomfort on hyperextension or extension-rotation. Radiographic changes of z-joint degeneration were not predictive of an analgesic response.[142]

An earlier study using a single, fluoroscopically guided block technique found some diagnostic maneuvers to be statistically more common in patients who respond to intraarticular z-joint injections. Such patients have pain aggravated by sitting and bending, and straight leg raising causes them to have back pain but not leg pain.[66] However, this study of 25 previously undiagnosed and untreated patients with low back pain did not control for placebo response to diagnostic intraarticular z-joint injections and was limited by its small sample size. The criteria used to diagnose z-joint pain were recently refuted by the use of controlled blocks.[151]

Another retrospective review using single blocks found prolonged relief from intraarticular steroids and local anesthetics in 67% of patients with localized paravertebral tenderness; 67% of patients with reproduction of symptoms with extension/rotation; 77% of patients with nondermatomal decrease in leg sensation; and 80% of patients with groin and upper thigh pain. These findings were based on retrospective review of 22 consecutive patients, using a scoring system that assigned 30 points for back pain associated with groin or thigh pain; 20 points for well-localized paraspinal tenderness; 30 points for reproduction of pain with extension and rotation; 20 points for significant radiographic changes; and 10 points for pain below the knee. All patients with scores of 60 points or more had relief for longer than 6 months.[88] This study suffers from the problems inherent in retrospective reviews and single blocks. The criteria used to diagnose z-joint pain were also recently refuted by the use of controlled blocks.[151]

## DIFFERENTIAL DIAGNOSIS

Disc disease, nerve root compression, sacroiliac joint syndrome, primary or secondary myofascial syndromes, and nonspinal disorders may mimic z-joint pain. In fact, anatomic changes to the z-joints are often accompanied by changes in the segmental disc and ligaments.[104] Painful nonspinal disorders such as gastrointestinal, genitourinary, cardiopulmonary, gynecologic, and peripheral joint disorders usually can be distinguished on clinical grounds and with supportive ancillary testing. A number of algorithms are useful in diagnosing nonspinal etiologies of spine pain.[44,170]

## DIAGNOSTIC STUDIES

Diagnostic studies can evaluate structural changes, functional or metabolic abnormalities, or nociceptive capabilities. Various diagnostic tests commonly used in the evaluation of spine pain are briefly addressed.

### Imaging Studies

No pathognomonic, diagnostic imaging studies are available for symptomatic z-joints. As in other causes of spine pain, the imaging studies must be closely correlated with clinical presentation. Pain is a subjective experience. The presence of an anatomic abnormality is not diagnostic of pain due to that abnormality. A cost-effective screening test with high specificity and sensitivity for z-joint pain is lacking. Cost constraints and the overall benign nature of z-joint pain may limit the search for such a test. However, because diagnostic tests are typically undertaken to exclude more ominous causes of spine pain, the spine clinician must be aware of the potential findings. Radiographs, CT, CT/myelography, bone scans, SPECT, and magnetic resonance imaging (MRI) scans provide additional diagnostic information when used in a judicious and logical manner. Imaging studies provide only anatomic information and cannot determine independently whether a particular structure is painful.[91,99,153,171]

Advanced spinal imaging often demonstrates signs of z-joint degeneration, even in asymptomatic individuals. For example, more than one-half of persons aged 40 or older have evidence of z-joint arthropathy on CT scans.[171] Whether such degenerative findings account for a given patient's pain complex requires clinical correlation, with selective analgesic injections of the suspected structures. Like the high incidence of z-joint abnormalities on advanced spinal imaging, the prevalence of disc abnormalities on CT or MRI scans increases with age.[99] Therefore, radiographic evidence of disc pathology is not a contraindication to z-joint injection procedures if the clinical evaluation provides sufficient cause to investigate the z-joints and not the discs.[50,131,142] Furthermore, the absence of degenerative or pathologic z-joint changes on plain radiographs, CT, MRI, bone scan, or SPECT scan does not exclude the potential for z-joint–mediated pain.[34,41,50,119,131,141,142,146,152,153]

**Diagnostic Injections:**

Because no reliable noninvasive tools exist for the accurate diagnosis of z-joint–mediated pain, and because the clinical features of z-joint pain, discogenic pain, ligamentous/muscular, and sacroiliac joint pain overlap, fluoroscopically guided z-joint injections of local anesthetics are commonly considered the gold standard for isolating or excluding the z-joints as the source of spine or extremity pain.[15,125] Either intraarticular or medial branch blocks can be used in the diagnostic work-up.[15,54,125] Physiologic analgesia is the underlying principle; pain relief after blockade of the nociceptive fibers implicates the blocked structure as the source of pain.[10,14,25,26] Therefore, analgesia after local anesthetic blocks of a z-joint or its nerve supply indicates that the pain likely emanates from the blocked joint(s).

Because analgesic blocks rely on a patient's subjective perception of pain, however, they are prone to false-positive responses. A patient's desire to obtain relief and a physician's enthusiasm for a procedure inadvertently encourage such false-positive responses. False-positive responses may be substantially minimized when a control injection is used. To avoid subjecting patients to inert injections as a control, comparative anesthetic blocks have been advocated.[10,14,25,26] The principle of comparative local anesthetic blocks is based on controlled, double-blind, randomized studies demonstrating that bupivacaine has a significantly longer duration of action than xylocaine.[129,144,167] Only patients who accurately report different durations of analgesia with the different anesthetics are considered to be true responders. Physiologic response to two different anesthetics—that is, pain relief of different durations corresponding to the known half-lives of the injected anesthetics—is thought to exclude a false-positive response to the injection.[150] If the intent of the z-joint procedure is purely diagnostic, anesthetic alone should be used.

**TREATMENT**

Controlled, prospective studies comparing treatment and natural history of z-joint pain are needed to guide selection of the most appropriate and cost-effective treatment program. Confirmation of the exact pain generator in acute lumbar and cervical pain is usually not required because most episodes of spine pain are self-limited.[3,163] Initial care is based on a presumptive diagnosis established by considering the mechanism of injury, pain patterns, physical findings, and imaging results. Conservative care of acute spine pain, including z-joint pain, may include oral nonnarcotic analgesics and anti-inflammatory medications, physical modalities, traction, instruction in body mechanics, education, selective strengthening, flexibility training, specialized manual physical therapy, aerobic conditioning, and time.

The authors advocate confirming a clinical suspicion of z-joint pain with diagnostic z-joint injection procedures only after a minimum of 4 weeks of appropriate, directed conservative care has failed to bring relief.[47,48,50] If pain substantially inhibits progress in physical therapy, earlier use of z-joint injection may help to focus therapies on a specific level and provide adequate analgesia to facilitate participation. Treatment of subacute and chronic spine pain is potentially more efficacious when an anatomic diagnosis is established and a multidisciplinary team approach is undertaken. Isolating the source of pain is critical to the development of scientific treatment protocols for spine pain of various origins. Ultimately, this approach will allow specific rather than empiric therapeutic interventions.

The following discussion of various noninvasive treatments for z-joint pain reflects the authors' opinions and is only a general construct for treatment. Specific, individual care should be based on a detailed clinical evaluation rather than a generic prescription derived from a standard algorithm. Unfortunately, there is no single prospective controlled study of the efficacy of any treatment for proven z-joint pain (via analgesic response to double blocks). Furthermore, no studies have assessed the efficacy of medication; physical therapy (modalities, flexibility, exercise); manual therapy (manipulation and other direct or indirect joint/soft tissue mobilization techniques); psychological intervention; or miscellaneous treatments used alone or in combination with potentially therapeutic z-joint blocks in patients with z-joint pain diagnosed by even single diagnostic blocks. The studies that evaluate treatment of spine pain of z-joint origin documented by analgesia after single diagnostic blocks assess the efficacy of isolated corticosteroid z-joint injections, posterior lumbar fusion, and radiofrequency denervation.[65,95,103,120,133,155,159,160]

General principles of rehabilitation apply to the treatment of z-joint–mediated spine pain. Flexibility and strength deficits should be identified and corrected. Education and training with respect to proper body mechanics, posture, and proprioception are essential. Early mobilization and physiologic stresses promote soft tissue healing through optimal alignment of collagen fibers[102] while preventing the deleterious effects of immobilization, including atrophy, weakening of ligaments, and impaired joint nutrition.[90] Rehabilitation goals for z-joint injuries include complete return of function, full pain-free range of motion, normal flexibility and strength, and education for prevention of future injury.

## Medications

Pain and inflammation can be reduced by the judicious use of nonsteroidal antiinflammatory drugs (NSAIDs). The antiprostaglandin effect of NSAIDs may control inflammatory response and provide pain relief. The duration of an NSAID's analgesic effect may be different from the duration of its antiinflammatory effect.[94] Some investigators have expressed concern that NSAIDs may interfere with the later stages of tissue repair and remodeling, in which prostaglandins help to mediate debris clean-up.[102] The dosage, timing, and potential side effects of NSAIDs should be evaluated. Patient responses to a particular NSAID cannot be predicted based on its chemical class or pharmacokinetics.[40]

In the authors' opinion, nonnarcotic analgesic medications should be used sparingly, and prolonged use of narcotic analgesics generally has no role in the treatment of z-joint pain. The so-called muscle relaxants act via general depression of the central nervous system rather than selectively on the skeletal muscle. The use of antidepressants in low doses may be helpful for some patients to augment sleep and to assist in pain control. Potential mechanisms of pain control from the antidepressants include controlling low central nervous system serotonin levels or enhancing naturally occurring analgesics such as endorphins and enkephalins.[71]

## Physical Therapy

### Physical Modalities
Various techniques are available to the physical therapist for control of further inflammation and pain. Acute injury is best treated by therapeutic cold, which decreases pain and muscle spasm and causes arteriolar and capillary blood flow to diminish, thus helping to control edema. The time required to cool an injured structure depends directly on the depth of intervening fat and may vary from 10–30 minutes.[64,111,112] Cryotherapy is easily applied to the spine at home or in the clinic and may be used in conjunction with other treatment techniques. In addition to providing pain relief and controlling inflammation, physical modalities have other benefits. Ultrasound stimulates tissue regeneration, promotes soft tissue repair, increases blood flow to damaged tissue to provide needed nutrients to healing tissue, aids in the removal of inflammatory byproducts, increases soft tissue distensibility, and decreases muscle spasm and pain.[35,62,73,182]

Electrical stimulation also may help to modulate acute pain and to decrease muscle spasm by inducing posttetanic relaxation and increasing circulation, which helps to remove inflammatory waste products.[137] Electrical stimulation techniques, including transcutaneous electrical nerve stimulation (TENS), high-voltage pulsed galvanic stimulation (HVPGS), interferential electrical stimulation, and minimal electrical noninvasive stimulation (MENS), have been reported to promote analgesia and muscle relaxation, resolution of edema, and wound healing as well as to retard inflammation and muscle atrophy.[137]

The application of electro-acuscope and low-energy lasers, which are newer and less traditional modalities for the management of pain associated with spine injuries, awaits well-controlled prospective studies to determine mechanisms of action and efficacy.[55]

### Braces
Joint protection techniques may help to reduce pain by minimizing repetitive movement into painful ranges of motion. A soft cervical collar or lumbar corset may be worn for as long as 10–12 days and then weaned as rapidly as possible to help avoid psychologic dependence and to prevent potential muscular weakness and decreased soft tissue flexibility. Weaning from a cervical collar should begin during the daytime, with continued use at night to prevent injury during sleep.[138,154] Once the patient has been completely weaned from daytime collar use, nighttime use also may be discontinued.

### Traction
Intermittent mechanical pelvic traction in a 90°–90° lying position or oscillatory inversion traction between 30° and 60° may unload the lumbar z-joints without overstretching the joint capsule, as does static traction.[37] However, the indiscriminate use of inversion traction has been associated with significant complications, including hyperextension, gastroesophageal reflux, headaches, and ruptured berry aneurysm. Active axial traction applied while the patient ambulates or performs other functional activities is referred to as "unloading" and is gaining popularity. Exercising in water with a flotation device is a form of unloading that is used successfully in sports rehabilitation.[37]

Applying the same principles to unload an injured spine appears to have merit but awaits rigorous scientific scrutiny.

## Manual Therapy

The role of manual therapy in documented z-joint pain remains empiric. The literature reviews manual techniques in the treatment of presumed z-joint pain. Controlled clinical trials comparing manipulations with placebo or more conservative treatments have produced variable results (with 32–92% experiencing relief) and generally provide short-lived relief.[5,27,45,81,87,139,164] Most studies have demonstrated improved outcome with manipulation compared with other treatment modalities for spine pain. However, the most efficacious treatment appears to be a protocol combining manual therapy and other therapies.[38,134]

Manual therapy may help to decrease pain and improve mobility and function to the point that the patient may begin to exercise in a painless manner. Manual techniques include massage of the soft tissues, manually sustained or rhythmically applied muscle stretching, traction applied in the longitudinal axis of the spine, passive joint mobilization, and, as the patient's pain begins to subside, specific or general high-velocity manipulation.[68,69,132] High-velocity manipulation may be helpful to treat painful dysfunctions that are aggravated by repetitive oscillatory movements.[67] Theoretically, the neurologic effects of manual therapy that may help to attenuate pain include restoration of axonal transport caused by mechanically induced deformation of spinal nerves,[68,106] stimulation of large-fiber joint afferents conveyed by joint receptors (dependent on the gate control theory),[68,178] and stimulation of clinically effective levels of endorphins.[68,165] Increased intraosseous pressure may cause pain and may be influenced by both joint position and intraarticular pressure. End-range passive mobilization techniques theoretically may help decrease intraarticular pressure and thereby reduce pain.[6,28,68,70,78,114]

Manual therapy may have other theoretic benefits. Repetitive passive joint oscillations carried out at the limit of the joint's available range may have a mechanical effect on joint mobility and improve vertebral motion restriction.[68,124,127,136,175] Mechanically controlled passive or active movements of joints may improve the remodeling of local connective tissue, the rate of tendon repair, and the gliding function within tendon sheaths during the repair process.[30,68,108,113,173] Passive joint motion has been shown to stretch joint capsules, lubricate tissues, and induce metabolic changes in soft tissue, cartilage, and bone.[68,72]

Soft tissue techniques, including lateral stretching, linear stretching, deep pressure, traction, and separation of muscle origin and insertion,[79,84] may help to decrease pain, muscle spasm, and soft tissue inflexibility as well as to improve circulation and remove inflammatory byproducts.[31,84] Myofascial techniques can be used to help stretch the noncontractile portion of the soft tissue.[166] Inhibition techniques such as positional release may help to modify increased muscle tone and thus to restore balanced muscular flexibility and strength.[100,101,107] Varying combinations of these techniques should be directed primarily at muscles that have become tight and painful secondary to the acute underlying facet pain. Treatment also should be directed to the muscles and other soft tissues chronically affected by poor posture to help restore their normal length and flexibility. Examples include muscles that are shortened, less flexible, and weak. The techniques also may be used to help restore normal flexibility, strength, and length to muscles that have been eccentrically lengthened and are weak.

## Exercise

To our knowledge, no research evaluating the effect of exercise therapy in proven z-joint pain has been published. Instead, generalizations are extrapolated from the treatment of nonspecific, nonradicular spine pain. Exercise prescriptions usually include flexibility, strengthening, aerobic conditioning, and educational components.

Active joint protection techniques are part of the initial phase of a cervicothoracic and lumbar stabilization program. Cervicothoracic and lumbar stabilization training is a specific type of therapeutic exercise that may help the patient (1) to gain dynamic control of cervicothoracic and lumbar spine forces, (2) to eliminate repetitive injury to the motion segments, and (3) to encourage healing of an injured segment. The underlying premise is that the motion segment and its supporting soft tissues react to minimize applied stress and thereby reduce the risk of injury. During the initial phase of stabilization training, the patient is taught how to find the neutral position or position of optimal function, which is the least painful cervicothoracic and lumbar spine position that minimizes segmental biomechanical stress. As the patient's condition improves, a series of flexibility and strengthening exercises is initiated to help correct postural dysfunction, inflexibilities, and muscle strength deficits and imbalances.[158]

Balanced lumbopelvic-lower extremity flexibility, in the opinion of some, often requires stretching of the hip flexors and lumbar extensors.[74] Achieving independent hip and lumbar spine motion is proposed to help eliminate excessive anterior pelvic tilt.[74] Increased anterior pelvic tilt causes increased lumbar lordosis and increased stress on the z-joints via segmental extension loading.[1,58,127] Adequate flexibility is believed to prevent excessive stress to the lower lumbar spine[83] and to improve mechanical functioning via symmetric distribution of forces. A slight flexion bias in the lumbosacral spine appears to be the position of comfort and helps to decrease lumbar z-joint loads and pain. Again, these opinions have not been scientifically proved in a population of patients with proven z-joint pain.

### Z-joint Injections

Z-joint injections may be part of a comprehensive program but should not be used as an isolated form of therapy.[47] Z-joint injections of local anesthetic provide diagnostic information.[15] The isolated therapeutic effect of intraarticular corticosteroids has not been proved, despite many open, noncontrolled clinical trials.[33,34,42,43,46,109,116,119,128,131] The semicontrolled trials[11,32,118] (that is, trials designed as randomized, controlled studies that did not meet all of the criteria established for the reporting of such trials[159]) reported minimal to no benefit from isolated z-joint injection. However, one well-designed study observed that administration of intraarticular corticosteroids in conjunction with other interventions has the potential for providing significant, lasting relief.[32] Co-interventions after z-joint injections may include physical therapy, joint mobilization, and manipulation. Further research is needed to confirm or refute the efficacy of such combined therapies.

### Fusion

Several uncontrolled studies have evaluated posterior fusion for lumbar z-joint pain relieved by single diagnostic z-joint blocks. No studies have proved that analgesic z-joint injections are predictive of pain relief from fusion, and some studies concluded that lumbar fusion is not helpful for z-joint pain.[65,95,160]

## CONCLUSION

The zygapophyseal joints are a source of low back pain. However, no noninvasive pathognomonic findings distinguish z-joint–mediated pain from other sources of spine pain. Physicians must apply their clinical judgment and knowledge of a patient's previous response to treatment to determine whether a z-joint may be a source of pain. The diagnosis of z-joint pain is therefore one of exclusion. Controlled, prospective studies comparing treatment and natural history of z-joint pain are needed to guide selection of the most appropriate and cost-effective treatment program. Initial care is based on a presumptive diagnosis established by considering the mechanism of injury, pain patterns, physical findings, and imaging results. Conservative care of z-joint pain may include oral nonnarcotic analgesics and antiinflammatory medications, physical modalities, traction, instruction in body mechanics, education, selective strengthening, flexibility training, specialized manual physical therapy, aerobic conditioning, and time. Zygapophyseal joint pain can be established only by using properly performed, fluoroscopically guided, contrast-enhanced anesthetic injection procedures with appropriate control injections. Interventions after z-joint injection procedures, such as physical or manual therapy, may prove to be synergistic with the immediate anesthetic and delayed corticosteroid effects.

## REFERENCES

1. Adams MA, Hutton HC: The effect of posture on the role of the apophyseal joints in resisting intervertebral compressive forces. J Bone Joint Surg 62B:358–362, 1980.
2. Adams MA, Hutton WC: The mechanical function of the lumbar apophyseal joints. Spine 8:327–330, 1983.
3. Anderson GBJ, Svensson H-O, Oden A: The intensity of work recovery in low back pain. Spine 8:880–884, 1983.
4. Aprill C, Bogduk N: The prevalence of cervical zygapophysial joint pain—A first approximation. Spine 17:744–747, 1992.
5. Arkuszewski Z: The efficacy of manual treatment in LBP: A clinical trial. Man Med 2:68–71, 1986.
6. Arnoldi C, Reimann I, Christensen S, et al: The effect of joint position in juxtaarticular bone marrow pressure. Acta Orthop Scand 51:893–897, 1980.
7. Ashton IK, Ashton BA, Gibson SJ, et al: Morphological basis for back pain: The demonstration of nerve fibers and neuropeptides in the lumbar facet joint capsule but not in the ligamentum flavum. J Orthop Res 10:72–78, 1992.
8. Avramov AI, Cavanaugh JM, Ozaktay CA, et al: The effects of controlled mechanical loading on group II, III and IV afferent units from the lumbar facet joint and surrounding tissue. An in vitro study. J Bone Joint Surg 74B:1464–1471, 1992.
9. Ball J: Enthesopathy of rheumatoid and ankylosing spondylitis. Ann Rheum Dis 30:213–223, 1971.
10. Barnsley L, Lord SM, Bogduk N: Comparative local anaesthetic blocks in the diagnosis of cervical zygapophyseal joint pain. Pain 55:99–106, 1993.
11. Barnsley L, Lord SM, Wallis BJ, Bogduk N: Lack of effect of intraarticular corticosteroids for chronic pain in the cervical zygapophyseal joints. N Engl J Med 330:1047–1050, 1994.
12. Beaman DN, Graziano GP, Glover RA, et al: Substance P innervation of lumbar spine facet joints. Spine 18:1044–1049, 1993.
13. Bland JH: Anatomy and biomechanics. In Disorders of the Cervical Spine. Philadelphia, W. B. Saunders, 1987, pp 9–63.
14. Boas RA: Nerve block in the diagnosis of LBP. Neurosurg Clin North Am 2:807–816, 1991.
15. Bogduk N: Back pain: Zygapophysial blocks and epidural steroids. In Cousins MJ, Bridenbaugh PO (eds): Neural Blockade in Clinical Anesthesia and Management of Pain, 2nd ed. Philadelphia, J. B. Lippincott, 1989, pp 935–954.
16. Bogduk N: The clinical anatomy of the cervical dorsal rami. Spine 7:319–330, 1982.
17. Bogduk N, Aprill C: On the nature of neck pain, discography and cervical zygapophysial joint blocks. Pain 54:213–217, 1993.
18. Bogduk N, Engel R: The menisci of the lumbar zygapophysial joints. A review of their anatomy and clinical significance. Spine 9:454–460, 1984.
19. Bogduk N, Jull G: The theoretical pathology of the acute locked back: A basis for manipulative therapy. Man Med 1:78–82, 1985.
20. Bogduk N, Long DM: Percutaneous lumbar medial branch neurotomy. A modification of facet denervation. Spine 5:193–200, 1980.
21. Bogduk N, Marsland A: On the concept of third occipital headache. J Neurol Neurosurg Psychiatry 49:75–780, 1986.
22. Bogduk N, Marsland A: The cervical zygapophysial joints as a source of neck pain. Spine 13:610–617, 1988.
23. Bogduk N, Twomey LT: Clinical Anatomy of the Lumbar Spine, 2nd ed. London, Churchill Livingstone, 1991.
24. Bogduk N, Valencia F: Innervation and pain patterns of the thoracic spine. In Grant R (ed): Physical Therapy of the Cervical and Thoracic Spine. Edinburgh, Churchill Livingstone, 1988, pp 27–37.

25. Bonica JJ: Local anesthesia and regional blocks. In Wall PD, Melzack R (eds): Textbook of Pain, 2nd ed. Edinburgh, Churchill Livingstone, 1989, pp 724–743.
26. Bonica JJ, Buckley FP: Regional analgesia with local anesthetics. In Bonica JJ (ed): The Management of Pain, vol II. Philadelphia, Lea & Febiger, 1990, pp 1883–1966.
27. Buerger A, Tobis J (eds): Approaches to the Validation of Manipulative Therapy. Springfield, IL, Charles C Thomas, 1977.
28. Bustrode C: Why are osteoarthritic joints painful? J R Nav Med Serv 62:5–16, 1976.
29. Campbell AJ, Wells IP: Pigmented villonodular synovitis of a lumbar vertebral facet joint. J Bone Joint Surg 64A:145–146, 1982.
30. Cantu R, Grodin A: Myofascial Manipulation: Theory and Clinical Application. Gaithersburg, MD, Aspen, 1992.
31. Cantu R, Grodin A: Soft tissue mobilization. In Basmajian JV, Nyberg R (eds): Rational Manual Therapies. Baltimore, Williams & Wilkins, 1993, pp 199–221.
32. Carette S, Marcoux S, Truchon R, et al: A controlled trial of corticosteroid injections into the facet joints for chronic low back pain. N Engl J Med 325:1002–1007, 1991.
33. Carrera GF: Lumbar facet joint injection in low back pain and sciatica: Preliminary results. Radiology 137:665–667, 1980.
34. Carrera GF, Williams AL: Current concepts in evaluation of the lumbar facet joints. Crit Rev Diagn Imaging 21:85–104, 1984.
35. Cole A, Eagleston R: The benefits of deep heat: Ultrasound and electromagnetic diathermy. Phys Sportsmed 22(2):77–88.
36. Cole AJ, Farrell JP, Stratton SA: Cervical spine athletic injuries: A pain in the neck. Phys Med Rehabil Clin North Am 5:37–68, 1994.
37. Cole AJ, Herring SA, Stratton SA, Narvaez J: Spine injuries in runners: A functional approach. J Back Musculoskel Rehabil 5:317–339, 1995.
38. Coxhead C, Inskip H, Meade T, et al: Multicentre trial of physiotherapy in the management of sciatic symptoms. Lancet 1:1065–1068, 1981.
39. Cyron BM, Hutton WC: The tensile strength of the capsular ligaments of the apophyseal joints. J Anat 132:145–150, 1981.
40. Dahl S: Nonsteroidal anti-inflammatory agents: Clinical pharmacology/adverse effects/usage guidelines. In Williams RF, Dahl SL (eds): Therapeutic Controversies in the Rheumatic Diseases. Orlando, FL, Grune & Stratton, 1987, pp 27–68.
41. Derby R, Bogduk N, Schwarzer A: Precision percutaneous blocking procedures for localizing spinal pain. Part 1: The posterior lumbar compartment. Pain Digest 3:89–100, 1993.
42. Destouet JM, Gilula LA, Murphy WA, Monsees B: Lumbar facet joint injection: Indication, technique, clinical correlation and preliminary results. Radiology 145:321–325, 1982.
43. Destouet JM, Murphy WA: Lumbar facet block: Indications and technique. Orthop Rev 14:57–65, 1985.
44. Deyo R: Early diagnostic evaluation of LBP. J Gen Intern Med 1:328–338, 1986.
45. Doran D, Newell D: Manipulation in treatment of LBP: A multicentre study. BMJ 2:161–164, 1975.
46. Dory MA: Arthrography of the lumbar facet joints. Radiology 140:23–27, 1981.
47. Dreyer S, Dreyfuss P: Low back pain and the zygapophysial (facet) joints. Arch Phys Med Rehabil 77:290–300, 1996.
48. Dreyer S, Dreyfuss P, Cole AJ: Zygapophysial (facet) joint injections. Phys Med Rehabil Clin North Am 6:715, 1995.
49. Dreyfuss P: Atlanto-occipital and lateral atlanto-axial joint injection techniques. Phys Med Rehabil State Art Rev 7:227–2371994.
50. Dreyfuss P, Dreyer SJ, Herring S: Lumbar zygapophysial (facet) joint injections. Spine 20:2040–2047, 1995.
51. Dreyfuss P, Lagattuta F, Kaplansky B, Heller B: Zygapophysial joint injection techniques in the spinal axis. Phys Med Rehabil State Art Rev 7:206–226, 1994.
52. Dreyfuss P, Michaelsen M, Fletcher D: Alanto-occipital and lateral atlanto-axial joint pain patterns. Spine 19:1125–1131, 1994.
53. Dreyfuss P, Rogers J, Dreyer S, Fletcher D: Atlanto-occipital joint pain: A report of three cases and description of an intra-articular joint block technique. Reg Anesth 1994.
54. Dreyfuss P, Schwarzer A, Lau P, Bogduk P: The target specificity of lumbar medial branch and L5 dorsal ramus blocks: A CT study. Spine (in press).
55. Dreyfuss P, Stratton S: The use of the low energy laser, electroacuscope, and neuroprobe in sports medicine: A current review. Physician Sportsmed 21(8):47–56, 1993.
56. Dreyfuss P, Tibiletti C, Dreyer S: Thoracic zygapophyseal joint pain: A review and description of an intra-articular block technique. Pain Digest 4:44–52, 1994.
57. Dreyfuss P, Tibiletti C, Dreyer S: Thoracic zygapophyseal joint pain patterns: A study in normal volunteers. Spine 19:807–811, 1994.

58. Dunlop RB, Adams MA, Hutton WC: Disc space narrowing and the lumbar facet joints. J Bone Joint Surg 66B:706–710, 1984.
59. Dussault RG, Nicolet VM: Cervical facet arthrography. Can Assoc Radiol J 36:79–80, 1985.
60. Dvorak J, Dvorak V: Biomechanics and functional examination of the spine. In Manual Medicine—Diagnostics, 2nd ed. New York, Thieme Medical Publishers, 1990, pp 1–34.
61. Dwyer A, Aprill C, Bogduk N: Cervical zygapophyseal joint pain patterns. I: A study in normal volunteers. Spine 15:453–457, 1990.
62. Dyson M: Therapeutic applications of ultrasound. In Nyberg WL, Ziskin MC (eds): Biological Effects of Ultrasound: Clinics in Diagnostic Ultrasound. New York, Churchill Livingstone, 1985, pp 121–133.
63. Eisentein SM, Parry CR: The lumbar facet arthrosis syndrome. J Bone Joint Surg 69B:3–7, 1987.
64. Eldred E, Lindsky D, Buchwald J: The effect of cooling on mammalian muscle spindles. Exp Neurol 2:144–157, 1960.
65. Esses SI, Moro JK: The value of facet blocks in patient selection for lumbar fusion. Spine 18:185–190, 1993.
66. Fairbank JCT, Park WM, McCall IW, O'Brien JP: Apophyseal injection of local anesthetic as a diagnostic aid in primary low-back pain syndromes. Spine 6:598–605, 1981.
67. Farrell J: Personal communication, April 1993.
68. Farrell J: Cervical passive mobilization techniques: The Australian approach. Phys Med Rehabil State Art Rev 4:309–334,1990.
69. Farrell JP, Soto J, Tichenor CJ: The role of manual therapy in spinal rehabilitation. In White A (ed): Spinal Medicine and Surgery: A Multidisciplinary Approach. St. Louis, Mosby, 1996.
70. Ferrel W, Nade S, Newbold P: Inter-relation of neural discharge; intraarticular pressure, and joint angle in the knee of the dog. J Physiol 373:353–365, 1986.
71. Fienmann C: Pain relief by antidepressants: Possible modes of action. Pain 23:1–8, 1985.
72. Frank C, Akeson W, Woo S, et al: Physiology and therapeutic value of passive joint motion. Clin Orthop 185:113–125, 1984.
73. Gann N: Ultrasound: Current concepts. Clin Manage 11:64–69, 1991.
74. Geraci M: Rehabilitation of pelvis, hip and thigh injuries in sports. Phys Med Rehabil Clin North Am 6:157–173, 1994.
75. Ghormley RK: Low back pain with special reference to the articular facets, with presentation of an operative procedure. JAMA 101:1773–1777, 1933.
76. Giles LG, Harvey AR: Immunohistochemical demonstration of nociceptors in the capsule and synovial folds of human zygapophyseal joints. Br J Rheumatol 26:362–364, 1987.
77. Giles LGF, Taylor JR: Innervation of lumbar zygapophyseal joint folds. Acta Orthop Scand 58:43–46, 1987.
78. Giovanelli-Blacker B, Elvey R, Thompson E: The clinical significance of measured lumbar zygo-apophyseal intra-capsular pressure variation. In Proceedings of Manipulative Therapists Association of Australia. Brisbane, Australia, 1985.
79. Glossary of Osteopathic Terminology. J Am Osteopath Assoc 80:552–567, 1981.
80. Glover JR: Arthrography of the joints of the lumbar vertebral arches. Orthop Clin North Am 8:37–42, 1977.
81. Godfrey C, Morgan P, Schatzker J: A randomized trial for LBP in a medical setting. Spine 9:301–304, 1984.
82. Goldthwait JE: The lumbosacral articulation: An explanation of many cases of lumbago, sciatica and paraplegia. Med Surg J (Boston) 164:365–372, 1911.
83. Gracovetsky S, Farfan H, Lamy C: The mechanism of the lumbar spine. Spine 6:249–262, 1981.
84. Greenman P: Principles of soft tissue and articulatory (mobilization without impulse) technique. In Principles of Manual Medicine. Baltimore, Williams & Wilkins, 1989, pp 71–87.
85. Grieve G: Common Vertebral Problems. Edinburgh, Churchill Livingstone, 1983.
86. Gronblad M, Korkala O, Konttinen YT, et al: Silver impregnation and immunohistochemical study of nerves in lumbar facet joint plical tissue. Spine 16:34–38, 1991.
87. Hadler N, Curtis P, Gillings A, Stinnett S: A benefit of spinal manipulation therapy as adjunctive therapy for acute LBP: A stratified control trial. Spine 12:702–706, 1987.
88. Helbig T, Lee CK: The lumbar facet syndrome. Spine 13:61–64, 1988.
89. Hemminghytt S, Daniels DL, Williams AL, et al: Intraspinal synovial cysts: Natural history and diagnosis by CT. Radiology 145:375–376, 1982.
90. Herring S: Rehabilitation of muscle injuries. Med Sci Sports Exerc 22:453–456, 1990.
91. Herzog R: Selection and utilization of imaging studies for disorders of the lumbar spine. Phys Med Rehabil Clin North Am 2:7–59, 1991.
92. Hirsch D, Ingelmark B, Miller M: The anatomical basis for low back pain. Acta Orthop Scand 33:1–17, 1963.
93. Hove B, Gyldensted C: Cervical analgesic facet joint arthrography. Neuroradiology 32:456–459, 1990.

94. Huskisson E: Non-narcotic analgesics. In Wall PD, Melzack R (eds): Textbook of Pain. Edinburgh, Churchill Livingstone, 1984, pp 505–513.
95. Jackson RP: The facet syndrome: Myth or reality? Clin Orthop 279:110–121, 1992.
96. Jackson RP, Jacobs RR, Montesano PX: Facet joint injection in low back pain: A prospective statistical study. Spine 13:966–971, 1988.
97. Jayson MIV: Degenerative disease of the spine and back pain. Clin Rheum Dis 2:557–584, 1976.
98. Jeffries B: Facet steroid injections. Spine State Art Rev 2:409–417, 1988.
99. Jensen M, Brant-Zwawadzki M, Obuchowski N: Magnetic resonance imaging of the lumbar spine in people without back pain. N Engl J Med 2:69–73, 1994.
100. Jones L: Spontaneous release by positioning. DO 4:109–116, 1964.
101. Jones L: Strain and Counterstrain. Newark, OH, American Academy of Osteopathy, 1981.
102. Kellett J: Acute soft tissue injuries—A review of the literature. Med Sci Sports Exerc 18:489–500, 1986.
103. King J, Lagger R: Sciatica viewed as a referred pain syndrome. Surg Neurol 5:46–50, 1976.
104. Kirkaldy-Willis W, Wedge J, Yong-Hing K, Reily J: Pathology and pathogenesis of lumbar spondylosis and stenosis. Spine 3:319–328, 1978.
105. Konttinen YT, Gronblad M, Korkala O, et al: Immunohistochemical demonstration of subclasses of inflammatory cells and active, collagen-producing fibroblasts in the synovial plicae of lumbar facet joints. Spine 15:387–390, 1990.
106. Korr I: Neurochemical and neurotrophic consequences of nerve deformation. In Glasgow EF, Twomey LT, Skull ER, et al (eds): Aspects of Manipulative Therapy. Melbourne, Churchill Livingstone, 1985, pp 64–71.
107. Kusunose R: Strain and counterstrain. In Basmajian JV, Nyberg R (eds): Rational Manual Therapies. Baltimore, Williams & Wilkins, 1993, pp 323–333.
108. Kvist M, Jarvenen M: Clinical, histochemical and biochemical features in repair of muscle and tendon injuries. Int J Sports Med 3:12–14, 1982.
109. Lau LSW, Littlejohn GO, Miller MH: Clinical evaluation of intra-articular injections for lumbar facet joint pain. Med J Aust 143:563–565, 1985.
110. Lawrence JS, Sharp J, Ball J, Bier F: Osteoarthritis. Prevalence in the population and relationship between symptoms and x-ray changes. Ann Rheum Dis 25:1–24, 1966.
111. Lehmann J: Therapeutic heat and cold. Clin Orthop 99:207, 1974.
112. Lehmann J, deLateur BJ: Diathermy and superficial heat and cold therapy. In Kottke EJ, Stillwell GK, Lehmann JF (eds): Krusen's Handbook of Physical Medicine and Rehabilitation. Philadelphia, W. B. Saunders, 1982, pp 275–350.
113. Lester JP, Windsor RE, Dreyer SJ: Medical Management of the Cervical Spine. New York, Churchill Livingstone, 1996.
114. Levick J: An investigation into the validity of subatmospheric pressure recordings from synovial fluid and their dependence on joint angle. J Physiol 289:55–67, 1979.
115. Lewin T, Moffet B, Viidik A: The morphology of the lumbar synovial intervertebral joints. Acta Morphol Netherland Scand 4:299–319, 1962.
116. Lewinnek GE, Warfield CA: Facet joint degeneration as a cause of low back pain. Clin Orthop 213:216–222, 1986.
117. Lewit K: The needle effect in the relief of myofascial pain. Pain 6:83–90, 1979.
118. Lilius G, Laasonen EM, Myllynen P, et al: Lumbar facet joint syndrome: A randomised clinical trial. J Bone Joint Surg 71B:681–190, 1989.
119. Lippit AB: The facet joint and its role in spine pain: Management with facet joint injections. Spine 9:746–750, 1984.
120. Lora J, Long D: So-called facet denervation in the management of intractable back pain. Spine 1:121–126, 1976.
121. Lynch MC, Taylor JF: Facet joint injection for low back pain. J Bone Joint Surg 68B:138–141, 1986.
122. Lysell E: Motion in the cervical spine. Acta Orthop Scand (Suppl 123), 1969.
123. Magora A, Schwartz TA: Relation between the low back pain syndrome and x-ray findings. Scand J Rehabil Med 8:115–125, 1976.
124. Maitland G: Vertebral Manipulation, 2nd ed. London, Butterworths, 1986.
125. Marks R, Houston T: Facet joint injection and facet nerve block—A randomized comparison in 86 patients. Pain 49:325–328, 1992.
126. McCall IW, Park WM, O'Brien JP: Induced pain referral from posterior lumbar elements in normal subjects. Spine 4:441–446, 1979.
127. Mennel J: Back Pain. Boston, Little, Brown, 1960.
128. Mooney V, Robertson J: Facet joint syndrome. Clin Orthop 115:149–156, 1976.
129. Moore D, Brindenbaugh P, et al: Bupivacaine for peripheral nerve block: A comparision with mepivacaine, lidocaine and tetracaine. Anesthesiology 32:460–463, 1970.
130. Moran R, O'Connell D, Walsh MG: The diagnostic value of facet joint injections. Spine 12:1407–1410, 1986.

131. Murtagh FR: Computed tomography and fluoroscopy guided anaesthesia and steroid injection in facet syndrome. Spine 13:686–689, 1988.
132. Nyberg R, Basmajian JV: Rationale for the use of spinal manipulation. In Basmajian JV, Nyberg R (eds): Rational Manual Therapies. Baltimore, Williams & Wilkins, 1993, pp 451–467.
133. Ogsbury JS, Simon RH, Lehman RAW: Facet "denervation" in the treatment of low back syndrome. Pain 3:257–263, 1977.
134. Otterbacher K, DiFabio R: Efficiency of spinal manipulation/mobilization therapy: A meta-analysis. Spine 10(9):833–837, 1985.
135. Panjabi M, Vasavada A, White A: Cervical spine biomechanics. Semin Spine Surg 5:10–16, 1993.
136. Paris S: Mobilization of the spine. Phys Ther 59:988–995, 1979.
137. Paterson DC, Carter RF, Tilbury RF, et al: The effects of varying current levels of electrical stimulation. Clin Orthop 169:303–312, 1982.
138. Press JM, Herring SA, Kibler WB: Rehabilitation of musculoskeletal disorders. In The Textbook of Military Medicine. Washington, DC, Borden Institute, Office of the Surgeon General, 1996.
139. Rasmussen G: Manipulation in LBP: A clinical trial. Manuelle Medizin 1:8–10, 1977.
140. Raymond J, Dumas JM: Intra-articular facet block: Diagnostic tests or therapeutic procedure? Radiology 151:333–336, 1984.
141. Raymond J, Dumas J, Lisbona R: Nuclear imaging as a screening test for patients referred for intra-articular facet block. Can Assoc Radiol J 35:291–292, 1984.
142. Revel ME, Listrat VM, Chevalier XJ, et al: Facet joint block for low back pain: identifying predictors of a good response. Arch Phys Med Rehabil 73:824–828, 1992.
143. Roy DF, Fleury J, Fontaine SB, Dussault RG: Clinical evaluation of cervical facet joint infiltration. Can Assoc Radiol J 36:118–120, 1988.
144. Rubin A, Lawson D: A controlled trial of bupivacaine: A comparison with lignocaine. Anaesthesia 23:327–331, 1968.
145. Rush J, Griffiths J: Suppurative arthritis of a lumbar facet joint. J Bone Joint Surg 71B:161–162, 1989.
146. Ryan PJ, Di Vadi L, Gibson T, Fogelman I: Facet joint injection with low back pain and increased facetal joint activity on bone scintigraphy with SPECT: A pilot study. Nucl Med Comm 13:401, 1992.
147. Schiowitz S: Biomechanics of joint motion. In DioGiovanna EL, Schiowitz S (eds): An Osteopathic Approach to Diagnosis and Treatment. Philadelphia, J. B. Lippincott, 1991, p 71.
148. Schwarzer AC, Aprill CN, Derby R, et al: Clinical features of patients with pain stemming from the lumbar zygapophysial joints: Is the lumbar facet syndrome a clinical entity? Spine 19:1132–1137, 1994.
149. Schwarzer AC, Aprill CN, Derby R, et al: The relative contributions of the disc and zygapophyseal joint in chronic low back pain. Spine 19:801–806, 1994.
150. Schwarzer AC, Aprill CN, Derby R, et al: The false-positive rate of uncontrolled diagnostic blocks of the lumbar zygapophysial joints. Pain 58:195–200, 1994.
151. Schwarzer AC, Derby R, Aprill CN, et al: Pain from the lumbar zygapophysial joints: A test of two models. J Spinal Disord 7:331–336, 1994.
152. Schwarzer AC, Scott AM, Wang S, et al: The role of bone scintigraphy in chronic low back pain: Comparison of SPECT and planar images and zygapophysial joint injection. Aust N Z J Med 22:185, 1992.
153. Schwarzer AC, Wang S, O'Driscoll D, et al: The ability of computed tomography to identify a painful zygapophysial joint in patients with chronic low back pain. Spine 20:907–912, 1995.
154. Shelokov A: Evaluation, diagnosis and initial treatment of general disc disease. Spine State Art Rev 5:167–176, 1991.
155. Silvers R: Lumbar percutaneous facet rhizotomy. Spine 15:36–40, 1990.
156. Sims-Williams H, Jayson MIV, Baddely H: Small spinal fractures in back patients. Ann Rheum Dis 37:262–265, 1978.
157. Stillwell DL: The nerve supply of the vertebral column and its associated structures in the monkey. Anat Rec 125:139–162, 1956.
158. Sweeney T, Prentice C, Saal J, et al: Cervicothoracic muscular stabilization techniques. Phys Med Rehabil State Art Rev 4:335–359, 1990.
159. The Standards of Reporting Trials Group: A proposal for structured reporting of randomized controlled trials. JAMA 272:1926–1931, 1994.
160. Tsang I: Perspective on LBP. Curr Opin Rheumatol 5:219–223, 1993.
161. Twomey LT, Taylor JR, Taylor MM: Unsuspected damage to lumbar zygapophyseal (facet) joints after motor vehicle accidents. Med J Aust 151:210–217, 1989.
162. Valencia F: Biomechanics of the thoracic spine. In Grant R (ed): Physical Therapy of the Cervical and Thoracic Spine. Edinburgh, Churchill Livingstone, 1988, pp 39–50.
163. Vallfors B: Acute, subacute and chronic low back pain: Clinical symptoms, absenteeism, and working environment. Scand J Rehabil Med 11(Suppl):1–98, 1985.
164. Waagen G, Haldeman S, Cook G, et al: Short-term trial of chiropractic adjustments for the relief of chronic low back pain. Man Med 2:63–67, 1986.

165. Ward R: Headache: An osteopathic perspective. J Am Osteopath Assoc 81:458–466, 1982.
166. Ward R: Myofascial release concepts. In Basmajian JV, Nyberg R (eds): Rational Manual Therapies. Baltimore, Williams & Wilkins, 1993, pp 451–467.
167. Watt M, Ross D, Atkinson R: A double-blind trial of bupivacaine and lignocaine. Anaesthesia 23:331–337, 1968.
168. Wedel DJ, Wilson PR: Cervical facet arthrography. Reg Anesth 10:7–11, 1985.
169. White AA, Panjabi MM: Clinical Biomechanics of the Spine, 2nd ed. Philadelphia, J.B. Lippincott, 1990, pp 102–103.
170. Wiesel S, Feffer H, Rothman R: A prospective evaluation of a standardized diagnostic and treatment protocol. Spine 9:199–203, 1984.
171. Wiesel SW, Tsourmas N, Feffer HL, et al: A study of computer assisted tomography I: The incidence of positive CAT scans in an asymptomatic group of patients. Spine 9:549–551, 1981.
172. Wilson PR: Thoracic facet joint syndrome—A clinical entity? Pain Suppl 4:S87, 1987.
173. Woo S, Gomez M, Amiel D, et al: The effects of exercise on the biomechanical and biochemical properties of swine digital flexor tendon. J Biomech Eng 103:51–56, 1981.
174. Woodring JH, Goldstein SJ: Fractures of the articular processes of the cervical spine. AJR 139:341–344, 1982.
175. Wright V, Dawson N: Biomechanics of joint function. In Holt PLJ (ed): Current Topics in Connective Tissue disease. Edinburgh, Churchill Livingston, 1975, p 115.
176. Wyke B: Articular neurology—A review. Physiotherapy 58:563–580, 1981.
177. Wyke B: Neurology of the cervical spinal joints. Physiotherapy 65:72–75, 1979.
178. Wyke B, Polacek P: Articular neurology: The present position. J Bone Joint Surg 57B:401, 1975.
179. Yahia LH, Garzon S: Structure on the capsular ligaments of the facet joints. Anat Anz 175:185–188, 1993.
180. Yang KH, King AI: Mechanism of facet load transmission as a hypothesis for low back pain. Spine 9:557–565, 1984.
181. Yu S, Sether L, Haughton VM: Facet joint menisci of the cervical spine: Correlative MR imaging and cryomicrotomy study. Radiology 164:79–82, 1987.
182. Ziskin MC, McDiarmid T, Michlovitz SL: Therapeutic ultrasound. In Michlovitz SL (ed): Thermal Agents in Rehabilitation. Philadelphia, F.A. Davis, 1990, pp 134–169.

# 5

# The Sacroiliac Joint: Principles of Treatment

ANDREW J. COLE, MD
PAUL DREYFUSS, MD
STEVEN A. STRATTON, PhD, PT, ATC

The sacroiliac joint (SIJ) can cause significant pain. However, it remains a controversial source of primary low back pain despite recent scientific studies that have validated it as a source of pain.[3,8,53,125] Its contribution to primary and secondary low back pain is often overlooked for a number of reasons. First, its anatomic location makes it difficult to examine. Second, many SIJ physical examination tests also place mechanical stresses on contiguous structures. Third, other anatomic structures may refer pain to the SIJ.[8]

Before 1934, the SIJ was considered the main source of low back pain. However, a study by Mixter and Barr[104] in 1934 focused attention on the intervertebral disc as the primary cause of low back pain. Attention has recently refocused on the SIJ as a primary or secondary cause of low back pain. Approximately 20% of low back and referred pain can be attributed to the SIJ.[97,125] Considerable confusion surrounds the role of the SIJ in pain production and its normal biomechanical function. Since 1930, research has focused on the basic anatomy and biomechanics of the SIJ rather than on rehabilitation.[9,15,36,139,142,148] SIJ pain is now treated with various aggressive conservative techniques that lack specific scientific validation.

Scientific scrutiny is currently focused on fluoroscopically guided, contrast-enhanced, intraarticular injection techniques. When performed properly, these techniques confirm that the SIJ is a source of pain[38,51,125] and also control the patient's pain so that rehabilitation can be advanced. Well-controlled outcome studies that measure the clinical efficacy of this adjunctive, diagnostic, and potentially therapeutic care option for SIJ pain do not exist. Considerable work remains to be done before the role of the SIJ in pain production is fully understood. Better diagnostic and therapeutic techniques can then be developed to help manage this source of pain.

## ANATOMY

The SIJ appears between the 10th–12th week of gestation[5,123] and continues to develop through childhood. It becomes C-shaped by adulthood. It is mobile[8,15] and has an

---

This chapter has been adapted with permission from Dreyfuss P, Cole AJ, Pauza K: Sacroiliac joint injection techniques. Phys Med Rehabil Clin North Am 7:785–813, 1995.

adult surface area of approximately 17.5 cm$^2$.[8,17] The joint has been described as having a long and short arm: the long arm faces posterolaterally and caudally, whereas the short arm faces posteriorly and cranially.[7] SIJ morphology changes with age.[15,120,147] The morphology of the SIJ also varies greatly with respect to size, shape, and contour from side to side among individuals.[34,141,143] Taken as a whole, the SIJ is classified as a synovial joint.[8,89] However, only one-fourth of its superior aspect is synovial, whereas inferiorly it is almost entirely synovial.[56] The synovial portion is most consistently located at S2 but may extend from S1–S3. The joint's synovial aspect is located in the anterior-inferior one-half to two-thirds of the joint.[128] The sacral cartilage is 2–3 times thicker (3 mm) than the iliac cartilage (1 mm).[15,120,123] The SIJ is also surrounded by a fibrous capsule. This capsule is well formed anteriorly but posteriorly may have multiple rents and tears.[8]

Accessory SIJ articulations may develop posterior to the articular surfaces between rudimentary transverse processes of the second sacral vertebrae and the ilium. These accessory SIJ articulations have a joint capsule and are saddle-shaped.[5,44,67,120,128,135] Although rarely seen before the fourth decade of life, these accessory articulations have an incidence of 8–35.8%. They may represent acquired fibrocartilage joints resulting from weight-bearing stresses. Their contribution to SIJ pain remains unknown.[8]

Until after puberty, the SIJ surface remains relatively flat.[8] By age 30, bony ridges develop on the articular surface of the ilium. The size and number of elevations and depressions within the joint increase during the third and fourth decades.[15,17] These elevations and depressions may represent adaptations to adolescent weight gain and help to enhance friction and stability of the joint.[141,143] Plain radiographs, MRI, and CT scans demonstrate progressive age-related degenerative changes. Age-related changes such as synovial articular surface erosions do not necessarily cause pain.[8,17,24,90,115,131] The synovial cleft narrows by 0.1–0.2 cm in people 50–70 years of age and by 0–0.1 cm in people older than 70 years.[115] Ankylosis has been reported[17,120] in individuals over 50 years old, especially men. However, recent studies refute the existence of absolute intraarticular ankylosis in the elderly.[115] Partial fibrous ankylosis and paraarticular synostosis may be more common than true ossification.

The interosseous ligament forms the posterior border of the SIJ because the posterior joint capsule is often rudimentary or absent. The interosseous ligament is the strongest ligament supporting the SIJ and is considered the strongest ligament in the body.[8,127,128] The anterior SIJ ligament is relatively weak. It represents a thickening of the joint capsule[8] (Fig. 1). The lumbosacral trunk (especially L4–S1) and obturator nerve are in close proximity to the anterior SIJ ligament.[42,75] The anterior SIJ ligament is also continuous with the anterior fibers of the iliolumbar ligament.[91] The iliolumbar, sacrotuberous, and sacrospinous ligaments are considered accessory ligaments. These three ligaments contribute some support to the SIJ.[146] The iliolumbar ligament consists of 2–5 distinct parts.[11,71,150] The iliolumbar ligament may prevent anterior translation and rotation of the L5 vertebral body.[11,21] SIJ stability may be enhanced by the thoracodorsal fascia and fibrous expansions of muscles adjacent to the SIJ that blend with the posterior SIJ ligaments.[144] These fascial connections may also allow forces from regional muscles, including the gluteus maximus and medius, to influence pelvic function.[139,142]

The synovial capsule and overlying ligaments contain unmyelinated free nerve endings that provide pain and thermal sensation to the SIJ. The capsule also receives encapsulated and complex unencapsulated nerve endings that provide pressure and position sense.[16,65,87,88,128] The ligaments and rudimentary joint capsule on the posterior aspect of the SIJ are innervated by the lateral branches of the posterior primary rami of L3–S3;[16,128] however, the major contributions are from the lateral branches of the posterior primary rami of L5–S2. The ligaments and joint capsule on the anterior aspect of the SIJ are innervated by L2–S2.[16,128] Although the major contributions are from L4–S1,

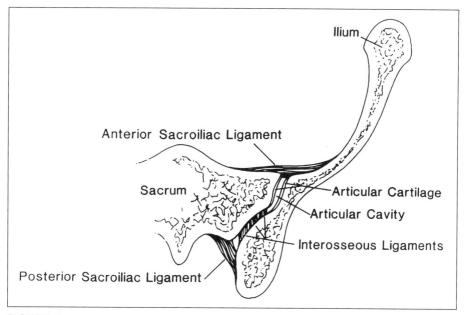

**FIGURE 1.**
The sacroiliac joint consists of a ligamentous compartment posteriorly and an articular compartment anteriorly. (From Bernard TN Jr, Cassidy JD: The sacroiliac joint syndrome—Pathophysiology, diagnosis, and management. In Frymoyer JW (ed): The Adult Spine: Principles and Practice. New York, Raven Press, 1991, p 2111, with permission.)

additional innervation may come from branches of the superior gluteal nerve (L4–S1).[128] L4 and L5 provide the most constant anterior nerve supply.[16,128] Recent research in adult cadaver dissection found that SIJ innervation may be distributed into four zones: (1) the superior ventral portion is mainly innervated by the ventral ramus of L5; (2) the inferior ventral portion is mainly supplied by the ventral ramus of S2 or branches from the sacral plexus; (3) lateral branches of the dorsal ramus of L5 innervate the superior dorsal portion; and (4) the inferior dorsal portion is innervated by nerves arising from a plexus composed of lateral branches of the dorsal rami of the sacral nerves.[79] S1 may provide the greatest contribution to the SIJ.[62] An autonomic nerve supply also has been postulated.[107,113] The nerve supply to the SIJ is not, however, always bilaterally symmetric.[2] The SIJ can create a myriad of referral zone patterns, most likely because of its multilevel, asymmetric innervation.[51,54] These referral patterns can confound even the most experienced clinician. Finally, an arthrokinetic reflex may also exist that employs articular mechanoreceptors to regulate regional muscle tone.[8,153]

Movement of the SIJ is involuntary and is caused by shear, compression, and other forces created by muscles that affect the SIJ indirectly. The surrounding muscles that produce secondary SIJ motion include the erector spinae, quadratus lumborum, psoas major and minor, piriformis, latissimus dorsi, oblique abdominals, and gluteal muscles. Of interest, although some of these muscles are considered the strongest in the human body, they create SIJ motion only indirectly. Indirect secondary SIJ motion is also caused by movement at other locations in the kinetic chain. For example, lower extremity muscles in the six compartments of the hip and thigh can indirectly influence motion of the SIJ.[91,137,138,140,142] Myofascial imbalances in any of these muscles due to central facilitation[58] may cause them to function in a shortened state that tends to inhibit their antagonists reflexively.[82] Dysfunctional movement patterns may theoretically result.[91] Body weight and postural changes also may create motion through the SIJ.[128]

## BIOMECHANICS

The entire spinal axis rests on a base formed by the SIJs. Loads transmitted from the lower extremities to the upper trunk are dissipated by the SIJs.[8] The SIJs lessen rapid changes in body weight transmission and absorb ground reaction and shear forces during ambulation and sitting.[2] The SIJ is essentially a triplanar shock absorber.[74] SIJ hypomobility diminishes the ability to dissipate these forces as effectively.[37] The SIJ is able to withstand 20 times less axial compression and two times less axial torsion than the lumbar spine. It can, however, tolerate six times more medially directed force than the lumbar spine.[8] The weaker SIJ anterior joint capsule and ligaments may be preferentially stressed during axial compression and torsion.[8] The precise types of normal SIJ motion are unclear. Various SIJ motions have been proposed, including gliding, rotation, tilting, nodding, and translation.[2,5] Alterations in lumbar spine mechanics have an affect on movement of the SIJ, hip, and pubic symphysis.[8] Motion of the SIJ is complex and likely does not occur around a single fixed axis.[2,5,8,25,43,58,144,149] Motion of the SIJ is usually limited to less than 4° of rotation and 1.6 mm of translation.[134] Any available SIJ motion decreases with age, in men between 40–50 years and in women after 50. During pregnancy, mobility is increased.[94,96] Complete ankylosis is rare.[133] Nutation and counternutation are considered the two most accepted types of motion at the SIJs. Nutation occurs with backward rotation of the ilium on the sacrum, whereas counternutation occurs with forward rotation of the ilium on the sacrum. It is unclear whether a change in the type or degree of motion can contribute to development of SIJ pain.[134]

## DYSFUNCTION

### Prevalence

The most common painful condition affecting the SIJ is SIJ dysfunction. SIJ dysfunction is also called SIJ mechanical pain or SIJ syndrome. The true prevalence of SIJ dysfunction-mediated pain is unknown, although three studies based on history and physical examination have revealed that the condition is probably more common than expected. The first study by Bernard et al.[9] reviewed a series of 1,293 patients with low back pain and demonstrated that SIJ dysfunction was the source of pain in 22.5%. Their second study demonstrated that minor trauma was responsible for 58% of the suffering from painful SIJ syndrome.[8] The third study, conducted by Greenman et al., evaluated 183 patients with failed back surgery syndrome. The authors found that 62.8% had leg-length inequality, sacral base unleveling, and concomitant SIJ dysfunction as contributing factors to their pain complex.[63]

Three recent studies based on fluoroscopically guided, contrast-enhanced, intra-articular injection have shed more light on the prevalence of SIJ dysfunction. Aprill evaluated 100 patients with low back pain with provocative/analgesic injection procedures. The preliminary data from his study demonstrated that the sole source of pain was found to be the zygapophyseal joint in 14%, the disc in 31%, and the SIJ in 15%.[3] Structures that contributed, at least in part, to low back pain included the zygapophyseal joint in 23%, the disc in 40%, and the SIJ in 23%.[3] No source of pain was identified in 29%.

In another investigation of 43 patients with chronic low back pain in whom maximal pain was below L5–S1, single diagnostic, fluoroscopically guided, contrast-enhanced SIJ blocks revealed an estimated prevalence of SIJ-mediated pain in 13–30%. Control intraarticular zygapophyseal joint injections were performed in all patients and discography in 21 of the 43. Greater than 75% relief of pain during the analgesic phase of the SIJ injection was used as the criterion for a positive response.[125]

In a study of 54 patients with unilateral low back pain and tenderness over the SIJ, the prevalence of SIJ-mediated pain was found to be 19%.[97] The study used two different intraarticular anesthetic blocks (lidocaine and bupivacaine); at least 75% pain reduction with each block was necessary for a positive response. Furthermore, at least 2 hours of relief had to be be reported after the bupivacaine block.

## History and Physical Examination

No specific or pathognomonic historical facts or physical examination tests accurately identify the SIJ as a source of pain.[40,97,125] Three studies have evaluated the accuracy of historical data and certain tests as predictors of SIJ dysfunction in patients with painful SIJ dysfunction as established by single or double anesthetic SIJ injections.[40,97,125] Definite SIJ pain can be determined only by appropriately performed fluoroscopically guided, contrast-enhanced injection procedures that control for false-positive responses by using an inert injectant or by performing two separate SIJ blocks with anesthetics of different durations of action on separate days (double-block technique). The patient should report adequate pain relief for a duration appropriate to the injected anesthetic. The double-block technique has been used to exclude false-positive responses during lumbar zygapophyseal joint blocks.[124]

Schwarzer's study found that an increase or decrease in pain with sitting, standing, walking, flexion, or extension did not discriminate pain of SIJ origin from other painful anatomic sources.[125] Furthermore, pain below the knee was found to be as common in patients with SIJ-mediated pain as in patients without SIJ-mediated pain.[125] Of groin, buttock, thigh, calf, and foot referral patterns, only groin pain was found to discriminate SIJ-mediated pain from other anatomic pain generators.[125]

Dreyfuss evaluated 85 patients with intraarticular, fluoroscopically guided, contrast-enhanced anesthetic SIJ injection in terms of various history and physical examination findings.[40] SIJ pain was diagnosed by pain relief of 90–100% after a contained intraarticular injection; by this criterion, 45 patients had SIJ pain, whereas 40 did not. Twelve physical examination tests were studied: (1) pain over the SIJ, (2) pain into the buttock, (3) pain into the groin, (4) pointing to the posterior sacroiliac spine as the source of pain, (5) Gillet test, (6) abnormal sitting position, (7) thigh thrust, (8) Patrick's test, (9) Gaenslen's test, (10) sacral thrust, (11) superior SIJ spring test, and (12) sacral sulcus tenderness. The study also evaluated whether pain increased, decreased, or remained unchanged after the following treatments or activities: antiinflammatory drugs, muscle relaxers, physical therapy, home exercise, local heat or cold, manipulation to the sacroiliac joint, walking, sitting, lying down, standing in place, wearing high heels, straining with a bowel movement, coughing and sneezing, and usual job activities. No historical fact, physical examination finding, or combination of findings could discriminate SIJ pain from other pain sources.[40]

Maigne used double anesthetic blocks to compare pain relief of more than 75% after intraarticular SIJ blocks with pain increased by lumbar flexion, lumbar extension, ipsilateral flexion, contralateral flexion, SIJ distraction test, SIJ compression test, sacral pressure test, Gaenslen's test, Patrick's test, resisted external hip rotation, and pubic symphysis pressure test. He also found no test to discriminate for SIJ pain.[97]

The remaining discussion of history and physical examination for painful SIJ dysfunction is based predominantly on the authors' and others clinical experience; scientific validation of these opinions is lacking. Future research efforts must further assess all possibly valuable history and physical examination findings against double-block intraarticular injections. Only then will the accuracy of noninvasive SIJ diagnostic tests be fully determined.

The astute clinician takes a thorough history and performs a focused physical examination to accurately assess the SIJ and its kinetic chain. Patients with SIJ pain may complain of pain that is sharp, aching, or dull. Variable patterns of pain referral may occur because of the SIJ's wide range of segmental innervation. Pain referral patterns also may depend on which part of the SIJ is affected. Saline and local anesthetic injections into the posterior SIJ ligaments have referred pain into the distal leg, mimicking pseudoradicular and sciatic pain.[8,68,73,75,76,80,129,130] In a recent SIJ injection study in asymptomatic subjects, the most constant referral zone was to a $3 \times 10$ cm area just inferior and lateral to the ipsilateral posterior-superior iliac spine.[52,53] Pain can be localized to the involved joint or may be referred to the buttocks, groin, posterior thigh, or distally beyond the knee and even into the foot.[125]

A history of trauma is common: a fall on the buttocks; a motor vehicle accident during which the knee hit the dashboard or a shoulder harness caused trunk rotation on impact; a rear-end motor vehicle accident with the ipsilateral foot on the brake at the time of impact; a broadside accident with a blow to the lateral aspect of the pelvic ring; a missed step while descending the stairs; or a foot that dropped into a hole or rut in the road while walking or running.[26–28] Painful SIJ dysfunction also may be caused by repetitive rotation through the lumbar spine, as in such sports as golf, pitching, and ice skating. Another common mechanism of painful SIJ dysfunction is lumbar rotation and axial loading, which may occur during ballet or ice skating.[8,51] Postures or motions that may predispose a worker to painful SIJ dysfunction may be discovered by taking a careful vocational history. Particularly vulnerable are workers who stand with their weight shifted onto one leg or flex and/or rotate the lumbar spine. Of interest, sidebending usually does not increase SIJ pain.[8] Although disputed by some, the risk of SIJ dysfunction may be increased in people with lumbar fusions or hip pathology.[59,109]

SIJ dysfunction may cause hamstring muscle strain.[22,23] Abdominal pain from SIJ dysfunction also has been reported at a point two inches lateral to the ipsilateral umbilicus on a line extending from the umbilicus to the anterior superior iliac spine.[14] Such abdominal pain may be referred from the iliopsoas muscle, which frequently becomes tight and painful as a result of underlying primary SIJ dysfunction.[132] SIJ pain is usually unilateral and tends to have a right-side bias in 45% of patients; 35% have left-sided pain, and 20% have bilateral pain.[8]

The relationship between the spinal axis and peripheral joints has been termed the *motion cascade*[29] and provides a framework that explains how a given spinal segmental or peripheral joint dysfunction creates a series of secondary deficits at sites both adjacent to and remote from the original problem. Because of the functional interdependence of the musculoskeletal system, the pelvis may contribute to adjacent or remote biomechanical dysfunction that also may become painful. The term *lumbopelvic-hip complex dysfunction* approximates the high level of mechanical interdependence in this region as well as its relationship with sites in other, more remote parts of the kinetic chain.[91]

A thorough, yet directed, physical examination should test for lumbar sources of pain before further assessment of the lumbopelvic-hip complex. This approach helps to avoid diagnostic confusion. Although the details of physical examination of the lumbar spine can be found in standard texts, two points deserve particular attention. In the presence of SIJ dysfunction, the supine straight-leg raise test may be falsely positive. Beyond 60° of straight-leg raising, SIJ movement[91] begins to occur. Therefore, in the setting of SIJ pain, a straight-leg raise may recreate SIJ referred pain in a radicular pattern that should not be confused with dural tension pain.[12,112,138,140] In addition, the straight-leg raise test may cause low back pain in the presence of SIJ dysfunction because of a dynamic change in innominate tilt with hip flexion.[12,112] Thus, any restriction in pelvic rotation caused by an SIJ dysfunction may lead to misinterpretation of the passive straight-leg raise test.[37] A second important point is that in the setting of isolated SIJ dysfunction, no neurologic signs should be present—although the patient may complain of "neurologic" symptoms.

Certain physical examination findings may suggest the SIJ as the source of pain. Gait analysis may reveal an antalgic gait with the trunk shifted toward the normal side.[51,120] The patient may assume an antalgic sitting posture to avoid excessive weight on the gluteal area of the painful side.[37,130] When the patient is asked to place one finger on the site of pain, they may point to the involved SIJ or the posterior-superior iliac spine.[50,51] On palpation, tenderness may be localized over the sacral sulcus and just medial to the posterior superior iliac spine.[8]

Various additional testing maneuvers have been developed to help diagnose painful SIJ dysfunction.[14,37,64,103] No definitive research shows any one method or category of methods to be superior as judged against standard, accepted diagnostic criteria such as false positive-controlled, fluoroscopically-guided, contrast-enhanced, intra-articular analgesic SIJ injections. The following is a list of additional physical examination test categories that are recommended by various authors to predict a painful SIJ dysfunction: (1) soft-tissue examination for zones of hyperirritability; (2) evaluation of fascial and/or musculotendinous restrictions; (3) length/strength muscle relationships; (4) postural analysis; (5) true leg length determination; (6) functional leg length determination;[5,36,91] (7) osteopathic evaluation, including static and dynamic osseous landmark evaluation (structural testing);[5,14,103] (8) dynamic osteopathic screening tests;[5,9,14,39,103] (9) evaluation of regional tissue texture changes; (10) provocative testing, including traditional orthopedic tests such as Gaenslen's or Patrick's test; (11) motion demand (articular spring) tests;[74] (12) ligament tension tests;[5] and (13) hip rotation testing.[8]

## Differential Diagnosis

There are a number of other causes of SIJ pain. SIJ fractures may be caused by trauma. Insufficiency stress fractures most frequently occur in elderly women with osteoporosis and may be misinterpreted as metastatic disease.[31] Such patients give a history of severe pain that is not associated with an acute traumatic event. Plain film findings can be easily overlooked, but bone scan usually reveals increased uptake at the fracture site. The increased uptake on bone scan creates an image in the shape of an "H," the so- called H-pattern[77] or Honda sign,[32] that is considered diagnostic of a sacral insufficiency fracture.[116] Multiple fracture sites, most commonly the vertebrae and ribs, strongly suggest the diagnosis of insufficiency fracture and obviate the need for bone biopsy.[122] Fatigue stress fractures are caused by abnormal muscular stress on normal bone.[32] Although rare, fatigue stress fractures have been reported in athletes and soldiers. They are thought to be due to significant repetitive microtrauma caused by impact loading from long periods of frequent physical exertion.[31,48,98,102]

SIJ infections usually result from hematogenous spread and are usually unilateral. Predisposing factors include pregnancy, trauma, endocarditis, intravenous drug abuse, and immunosuppression.[8,41,72] Infection may cause distention of the anterior joint capsule and create pain in the distribution of the irritated lumbar and sacral nerve roots.[8,121] Pyogenic sacroiliitis is relatively rare in adults and even rarer in children. Pyogenic sacroiliitis accounts for 1.5% of joint infections in children.[93] Unlike peripheral joint sepsis, the diagnosis of SIJ infection in children may be difficult and delayed. Bone scan helps to make an early diagnosis in suspected cases[13,114] and allows early intervention with antibiotics.[1]

SIJ inflammation may be due to metabolic, traumatic, arthritic, or infectious causes. Ankylosing spondylitis causes bilateral, symmetrical SIJ inflammation and may result in SIJ fusion. Psoriatic arthritis and Reiter's disease also may involve the SIJs bilaterally[8,19] Rheumatoid arthritis rarely involves the SIJs except late in the course of long-standing disease.

Degenerative joint disease eventually affects all SIJs. Joint space narrowing, subchondral sclerosis, periarticular ankylosis, intraarticular gas formation, and osteophyte formation occur. Degenerative changes are frequently seen in patients over 30, but their radiographic presence does not correlate with pain.

Metabolic processes, including deposition diseases such as calcium pyrophosphate deposition disease (CPDD), gout, ochronosis, and acromegaly, may affect the SIJ. These processes may lead to early degeneration, inflammation, and pain.[84]

Other possible causes of SIJ pain include primary sacroiliac tumors, which are rare and usually synovial villoadenomas;[119] iatrogenic instability, which may be caused by overzealous iliac bone harvesting for surgical graft material or by resection of pelvic tumors; and osteitis condensans ilii, which has a prevalence of 2.2% and is usually bilateral and self-limiting. It occurs primarily in young multiparous women. Increased bone density is visualized on the inferior iliac side of the SIJ in a well-defined triangular area.[17,19]

Pain may be referred to the SIJ from conditions affecting other tissues near the SIJ, such as lumbar radiculopathy, lumbar zygapophyseal joint pain, Maigne's syndrome, contained discogenic disease, hip disease, or multifidi/gluteal trigger points.[8,9] In this setting, the SIJ may be inappropriately assumed to be the primary source of pain when, in fact, it is only secondarily involved by referral. Pregnancy causes relative hypermobility of the SIJ due to increased levels of relaxin, which causes relaxation of the soft tissues supporting the SIJ. A painful sacroiliac ligament sprain may occur.[105] Reactive sacroiliitis may develop as a late sequela of pelvic inflammatory disease (PID). Slightly more than 50% of patients with a history of severe PID and lumbosacral pain may develop sacroiliitis as demonstrated by bone scan. Approximately 30% of such patients may demonstrate abnormalities on plain film.[106]

## IMAGING

When necessary, radiographic testing may help to diagnose infection, fracture, neoplasm, inflammation, and metabolic or traumatic conditions. Treatment plans can then be formulated accordingly. Unlike infection, fracture, neoplasm, inflammation, and metabolic or traumatic conditions, all of which have specific radiographic findings, SIJ dysfunction is a diagnosis of exclusion.[8] Usually, plain films are the initial imaging study. However, the anatomic complexity of the SIJ may make interpretation of plain films difficult, and more advanced imaging such as computed tomography (CT), magnetic resonance imaging (MRI), bone scan, and single photon emission computed tomography (SPECT) may become necessary.[70]

### Plain Films

A standard anteroposterior view of the pelvis is usually the first film taken, although a modified Ferguson view may yield additional details. The modified Ferguson view is considered accurate in 85% of cases.[19] Plain film images are the most cost-effective radiographic study of the SIJ. Radiographic changes are usually first seen on the iliac side of the SIJ because of the thinness of the cartilage relative to the sacral side. The first sign of abnormality that can be visualized on plain films is loss of the normal white cortical line that outlines the SIJ. Note also should be taken of (1) joint space width (too wide, too narrow, irregular); (2) presence and type of erosions; (3) sclerosis; (4) bony bridging (ankylosis vs. osteophyte formation); and (5) whether the observed changes are unilateral, bilaterally symmetrical, or bilaterally asymmetrical.[19]

There are no pathognomonic plain film findings of SIJ dysfunction. Conversely, at least 24.5% of asymptomatic patients older than 50 years have SIJ abnormalities on plain film.[24,81]

## Magnetic Resonance Imaging

MRI provides exquisite soft tissue detail of muscle, cartilage, and ligamentous structures around the SIJ.[118] MRI is also particularly helpful in identifying early inflammatory conditions and soft tissue tumors affecting the SIJ.[8] One study has demonstrated that MRI has 100% predictability and thus is the best single test for confirming active inflammatory sacroiliitis.[4]

## Computed Tomography

The CT scan best identifies bony abnormalities of the SIJ but also provides some soft tissue detail.[49] Lawson et al. found CT to be superior to plain films for detection of early SIJ erosive changes and joint space narrowing. When a discrepancy was found between plain film and CT findings, the abnormalities were either only demonstrated or better demonstrated by CT.[90] Recently a limited, low-dose, three-scan CT was shown to be as accurate as a complete CT series for examination of the SIJ. This scan also requires less imaging time and radiation exposure than a full CT series and may be an effective alternative to plain films for assessing SIJ pain.[57]

## Bone Scan

Bone scan can identify increased mechanical stress to the SIJ, stress fractures, occult fracture, infection, metabolically active degeneration, and neoplasms. An abnormality may be found with bone scan even when other imaging modalities are normal. For example, a bone scan may demonstrate bilateral SIJ disease, even though previous imaging detected only unilateral disease.[18,19] Preliminary research suggests that a bone scan may be positive in the presence of SIJ dysfunction. However, more often than not, a bone scan is normal.[31,33,35,61,101,109,110,136] SPECT scanning has been shown preliminarily to be of no value in patients with symptomatic SIJ dysfunction as diagnosed by relief after intraarticular blocks.[126] SPECT scanning is both sensitive and specific for the detection of established sacroiliitis and may help to identify inflammatory disease at other sites in the spine.[70]

## REHABILITATION TECHNIQUES AND PRINCIPLES

Treatment of SIJ dysfunction must include the entire lumbopelvic complex and lower extremity kinetic chain. Numerous treatment techniques from various schools, including osteopathic, manual, and chiropractic medicine, have evolved to help rehabilitate SIJ dysfunction. No research validates one treatment protocol as superior. In fact, no prospective, controlled studies evaluate the effectiveness of any treatment for patients with SIJ-mediated pain as confirmed by pain relief after intraarticular SIJ blocks. The most effective rehabilitation programs probably integrate aspects of treatment from each school to provide the most cost-effective care. Whichever approach is taken, the authors believe that the rehabilitation program must progress beyond absence of symptoms, because anatomic and functional changes that may increase the chance of reinjury may persist. In fact, the single best predictor for new injury is a history of previous injury.[6,10,30,46,95,117]

Kibler's theoretical construct for treatment of musculoskeletal injuries[85] can be used to develop a treatment strategy for SIJ dysfunction. The *vicious cycle of tissue overload injury* is a functionally based model that requires the clinician to evaluate and treat not only the primary site of dysfunction but also all other related secondary sites of dysfunction in the entire kinetic chain. It defines all aspects of a patient's total injury complex. According to Kibler et al., five complexes are associated with the cycle.[85] *Tissue injury complex* describes the group of anatomic structures that have sustained damage. The *clinical symptom complex* consists of all symptoms and signs that result from the injury. The *tissue overload complex* encompasses the group of tissues subjected to tensile overload. The *functional biomechanical deficit complex* is the constellation of inflexibilities and/or muscle strength imbalances that can alter normal biomechanics. Finally, the *subclinical adaptation complex* describes all of the substitute activities that are used to compensate for the altered biomechanics.

The rehabilitation program for SIJ dysfunction can be divided into acute, subacute, recovery, and maintenance phases. The tissue injury and clinical symptom complexes are treated during the acute phase of rehabilitation. Nonsteroidal antiinflammatory drugs help to reduce pain and inflammation,[78] therapeutic cold decreases pain and muscle spasm,[45,92] and electrical stimulation modulates acute pain and decreases muscle spasm by inducing posttetanic relaxation and increasing circulation to remove inflammatory byproducts.[148,151] Patient education begins in this phase and continues throughout the course of treatment. A home program is also provided during the acute phase and is expanded as the patient progresses through the rehabilitation program. SIJ motion and pain may be reduced by using an SIJ belt, which is worn most effectively directly superior to the greater trochanter.[137,139]

During the subacute phase, moist heat,[92] inhibitive techniques (positional release,[107] functional technique[83]), muscle flexibility exercises, and mobilization techniques (muscle energy technique,[103] direct articulation oscillation techniques[47]) may help to reduce pain. If there are no contraindications,[69] such as joint or nerve pathology, manipulation using a high-velocity, low-amplitude, short-lever arm thrust technique may be employed.[108]

The efficacy of manipulation for the diagnosis of SIJ pain based solely on history and physical examination has been demonstrated in two allopathic, uncontrolled manipulation studies. Ninety percent of patients with chronic SIJ syndrome were effectively treated with a daily regimen for 2–3 weeks. A maintenance exercise program was believed to be important to prevent recurrences.[20,86] The SIJ may be affected by a leg length inequality of more than one-half inch. Many clinicians consider correcting a leg length discrepancy of more than one-half inch.[22]

The recovery phase of rehabilitation addresses tissue overload and functional biomechanical deficits. Mobility of the lumbar spine, sacroiliac joint, pelvis, and hip is assessed with an articular examination. Manual therapy, including joint and soft tissue techniques, help to eliminate vertebral motion and pelvic restrictions as well as to improve soft tissue flexibility and extensibility of the lumbar, pelvic, and hip complexes.[29,66,100,145] Postural correction exercises, strengthening of weakened muscles, and strength training of multiplanar coordinated movements help to normalize posture.[99,100,111] Strength and flexibility training help to correct compensatory movement patterns created by soft tissue adaptation.[82,99,100,111] Such training techniques also improve motor control during activities such as walking forward or backward, trunk rotation, squatting, and sit-to-stand movements. An aerobic conditioning program completes this phase of rehabilitation.[152]

The maintenance phase provides a home program that maintains soft tissue flexibility balance and strength in all three cardinal planes. The aerobic conditioning program is advanced in this phase.[152]

No scientifically validated exercise programs have been designed for patients with SIJ pain. There are theoretical advantages to strengthening certain muscles, such as the erector spinae, gluteus maximus; and long head of the biceps femoris, that may secondarily enhance the stability of the joint via fascial connections to the SIJ complex.[139]

In patients with the pelvic crossed syndrome, there are also theoretical advantages to stretching certain soft tissue groups that may create pelvic rotational dysfunction.[60]

## AN INTEGRATED APPROACH

Figure 2 presents an integrated approach used by the authors for the management of patients with SIJ pain.[26,27,38] This particular approach has not been validated over other approaches and reflects the biases and experience of the authors. Scientific knowledge was used when possible to influence the decision-making process. Clinical assessments and patient opinions or preferences should determine how to use this algorithm; it should not dictate how a patient is treated.

The amount of pain relief at each juncture in the decision-making process decreases the longer treatment continues. This reflects the fact that the chance of complete recovery decreases as treatment duration increases.

Patients with presumed SIJ pain are entered into the treatment sequence and receive two weeks (with three sessions per week) of aggressive conservative care for primary SIJ dysfunction as well as any secondary sites of pain and dysfunction. Physician reassessment occurs approximately two weeks after aggressive conservative care begins. Patients whose pain and underlying biomechanical deficits have improved by 95% or more are discharged with a home maintenance program. If improvement is less than 95%, aggressive conservative care is modified and continued for another two weeks. Patients whose pain and underlying biomechanical deficits have improved by 90% or more within two weeks of additional treatment are discharged with a home maintenance program. If the patient's relief is less than 90%, the first fluoroscopically guided, contrast-enhanced, intraarticular injection with local anesthetic and corticosteroid is performed. If the patient is unable to tolerate any portion of the initial aggressive conservative care program, the treatment is immediately modified and care continued.

If the patient obtains less than 90% relief from the first fluoroscopically guided, contrast-enhanced, intraarticular injection, the presumption is that the pain does not emanate predominantly from the intraarticular portion of the SIJ. In this case, other diagnostic injection procedures, such as zygapophyseal joint blocks, medial branch blocks, nerve root blocks, and discography, may be performed until the source of pain is localized so that appropriate treatment can be instituted. If these diagnostic injection procedures fail to identify the pain source, it may be presumed to be the posterior SIJ ligament complex. Posterior ligament blocks are then performed with both local anesthetic and steroid. Patients with less than 90% relief should be evaluated for other sources of pain. If pain relief is 90% or more, aggressive conservative care should continue for 1–2 weeks. If the patient has less than 90% relief, prolotherapy may be considered. If relief is 90% or greater, the patient can be discharged with a home program.

If the patient has 90% or greater relief from the first fluoroscopically guided, contrast-enhanced, intraarticular injection, a substantial portion of pain probably emanates from the intraarticular portion of the SIJ. Aggressive conservative care should be initiated immediately and continued for up to two weeks. If relief is 90% or greater, the patient can be discharged with a home program. If relief from the two-week period of aggressive conservative care is less than 90%, the patient either had a false-positive response to the first injection procedure or suffers from recalcitrant intraarticular SIJ pain. In the second case, aggressive conservative management should be modified, and if the patient has 90% or greater relief, discharge with a home program is appropriate. If the patient's relief is less than 90%, the second fluoroscopically guided, contrast-enhanced intraarticular injection with local anesthetic and steroid is performed. If the patient is unable to tolerate the aggressive conservative care program that was initiated

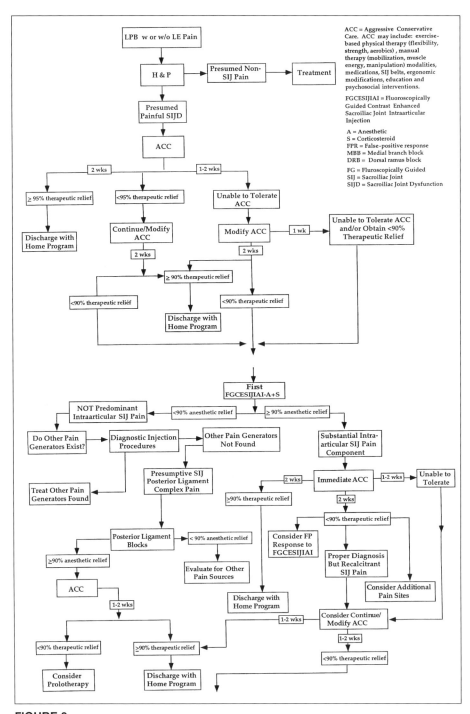

**FIGURE 2.**
Algorithm for managing sacroiliac joint pain. (From Cole AJ, Dreyfuss P, Stratton SA:The sacroiliac joint: A functional approach. In Critical Reviews in Physical and Rehabilitation Medicine. New York, Begell House, in press, with permission.)

*(Continued on following page.)*

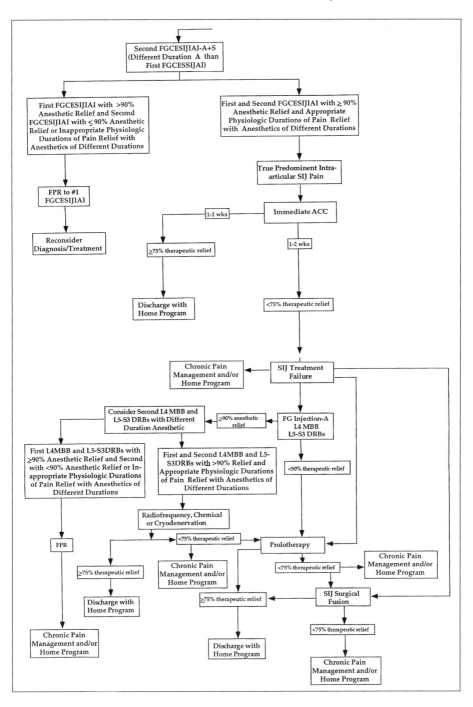

after the first injection procedure, aggressive conservative care should be modified. Patients who have 90% or greater relief with the modified approach should be discharged with a home program. If the patient's relief is less than 90%, a second injection with local anesthetic and steroid should be performed.

The second injection should use an anesthetic with a different duration of action. If the first injection produced 90% or more anesthetic phase relief and the second injection produced less than 90% anesthetic phase relief or the patient had inappropriate physiologic durations of pain relief with anesthetics of different duration, a false-positive response occurred to the first injection. In this case, the diagnosis of intraarticular SIJ pain should be reconsidered and treatment modified accordingly.

If both the first and second injections produced 90% or greater physiologic relief, predominantly intraarticular SIJ pain is assumed. Aggressive conservative care is begun immediately and continued for up to two weeks. Patients who have 75% or greater relief are discharged with a home program. If, however, they have less than 75% relief, SIJ treatment has failed, and the patient should be entered into a chronic pain management program, discharged with a home program, or undergo a trial of prolotherapy, surgical fusion of the SIJ, or fluoroscopically-guided local anesthetic injection of the L4 medial branches and L5–S3 dorsal rami.

If fluoroscopically guided local anesthetic injections of the L4 medial branches and L5–S3 dorsal rami produce 90% or greater anesthetic phase relief, a second set of similar injections may be considered using an anesthetic of different duration. If the first injection produced 90% or greater anesthetic phase relief and the second injection produced less than 90% anesthetic phase relief or the patient had inappropriate physiologic durations of pain relief with anesthetics of different durations, a false-positive response is assumed. The patient is placed in a chronic pain management program and/or discharged with a home program. If, however, both the first and second injections of the L4 medial branches and L5–S3 dorsal rami produced 90% or greater anesthetic phase relief and the patient had an appropriate physiologic duration of pain relief with anesthetics of different durations, denervation of the same nerves can be performed with radiofrequency, phenol, or cryotherapy. Patients who have 75% or greater relief with this procedure can be discharged with a home program. If relief is less than 75%, they can be entered into a chronic pain management program and/or discharged with a home program or prolotherapy can be performed (see below for further description).

If the patient had less than 90% relief from the first set of injections of the L4 medial branches and L5–S3 dorsal rami, prolotherapy can be performed. Patients who have 75% or greater relief with prolotherapy should be discharged with a home program. If relief is less than 75%, they can be entered into a chronic pain management program and/or home program or surgical fusion of their SIJ can be performed. If pain relief with the surgical fusion is 75% or greater, the patient can be discharged with a home program; if relief is less than 75%, the patient can be entered into a chronic pain management program and/or discharged with a home program.

Patients may receive psychologic intervention at any point in the treatment process if the physician believes that it may improve treatment progress.

## CONCLUSION

The SIJ is a primary source of back pain. It also may become a secondary site of pain when dysfunction occurs anywhere along its kinetic chain. No historical facts or physical examination findings have been scientifically proved to be diagnostic for painful SIJ dysfunction. Fluoroscopically guided, contrast-enhanced, intraarticular SIJ injections are currently the only method available to determine definitively that pain emanates from the SIJ. These diagnostic and potentially therapeutic injections become necessary only when a patient receives no benefit, plateaus, or makes minimal progress with aggressive conservative care. Further research is needed to determine which treatment or combination of treatment strategies best serves the patient with SIJ pain.

**Acknowledgment.**    The authors thank Marcus Calahan for his assistance in preparation of the manuscript.

## REFERENCES

1. Abbott GT, Carty H: Pyogenic sacroilitis, the missed diagnosis? Br J Radiol 66:120–122, 1993.
2. Alderink GJ: The sacroiliac joint: Review of anatomy, mechanics and function. J Orthop Sports Phys Ther 13:71–84, 1991.
3. Aprill C: The role of anatomically specific injections into the sacroiliac joint. Presented at the First Interdisciplinary World Congress on Low Back Pain and its Relation to the Sacroiliac Joint, San Diego, November 5–6, 1992.
4. Battafarano DF, West SG, Rak KM, et al: Comparison of bone scan, computed tomography, and magnetic resonance imaging in the diagnosis of active sacroilitis. Semin Arthritis Rheum 23(3):161–176, 1993.
5. Beal MC: The sacroiliac problem: Review of anatomy, mechanics, and diagnosis. J Am Osteopath Assoc 81:667–679, 1982.
6. Bender J, et al: Factors affecting the occurrence of knee injuries. J Assoc Phys Ment Rehabil 18:139, 1964.
7. Bernard TN: Sacroiliac joint injection. In Proceedings of the First Interdisciplinary World Congress on Low back Pain and its Relation to the Sacroiliac Joint, San Diego, November 5–6, 1992, pp 401–403.
8. Bernard TN Jr, Cassidy JD: The sacroiliac joint syndrome—pathophysiology, diagnosis, and management. In Frymoyer JW (ed): The Adult Spine: Principles and Practice. New York, Raven Press, 1991, pp 2107–2130.
9. Bernard TN Jr, Kirkaldy-Willis WH: Recognizing specific characteristics of non-specific low back pain. Clin Orthop 217:266–280, 1987.
10. Blyth CS, Mueller FU: Football injury survey. Part 1: When and where players get hurt. Phys Sports Med 2:45, 1974.
11. Bogduk N, Twomey LT: Clinical Anatomy of the Lumbar Spine, 2nd ed. Churchill Livingstone, New York, 1991, pp 40–42.
12. Bohannon RW, Gajdosik R, LeVeau BF: Contribution of pelvic and lower limb motion to increases in the angle of passive straight leg raising. Phys Ther 65:474–476, 1985.
13. Bohay DR, Gray JM: Sacroiliac joint pyarthrosis. Orthop Rev Jul:817–823, 1993.
14. Bourdillon JF: Spinal Manipulation, 3rd ed. London, William Heinemann, 1982.
15. Bowen V, Cassidy JD: Macroscopic and microscopic anatomy of the sacroiliac joint from embryonic life until the eighth decade. Spine 6:620–628, 1981.
16. Bradley KC: The anatomy of backache. Aust NZ J Surg 44:227–232, 1974.
17. Brooke R: The sacroiliac joint. J Anat 58:299–305, 1924.
18. Brower AC: The sacroiliac joint. In Arthritis in Black and White. Philadelphia, W.B. Saunders, 1988, p 10.
19. Brower AC: Disorders of the sacroiliac joint. Surg Rounds Orthop 13:47–54, 1989.
20. Cassidy JD, Kirkaldy-Willis WH, McGregor M: Spinal manipulation for the treatment of chronic low back and leg pain: An observational study. In Buerger AA, Greenman PE (eds): Empirical Approaches to the Validation of Spinal Manipulation. Springfield, IL, Charles C Thomas, 1985, pp 119–148.
21. Chow DHK, Luk KDK, Leong JCY, Woo CW: Tortional stability of the lumbosacral junction: Significance of the iliolumbar ligament. Spine 14:611–615, 1989.
22. Cibulka MT, Koldehoff RM: Leg length disparity and its effect on sacroiliac joint dysfunction. Clin Manage 6:10–11, 1986.
23. Cibulka MT, Rose SJ, Delitto A, et al: Hamstring muscle strain treated by mobilizing the sacroiliac joint. Phys Ther 66:1220–1223, 1986.
24. Cohen AS, McNeill JM, Calkins E, et al: The "normal" sacroiliac joint: Analysis of 88 sacroiliac roentgenograms. Am J Roent Radium Ther 100:559–563, 1967.
25. Colachis SC, Worden RE, Bechtol CD, et al: Movement of the sacroiliac joint in the adult male: A preliminary report. Arch Phys Med Rehabil 44:490–498, 1963.
26. Cole AJ, Dreyfuss P, Pauza K: Sacroiliac joint injection techniques. In Vleeming A, Mooney V, Snijders C, Dorman T (eds): Proceedings of the Second Interdisciplinary World Congress on Low Back Pain: The Integrated Function of the Lumbar Spine and Sacroiliac Joints. San Diego, 1995, pp 567–597.
27. Cole AJ, Dreyfuss P, Stratton SA: The sacroiliac joint: A review. Crit Rev Conc (In press).
28. Cole AJ, Herring SA, Stratton SA, et. al: Spine injuries in runners: A functional approach. J Back Musculoskel Rehabil 5:317–339, 1995.
29. Cole AJ, Herring SA: Role of the physiatrist in management of musculoskeletal pain. In Tollison CD (ed): The Handbook of Pain Management, 2nd ed. Baltimore, Williams & Wilkins, 1994, pp 85–95.
30. Cole AJ, Herring SA: Rehabilitation and return to play. In Sallis RE, Massimino F (eds): American College of Sports Medicine's Essentials of Sports Medicine. St. Louis, Mosby, 1996.

31. Cooper KL, Beaubout JW, Swee RG: Insufficiency fractures of the sacrum. Radiology 156:15–20, 1985.

32. Daffner RH, Pavlov H: Stress fractures: Current concepts. AJR 159:245–252, 1992.

33. Davis P, Lente BC: Evidence for sacroiliac disease as a common cause of low backache in women. Lancet ii:496–497, 1978.

34. Dijkstra PJ, Vlemming A, Stoeckart R: Complex motion tomography of the sacroiliac joint. Rontgenstr Fortschr 150:635–642, 1989.

35. Dodig D, Domljan Z, Popovic S, et al: Effect of imaging time on the values of the sacroiliac index. Eur J Nucl Med 14:504–506, 1988.

36. DonTigny RL: Function and pathomechanics of the sacroiliac joint: A review. Phys Ther 65:35–44, 1985.

37. DonTigny RL: Anterior dysfunction of the sacroiliac joint as a major factor in the etiology of idiopathic low back pain syndrome. Phys Ther 70:250–265, 1990.

38. Dreyfuss P, Cole AJ, Pauza K: Sacroiliac joint injection techniques. Phys Med Rehabil Clin North Am 7:785–813, 1995.

39. Dreyfuss P, Dreyer S, Griffin J, et al: Positive sacroiliac joint screening tests in asymptomatic adults. Spine 19:1138–1143, 1994.

40. Dreyfuss P, Michaelsen M, Pauza K, et al: The value of medical history and physical examination in diagnosing sacroiliac joint pain. Spine 21:2594–2602, 1996.

41. Dunn EJ, Bryan DM, Nugent JT, Robinson RA: Pyogenic infections of the sacroiliac joint. Clin Orthop 118:113–117, 1976.

42. Ebraheim NA, Padanilam TG, Waldrop JT, et al: Anatomic consideration in the anterior approach to the sacro-iliac joint. Spine 19:721–725, 1994.

43. Egund N, Olsson TH, Schmid H, Selvik G: Movements in the sacroiliac joints demonstrated with roengen stereophotogrammetry. Acta Radiol Diagn 19:833–946, 1978.

44. Ehara S, El-Khoury GY, Bergman RA: The accessory sacroiliac joint: A common anatomic variant. Am J Roent Radium Ther 150:857–859, 1988.

45. Eldred E, Lindsky D, Buchwald J: The effect of cooling on mammalian muscle spindles. Exp Neurol 2:144–157, 1960.

46. Elkstrand J, Gillquist J: Soccer injuries and their mechanisms: A prospective study. Med Sci Sports Exerc 15:267, 1983.

47. Farrell JP, Jensen GM: Manual therapy: A critical assessment of role in the profession of physical therapy. Phys Ther 72:11–20, 1992.

48. Fink-Bennett DM, Benson MT: Unusual exercise-related stress fractures. Two case reports. Clin Nucl Med 9:430–434, 1984.

49. Firooznia H, Golimbu C, Rafii M, et al: Computed tomography of the sacroiliac joints: Comparison with complex-motion tomography. J Comput Assist Tomogr 8:31–39, 1984.

50. Fortin JD: Personal observation, 1993.

51. Fortin JD: Sacroiliac joint dysfunction—A new perspective. J Back Musculoskel Rehabil 3:31–43, 1993.

52. Fortin JD, Aprill CN, Ponthieux B, et al: Sacroiliac joint: Pain referral maps upon applying a new injection/arthrography technique. Part II: Clinical evaluation. Spine 19:1483–1489, 1994.

53. Fortin JD, Dwyer AD, West S, Pier J: Sacroiliac joint: Pain referral maps upon applying a new injection/arthrography technique. Part I: Asymptomatic volunteers. Spine 19:1475–1482, 1994.

54. Fortin JD, Tolchin RB: Sacroiliac joint provocation and arthrography. Arch Phys Med Rehabil. 74:1259, 1993.

55. Freiberg AH, Vinke TH: Sciatica and the sacroiliac joint. Clin Orthop 16:126–134, 1974.

56. Friedman L, Silverberg P, Butler R, et al: CT evaluation of the sacroiliac joint with development of a miniseries. In Proceedings from Low Back Pain and its Relation to the Sacroiliac Joint, San Diego, 1992, pp 285–293.

57. Friedman L, Silberberg PJ, Rainbow A, Butler R: A limited, low-dose computed tomography protocol to examine the sacroiliac joints. Can Assoc Radiol J 44(4):267–272, 1993.

58. Frigerio NA, Stowe RR, Howe JW: Movement of the sacroiliac joint. Clin Orthop 100:370–377, 1974.

59. Frymoyer JW, Howe J, Kuhlmann D: The long-term effects of spinal fusion on the sacroiliac joints and ileum. Clin Orthop 134:196–201, 1978.

60. Geraci MC: Rehabilitation of pelvis, hip and thigh injuries in sports. Phys Medi Rehabil Clin North Am 6:157–173, 1994.

61. Goldberg RP, Genant HK, Shimshak R, et al: Applications and limitations of quantitative sacroiliac joint scintigraphy. Radiology 128:683–686, 1978.

62. Greenman PE: Clinical aspects of sacroiliac function in walking. J Man Med 5:25–130, 1990.

63. Greenman PE: Sacroiliac dysfunction in the failed low back pain syndrome. In Proceedings for the First Interdisciplinary World Congress on Low Back Pain and its Relation to the Sacroiliac Joint, San Diego, 1992, pp 329–352.

64. Grieve GP: Mobilization of Spine. London, Churchill Livingstone, 1984, pp 79–85.

65. Grob KR, Neuhuber WL, Kissling RO: Innervation of the sacroiliac joint of the human [German]. Zeitschr Rheumatol 54(2):117–122, 1995.
66. Grodin A, Cantu R: Soft tissue mobilization. In Basmajian JV, Nyberg R (eds): Rational Manual Therapies, Baltimore, Williams & Wilkins, 1993, pp 199–222.
67. Hadley LA: Accessory sacro-iliac articulations. J Bone Joint Surg 34A:149–155, 1952.
68. Haggart GE: Sciatic pain of unknown orgin: Effective method of treatment. J Bone Joint Surg 20A:851–59, 1938.
69. Haldeman S, Phillips RB: Spinal manipulative therapy in the management of low back pain. In Frymoyer JW (ed): The Adult Spine: Principles and Practice. New York, Raven Press, 1991, pp 1581–1605.
70. Hanly JG, Barnes DC, Mitchell MJ, et al: Single photon emission computer tomography in the diagnosis of inflammatory spondyloarthropathies. J Rheumatol 20:2062–2068, 1993.
71. Hanson P, Sonesson B: The anatomy of the iliolumbar ligament. Arch Phys Med Rehabil 75:1245–1246, 1994.
72. Hauge MD, Cooper KL, Litin SC: Insufficiency fractures of the pelvis that stimulate metastatic disease. Mayo Clin Proc 63:807–812, 1988.
73. Hershey CD: The sacro-iliac joint and pain of sciatic radiation. JAMA 122:983–986, 1943.
74. Hesch J, Aisenbrey JA, Guarino J: Manual therapy evaluation of the pelvic joints using palpatory and articular spring tests. In Proceedings for the First Interdisciplinary World Congress on Low Back Pain and its Relation to the Sacroiliac Joint. San Diego, 1992, pp 435–459.
75. Hiltz DL: The sacroiliac joint as a source of sciatica: A case report. Phys Ther 56:1373, 1976.
76. Hirsch C, Ingelmark BE, Miller M: The anatomical basis for low back pain. Acta Orthop Scand 33:1–17, 1963.
77. Holder LE: Bone scintigraphy in skeletal trauma. Radiol Clin North Am 31:739–781, 1993.
78. Huskisson E: Non-narcotic analgesics. In Wall PD, Melzach R (eds): Textbook of Pain. New York,Churchill Livingstone, 1984, pp 505–513.
79. Ikeda R: Innervation of the sacroiliac joint. Macroscopical and histological studies [Japanese]. J Nippon Med School. 58:587–596, 1991.
80. Inmann VT, Saunders JB: Referred pain from skeletal structures. J Nerv Ment Dis 99:660–667, 1944.
81. Jajic I, Jajic Z: The prevalence of osteoarthritis of the sacroiliac joints in an urban population. Clin Rheumotol 6:39–41, 1987.
82. Janda V: Muscle weakness and inhibition (pseudoparesis) in back pain syndromes. In Grieve GP (ed): Modern Manual Therapy of the Vertebral Column. Edinburgh, Churchill Livingstone, 1986, p 197.
83. Johnston WL: Funtional technique. In Basmajian JV, Nyberg R (eds): Rational Manual Therapies. Baltimore, Williams & Wilkins, 1993, pp 335–346.
84. Kerr R: Radiologic case study. Sacroiliac joint involvement by gout and hyperparathyroidism. Orthopedics 11:185–187, 190, 1988.
85. Kibler BW, Chandler TJ, Pace BK: Principles of rehabilitation after chronic tendon injuries. Clin Sports Med 11:661–671, 1992.
86. Kirkaldy-Willis WH, Cassidy JD: Spinal manipulation in the treatment of low back pain. Can Fam Physician 31:535–539, 1985.
87. Korr IM: Proprioceptors and somatic dysfunction. J Am Osteopath Assoc 74:638–650, 1975.
88. Lamb DW: The neurology of spinal pain. Phys Ther 59:971–973, 1979.
89. Lavignolle B, Vital JM, Senegas J, et al: An approach to the functional anatomy of the sacroiliac joints in vivo. Anat Clin 5:169–176, 1983.
90. Lawson TL, Foley WD, Carrera GF, Berland LL: The sacroiliac joints: Anatomic, plain roentgenographic, and computed tomographic analysis. J Comput Assist Tomogr 6:307–314, 1982.
91. Lee D: The relationship between the lumbar spine, pelvic girdle, and hip. In Course Proceedings for the First Interdisciplinary World Congress on Low Back Pain and its Relation to the Sacroiliac Joint, San Diego, 1992, pp 464–478.
92. Lehmann J, deLateur BJ: Diathermy and superficial heat and cold therapy. In Kottke EJ, Stillwell GK, Lehmann JF (eds): Krusen's Handbook of Physical Medicine and Rehabilitation. Philadelphia, W.B. Saunders, 1982, pp 275–350.
93. Lourie G, Pruzansky M, Reiner M, et al: Pyarthrosis of the sacroiliac joint presenting as lumbar radiculopathy—A case report. Spine 11:638–640, 1986.
94. Lynch FW: The pelvic articulations during pregnancy, labor, and puerperium: An x-ray study. Surg Gynecol Obstet 30:575, 1920.
95. Lysens M, et al: The predictability of sports injuries. Sports Med 1:6, 1984.
96. MacDonald GR, Hunt TL: Sacro-iliac joint: Observations on the gross and histological changes in the various age groups. Can Med Assoc J 66:157–163, 1952.
97. Maigne JY, Aivaliklis A, Pfefer F: Results of sacroiliac joint double block and value of sacroiliac pain provocation tests in 54 patients with low back pain. Spine 21:1889–1892, 1996.
98. Marymont JV, Lynch MA, Henning CE: Exercise-related stress reaction of the sacroiliac joint. An unusual cause of low back pain in athletes. Am J Sports Med 14:320–323, 1986.

99. May P: Movement awareness and stabilization training. In Basmajian JV, Nyberg R (eds): Rational Manual Therapies. Baltimore, Williams & Wilkins, 1993, pp 347–258.

100. McClure M: Flexibility training. In Basmajian JV, Nyberg R (eds): Rational Manual Therapies. Baltimore, Williams & Wilkins, 1993, pp 359–386.

101. Mieray D, Yong-Hing K, Wilkinson AA, et al: Scintigraphic analysis of sacroiliac pain: Toward a diagnostic criteria for SI syndrome. Presented at the Annual Meeting of the North American Spine Society, Boston, 1992.

102. Milgrom C, Chisen R, Giladi M, et al: Multiple stress fractures: A longitudinal study of a soldier with 13 lesions. Clin Orthop 192:174–179, 1985.

103. Mitchell FL Jr, Moran PS, Pruzzo NA: An evaluation and treatment manual of osteopathic muscle energy techniques. Valley Park, Mitchell, Moran, & Pruzzo Associates, 1979, pp 49–62, 109–155.

104. Mixter WJ, Barr JS: Rupture of the intervertebral disc with involvement of the spinal canal. N Engl J Med 211:210, 1934.

105. Mooney V: Understanding, examining for, and treating sacroiliac pain. J Musculoskel Med 10:37–49, 1993.

106. Mozas J, Castilla JA, Alarcon JL, et al: Reactive sacroiliitis as late sequela after severe pelvic inflammatory disease verified by laparoscopy or laparotomy. Acta Obstet Gynecol Scand 73:324–327, 1994.

107. Norman GF, May A: Sacroiliac conditions simulating intervertebral disk syndrome. West J Surg Obstet Gynecol 64:641–642, 1956.

108. Nyberg R: Manipulation: Definitions, types application. In Basmajian JV, Nyberg R (eds): Rational Manual Therapies. Baltimore, Williams & Wilkins, 1993, pp 21–48.

109. Onsel C, Collier BD, Metin K, et al: Increased sacroiliac joint uptake after lumbar fusion and/or laminectomy. Clin Nuclear Med 17:283–287, 1992.

110. Paquin J, Rosenthall L, Esdaile J, et al: Elevated uptake of 99M technetium methylene diphosphonate in the axial skeleton. I: Ankylosing spondylitis and Reiter's disease: Implications for quantitative sacroiliac scintigraphy. Arthritis Rheum 26:217–220, 1983.

111. Pardy W: Strength training. In Basmajian JV, Nyberg R (eds): Rational Manual Therapies. Baltimore, Williams & Wilkins, 1993, pp 387–424.

112. Perl ER: The straight leg raising sign: A review. J Orthop Sports Phys Ther 2:127, 1981.

113. Pitkin HC, Pheasant HC: Sacroarthrogenetic telalgia. 1: A study of referred pain. J Bone Joint Surg 18A:111–133, 1936.

114. Reilly JP, Gross RH, Emans JB, et al: Disorders of the sacroiliac joint in children. J Bone Joint Surg 70A:31-40, 1988.

115. Resnick D, Niwayama G, Georgen TG: Degenerative disease of the sacroiliac joint. Invest Radiol 10:608–621, 1975.

116. Ries T: Detection of osteoporotic sacral fractures with radionuclides. Radiology 146:783–785, 1983.

117. Robey JM, Blyth CS, Mueller FD: Athletic injuries: Application of epidemiologic methods. JAMA 217:184, 1971.

118. Sandrasegaran K, Saifuddin A, Coral A, Butt WB: Magnetic resonance imaging of septic sacroiliitis. Skeletal Radiol 23:289–292, 1994.

119. Sarma NH: Pigmented villonodular synovitis of sacral joint-report of a case. Cent Afr J Med 31:156–157, 1985.

120. Sashin D: A critical analysis of the anatomy and the pathological changes of the sacroiliac joints. J Bone Joint Surg 12A:891–910, 1930.

121. Schaad UB, McCracken GH, Nelson JD: Pyogenic arthritis of the sacroiliac joint in pediatric patients. Pediatrics 66:375–379, 1980.

122. Schneider R, Yacovone J, Ghelman B: Unsuspected sacral fractures: Detection by radionuclide bone scanning. AJR 144:337–341, 1985.

123. Schunke GB: Anatomy and development of the sacroiliac joint in man. Anat Rec 72:313–331, 1938.

124. Schwarzer AC, Aprill CN, Derby R, et al: Clinical features of patients with pain stemming from the lumbar zygapophysial joints: Is the lumbar facet syndrome a clinical entity? Spine 19:1132–1237, 1994.

125. Schwarzer AC, Aprill CN, Bogduk N: The sacroiliac joint in chronic low back pain. Spine 20:31–37, 1995.

126. Slipman C, Sterenfeld EB, Pauza K, et al: The value of single photon emission computed tomography in the diagnosis of sacro-iliac joint syndrome. Arch Phys Med Rehabil 74:1242, 1993.

127. Slocum L, Terry RJ: Influence of the sacrotuberous and sacrospinous ligaments in limiting movements at the sacroiliac joint. JAMA 87:307–309, 1926.

128. Solonen KA: The sacroiliac joint in light of anatomical, roentgenological, and clinical studies. Acta Orthop Scand (Suppl) 27:1–127, 1957.

129. Steindler A: Differential diagnosis of pain low in the back: Allocation of source of pain by procaine hydrochloride method. JAMA 110:106–113, 1938.

130. Steindler A: The interpretation of sciatic radiation and the syndrome of low-back pain. J Bone Joint Surg 22A:28–34, 1940.

131. Stewart TD: Pathological changes in aging sacroiliac joints: A study of dissecting-room skeletons. Clin Orthop Rel Res 183:188–196, 1984.
132. Stratton SA: Personal communication, 1995.
133. Sturesson B: Mobility of the pelvis measured in living persons. In Course Proceedings for the First Interdisciplinary Conference on Low Back Pain and its Relation to the Sacroiliac Joint, San Diego, 1992, pp 181–183.
134. Sturesson B, Selvik G, Uden A: Movements of the sacroiliac joints—A roentgen stereophotogrammetric analysis. Spine 14:162–165, 1989.
135. Trotter M: Accessory sacro-iliac articulations. Am J Phys Anthropol 22:247–261, 1937.
136. Vesterskold L, Axelsson B, Jacobsson H: A method for combined quantitative pertechnetate and bone scintigraphy of the sacro-iliac joints. Scand J Rheumatol 14:324–328, 1985.
137. Vleeming A, Buyruk HM, Stoeckart R, et al: Towards an integrated therapy for peripartum pelvic instability: A study based on the biomechanical effects of pelvic belts. Am J Obstet Gynecol 166:1243–1247, 1992.
138. Vleeming A, Stoeckart R, Snijders CJ: The sacrotuberous ligament: A conceptual approach to its dynamic role in stabilizing the sacroiliac joint. Clin Biomech 4:201–203, 1989.
139. Vleeming A, Stoeckart R, Snijders CJ: General Introduction. In Course Proceedings of Low Back Pain and its Relation to the Sacroiliac Joint, San Diego, 1992, pp 3–64.
140. Vleeming A, Van Wingerden JP, Snijders CJ, et al: Load application to the sacrotuberous ligament: Influences on sacroiliac joint mechanics. Clin Biomech 4:204–209, 1989.
141. Vleeming A, Stoeckart R, Volkers ACW, et al: Relation between form and function in the sacroiliacal joint. Part I: Clinical anatomical aspects. Spine 15:133–135, 1990.
142. Vleeming A, Van Wingerdan JP, Dijkstra PF, et al: Mobility in the sacroiliac joints in the elderly: A kinematic and radiographic study. Clin Biomechan 7:170–176, 1992.
143. Vleeming A, Volkers ACW, Snijders CJ, et al: Relation between form and function in the sacroiliac joint. Part II: Biomechanical aspects. Spine 15:133–135, 1990.
144. Walker JM: The sacroiliac joint: A critical review, Phys Ther 72:903–916, 1992.
145. Ward RC: Myofascial release concepts. In Basmajian JV, Nyberg R (eds): Rational Manual Therapies. Baltimore, Williams & Wilkins, 1993, pp 223–242.
146. Weisl H: Ligaments of sacro-iliac joint examined with particular reference to their function. Acta Anat 20:201–213, 1954.
147. Weisl H: The articular surfaces of the sacroiliac joint and their relation to movement of the sacrum. Acta Anat 22:1–14, 1954.
148. White AA, Edwards WT, Liberman D, et al: Biomechanics of lumbar spine and sacroiliac articulation: Relevance to idiopathic low back pain. In White AA, Gordon SL (eds): American Academy of Orthopedic Surgeons Symposium on Idiopathic Low Back Pain. St. Louis, Mosby, 1982, pp 269–322.
149. Wilder DG, Pope MH, Frymoyer JW: The functional topography of the sacroiliac joint. Spine 5:575–579, 1980.
150. Williams PL, Warwick R: Gray's Anatomy, 36th ed. Edinburgh, Longman, 1980.
151. Windsor RE, Lester JP, Herring SA: Electrical stimulation in clinical practice. Physician Sportsmed 21:85–93, 1993.
152. Wolf LB: Aerobic exercise. In Basmajian JV, Nyberg R (eds): Rational Manual Therapies. Baltimore, Williams & Wilkins, 1993, pp 425–440.
153. Wyke B: The neurology of joints. Ann R Coll Surg Engl 41:25–50, 1967.

# 6

# Myofascial Pain

ANDREW A. FISCHER, MD, PhD

Several recent developments have changed profoundly the basic diagnostic criteria of myofascial muscle pain syndromes and their management. Specific diagnostic criteria for myofascial pain have been verified by new experimental data (kappa values)[24,30] and quantified by pressure algometry.[4] The diagnosis of fibromyalgia also needs to be quantified by algometry.[6] New therapeutic approaches include improved techniques for trigger point injections and other local injections for pain management. Preinjection blocks (PIBs) represent a new approach to prevention of pain caused by needle penetration of tender areas.[7,8,17,19] Myofascial pain plays an important role in diagnosis and management of musculoskeletal pain, particularly soft tissue disorders.[1,3,11,12,15,18,20–22,25–36]

Tender spots, with maximal pain located in the most tender area, are the most frequent causes of pain in soft tissue disorders.[6,7] In the author's experience, muscle spasm is the second most frequent cause of muscular pain in soft tissue injuries. Muscle spasm has been defined as an involuntary contraction, usually painful, that cannot be relieved completely by voluntary effort.[1,6,7] Trigger points are small, exquisitely tender spots that shoot pain into a distant area called the reference or referred pain zone (RPZ).[20–22,35,36] Tender spots and trigger points are most often located in muscles but may occur in any kind of soft tissue disorders or injury, such as sprained ligaments, periostitis, tendinitis, or bursitis. Specific RPZs have been described for myofascial trigger points located in muscles[27,28,31,35,36] as well as in ligaments.[16] The significance of RPZs for clinical management is obvious, because effective treatment depends on identifying exactly where the pain originates. Treatment limited to the RPZ, which is the area of the patient's complaint, fails to induce long-term and complete relief. Only treatment of trigger points, which are the cause of pain, is effective.[20,21,35,36]

## DEFINITION OF MYOFASCIAL PAIN SYNDROMES AND FIBROMYALGIA

The term *myofascial pain* is used for two completely different categories of conditions.[29] A narrower definition of myofascial pain is limited to trigger points and tender spots located in muscles. In general, trigger points can be defined as small, exquisitely tender areas that spontaneously or on activation by pressure or needle penetration shoot pain into a distant part of the body (RPZ). Some trigger points—for example, those in the sternocleidomastoid muscle—also produce autonomous nervous system (sympathetic) dysfunction such as lacrimation or coryza. Myofascial trigger points are located within a taut band that consists of a group of muscle fibers distinguished by hard consistency, tenderness, and hyperirritability. Taut bands are manifested by a twitch response to snapping or, more reliably, penetration by a needle. Tender spots demonstrate the same local findings as trigger points, including a taut band, except that pain does not shoot to a distant region but is perceived in the area of the tender spot.[6,10]

In broader terms, myofascial pain syndromes include conditions other than trigger points that cause muscle pain, such as tender spots, muscle spasm and tension, and muscle deficiency manifested by decreased flexibility or strength. Fibromyalgia, along with other diffuse muscle tenderness, represents a separate category.

## DIFFERENTIAL DIAGNOSIS OF MUSCLE PAIN SYNDROME

Muscle spasm is an involuntary local contraction that extends over the entire muscle, whereas a taut band involves only a portion of muscle fibers. Spasm cannot be relieved completely by voluntary effort.[1,6,7] The spasm is a reflex reaction to an irritative focus.[3] Muscle tension, or the inability to relax certain muscles because of psychologic stress and tension, affects specifically susceptible muscles such as the upper trapezii, cervical and lumbar musculature, and muscles that move the pelvic floor and temporomandibular joint.[20–22] Muscle deficiency is characterized by loss of flexibility (i.e., tightness of the afflicted muscles) as well as weakness and/or loss of endurance.[20–22] Fibromyalgia is a disorder of pain modulation that causes generally decreased tolerance to pain.[6,37] It manifests by diffuse pain and tenderness that extend to many muscles and also affect nonmuscular tissues. In sharp contrast, muscle pain syndromes are characterized by focal tenderness limited to muscle tissue only and not extending to the involved region. It has been proved that manual pressure is an unreliable method of detecting tender points, which are diagnostic for fibromyalgia.[6] Physicians are unable to apply exactly 4 kg of pressure, which is required by the diagnostic criterion. Quantification of pressure by algometry is therefore necessary.[6] In addition to widespread pain, diagnosis of fibromyalgia requires that 11 of 18 specific tender points are painful at a pressure of 4 kg (Table 1).[37] Painful inflammatory muscle diseases (e.g., myositis) connected with specific muscle conditions and polymyalgia rheumatica are not categorized as myofascial pain. The common denominator of myofascial pain syndromes is negative laboratory findings, particularly absence of inflammation.

**TABLE 1.**
Differential Diagnosis of Focal (Point) Tenderness (Pressure Pain Sensitivity)

1. **Tender spots:** tenderness limited to a point (< 2 cm in diameter). Pressure threshold is lower by 2 kg/cm2 relative to normosensitive (nontender) tissue. Tender spots cause pain in the area of maximal point tenderness.

2. **Trigger points:** small, exquisitely tender spots that may shoot pain into a distant area (specific referred pain zone). Trigger points may be located in ligaments, pericapsular tissues, tendons (sheets), bursae, other soft tissues, or periosteum.

3. **Myofascial trigger points:** point tenderness within muscle tissue, usually located in a taut band, formed by a group of contracted muscle fibers and/or fibrotic tissue. Pain shoots into the reference pain zones that are specific for the trigger point. A **taut band** is a group of tender muscle fibers that demonstrate hard consistency on palpation. Taut bands may produce a "twitch reaction" on snapping or needle entry, indicating their hyperirritability. They may consist of a group of constantly contracted or damaged muscle fibers. The tight muscle fibers usually surround a core of fibrotic tissue band, particularly in the chronic stage.

4. **Tender points in fibromyalgia:** tenderness at a pressure of 4 kg over 11 of 18 specific points, which are diagnostic for fibromyalgia. The 18 points diagnostic for fibromyalgia include also nonmuscular tissues. Diffuse tenderness over muscles is present also beyond the tender points.

From Fischer AA: New developments in diagnosis of myofascial pain and fibromyalgia. Phys Med Rehabil Clin North Am 8:1–21, 1997, with permission.

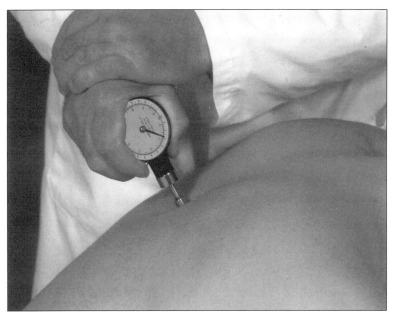

**FIGURE 1.**
Algometer for quantification of tenderness and diagnosis of trigger points and fibromyalgia.

## QUANTIFICATION OF TENDERNESS AND DIAGNOSIS BY ALGOMETRY

The degree of point tenderness, which is the diagnostic hallmark of trigger points and tender spots, can be quantified by a pressure algometer (Fig. 1).[4,6,17] Tenderness, or pressure pain threshold (PPT), is the only consistent finding and the most reliable and reproducible criterion for diagnosis of myofascial trigger points and tender spots.[30] Criteria for myofascial trigger points also include palpation of taut bands and elicitation of twitch responses.[27,30] As indicated in Table 1, tender spots and trigger points reach an abnormal level of tenderness if algometry shows a decrease in PPT by 2 kg/cm$^2$ relative to normosensitive control tissue.[4] The physiologic basis of tenderness is sensitization of nerve endings by inflammatory substances.[23] Table 2 summarizes the symptoms of myofascial trigger points.

**TABLE 2.**
Symptoms of Trigger Points

1. Pain
2. Limited range of motion, morning stiffness
3. Weakness; strength limited by trigger point threshold of pain
4. Autonomic disturbances: excessive lacrimation, nasal secretion, pilomotor activity, changes in sweat patterns
5. Proprioceptive dysfunction: disturbed weight perception, spatial disorientation, postural dizziness
6. Depression
7. Sleep disturbance: nonrestorative sleep causing morning fatigue

Based on Simons DG: Myofascial pain syndromes due to trigger points. In Goodgold J (ed): Rehabilitation Medicine. St. Louis, Mosby, 1988, pp 686–723; Travell JG, Simons DG: Myofascial Pain and Dysfunction: The Trigger Point Manual, vol I. Baltimore, Williams & Wilkins, 1983; and Travell JG, Simons DG: Myofascial Pain and Dysfunction: The Trigger Point Manual. The Lower Extremities, vol II. Baltimore, Williams & Wilkins, 1992.

**TABLE 3.**
Classification of Trigger Points and Tender Spots

| | |
|---|---|
| I. Types of trigger points, according to involved tissue | |
| Muscle or fascia (myofascial) | Skin (cutaneous), periosteum |
| Ligaments (sprain, strain) | Pericapsular or other soft tissue |

II. Trigger point activity
Active—pain is present spontaneously, at rest or with mild activity
Latent—no spontaneous pain; pain is induced by palpation, needle insertion, or unusually high
level of activity

III. Myofascial trigger points, mechanism of occurrence
1. Primary—not caused by other trigger points
Associated trigger points:
2. Secondary—from overloading of an antagonist or synergist to muscle containing primary
trigger point
3. Satellite trigger point: occur in the reference pain zone of a trigger point

IV. Duration of trigger point
Acute trigger points: acute onset by overload trauma; hours or days after onset; intensive pain
Chronic trigger points: duration extends to weeks, months, or years; symptoms may be mild or
severe; trigger points spread, induce secondary and satellite trigger points and progress to
more severe intensity
Recurrent trigger points: latent trigger points that occasionally become activated by overuse,
tension, change of weather, or other factors (endocrine, metabolic, vitamin deficiency)

Based on Simons DG: Myofascial pain syndromes due to trigger points. In Goodgold J (ed): Rehabilitation Medicine. St. Louis, Mosby, 1988, pp 686–723; Travell JG, Simons DG: Myofascial Pain and Dysfunction: The Trigger Point Manual, vol I. Baltimore, Williams & Wilkins, 1983; and Travell JG, Simons DG: Myofascial Pain and Dysfunction: The Trigger Point Manual. The Lower Extremities, vol II. Baltimore, Williams & Wilkins, 1992.

When the patient is asked to indicate with one finger where the pain is worst, the location usually corresponds exactly to the point of maximal tenderness. The proper expression for the condition is tender spots, as diagnosed by palpation. Rarely does the patient point to an RPZ or an associated trigger point.[6,10] Table 3 presents a classification of trigger points and tender spots according to location, activity, mechanism of occurrence, and duration.[25,27,35,36] Table 4 lists conditions in which tender spots or trigger points are the immediate cause of pain. Needling and infiltration of trigger points or tender spots, as described later, effectively relieve pain in these conditions by breaking up and healing the abnormal tissue.[6–10]

## TREATMENT OF MYOFASCIAL PAIN SYNDROME, TRIGGER POINTS, TENDER SPOTS, AND MUSCLE SPASM

Treatment of pain syndromes involving trigger points or tender spots consists of two steps:

1. Treatment of the trigger point and taut band, which relieves pain and eliminates pathology underlying the trigger points or tender spots (abnormal tissue).

2. Identification and removal or treatment of the cause(s) of trigger points as well as perpetuating factors.

Successful treatment of tender spots and trigger points must focus on the maximally tender spot and taut band; therefore, it is of critical importance to identify the immediate cause of pain. This goal may be achieved in three simple steps:[7,10]

1. Ask the patient to indicate with one finger where the pain is most intense.

2. Find the maximally tender point by palpating with fingertips. Press the point with one fingertip, and ask the patient, "Is this the pain you are complaining of?" The patient's recognition of pain indicates that this particular point is the immediate cause of complaints. The degree of tenderness can be quantified by algometry.

**TABLE 4.**
Conditions in Which Trigger Points or Tender Spots May Be the Immediate Cause of Pain

Headaches—temporal, occipital

Tension headaches

Degenerative disc disease and radiculopathy—myotomal distribution of trigger points

Sciatica—piriformis syndrome

Neuralgia (e.g., brachial)

Osteoarthritis—pericapsular and ligament tender spots

Tennis elbow—epicondylitis

Subacromial bursitis—causes tender spots or trigger points in deltoid and subdeltoid muscles

Trochanteric bursitis—causes tender spots or trigger points in glutei

Capsulitis, tendinitis (e.g., bicipital)

Visceral—pleurodynia, pleurisy

Endocrine disorders

Chest pain—of cardiac origin; may cause tender spots or trigger points in chest muscles

Myalgia

**Note:** Frequently injury (ligament sprain) or inflammation (bursitis) induces tender spots or trigger points in the adjacent muscles, which become the immediate cause of pain. Treatment limited to muscle pain leaves the original pathology intact and causes recurrence of tender spots, trigger points, and pain.

From Fischer AA: New developments in diagnosis of myofascial pain and fibromyalgia. Phys Med Rehabil Clin North Am 8:1–21, 1997, and Fischer AA: New approaches in treatment of myofascial pain. Phys Med Rehabil Clin North Am 8:16–17, 1997.

3.  Alleviate the pain by inactivation of the tender spot or trigger point. Such alleviation confirms the findings of the two previous steps. Inactivation can be achieved by several methods.[6–10,17,22,25,27,35,36] The most effective is needling of the tender area, including the taut band, usually in combination with infiltration with lidocaine.[7] Needling with infiltration by saline in patients who are allergic to lidocaine is also effective and relieves pain as well as diminishes local tenderness.

Noninvasive techniques to inactivate trigger points include acupressure with thumb for about 1 minute, which causes temporary ischemia and numbing of the tender spot or trigger point. More effective is spray with a vapocoolant (e.g., ethyl chloride or fluorimethane) combined either with active relaxation exercises[10,20–22,25] or passive stretching.[27,35,36] The techniques of spray with active movement or stretch are described below.

In the author's experience, one of the most effective methods of inactivating trigger points is reciprocal inhibition, or relaxation by activation of antagonist muscles (RAA technique).[7,10] The treated muscle is under maximal stretch (at the end of range of motion). The most effective relaxation is achieved by a combination of eye movement (looking downward), deep exhalation, and application of mild resistance to the antagonist of the muscles to be relaxed. This method may be followed by slow stretching.

Table 5 lists causes or perpetuating factors of trigger points and tender spots.

## INJECTION TECHNIQUES FOR MANAGEMENT OF SOFT TISSUE PAIN

The only modality that brings instantaneous, complete, and lasting relief of pain in soft tissue disorders is injection[7–10] or, more precisely, infiltration (i.e., slow diffuse dispersion of a local anesthetic into the entire abnormal tissue in contrast to sudden deposition of a substance into a point). Needling—the repetitive insertion and withdrawal of the injection needle—has the unique effect of breaking up the edematous, inflamed, or (in later stages) fibrotic (scar) tissue. Needling and infiltration (N and I) constitute a

**TABLE 5.**
Causes of Trigger Points and Perpetuating Factors

| |
|---|
| Local—mechanical |
|   1. Acute injuries: sprain, whiplash |
|   2. Sport injuries: tennis, golf, pitcher's elbow, shoulder |
| Chronic repetitive microtrauma |
|   1. Industrial work |
|   2. Typewriter, computer |
| General factors: hypothyroidism, estrogen deficiency?, metabolic electrolyte disorders, vitamin deficiencies, infections |

From Travell JG, Simons DG: Myofascial Pain and Dysfunction: The Trigger Point Manual, vol I. Baltimore, Williams & Wilkins, 1983, and Travell JG, Simons DG: Myofascial Pain and Dysfunction: The Trigger Point Manual. The Lower Extremities, vol II. Baltimore, Williams & Wilkins, 1992.

specific technique to eliminate the tissue abnormality that causes pain, sensitization, and functional limitations. Table 6 reviews different effective injection techniques.

Tender spots and trigger points are best treated by a specific technique of N and I that is not limited to the maximally tender point but extends over the entire taut band and particularly over its insertion to bones (enthesopathy).[7–10,20–22] Different techniques for N and I have been described in detail.[7–10,20–22,35,36]

Figure 2 shows the physical findings over the trigger point and the taut band in which it is located as well as the effect of preinjection block (PIB). Palpation reveals a relatively thick taut band. Within the band an exquisitely tender spot or trigger point can be palpated. The upper part of Figure 2 also shows a preinjection block (PIB) technique called "coating." The block is administered along both sides of the taut band, avoiding the most tender and painful parts, which would cause pain on needle penetration. The left side of the figure shows the penetration of the needle next to the taut band at its proximal end. From the same needle penetration, infiltration is performed along the taut band, depositing 0.5–1 ml of 1% lidocaine at each stop as indicated by the circles. The lower part of Figure 2 shows how the taut band and tender spots or trigger point shrink after the PIB. Evidently the neurogenic component of the taut band and trigger point has been relieved by the PIB. At the same time the tenderness of the taut band decreases, as documented by an increased pressure pain threshold on algometry. At this stage the remaining part of the taut band offers fibrotic resistance on palpation and needle penetration. The lower part of Figure 2 also demonstrates the technique of N

**TABLE 6.**
Injection Techniques for Soft Tissue Pain

| |
|---|
| I. Preinjection blocks (PIBs) prevent pain caused by penetration of sensitive tissue (tender spots, trigger points, sprains, reflex sympathetic dystrophy, muscle spasm). PIBs by themselves relieve pain. |
|     1. Coating block |
|     2. Paraspinous block |
|     3. Subcutaneous block |
|     4. Peripheral nerve block |
|   For elimination of local pathology and sensitization, needling and infiltration of the tender, abnormal areas are necessary. |
| II. Needling and infiltration of abnormal and tender areas |
|     1. Tender spots and trigger points or surrounding area |
|     2. Sprains and injuries to muscles, ligaments, or other soft tissues |
|     3. Irritative focus that causes pain and muscle spasm, bursitis, tendinitis, injuries, fasciitis |
|     4. Repetitive stress disorders (cumulative trauma disorders) |
|     5. Reflex sympathetic dystrophy |
| III. Diffuse somatic block to relieve muscle spasm |

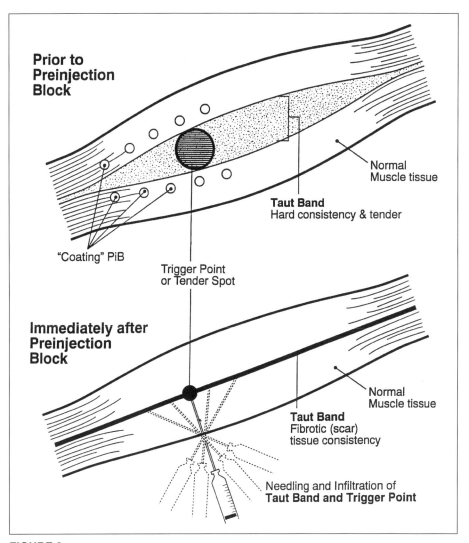

**Prior to Preinjection Block**

"Coating" PiB

Trigger Point or Tender Spot

Normal Muscle tissue

**Taut Band** Hard consistency & tender

**Immediately after Preinjection Block**

Normal Muscle tissue

**Taut Band** Fibrotic (scar) tissue consistency

Needling and Infiltration of **Taut Band and Trigger Point**

**FIGURE 2.**
Preinjection block (PIB) technique called coating block and its effect in relieving the neurogenic component of taut band and trigger points. After PIB the remaining core of the taut band consists of fibrotic resistance. The lower part shows how the fibrotic tissue core is broken up by needling and infiltration (N and I) with 1% xylocaine. After N and I most patients experience no pain, and palpatory findings (tightness, tenderness) become normal.

and I, which extends over the entire taut band. Infiltration is performed with about 0.1–0.2 ml of 1% lidocaine at each needle stop. For best results the attachment of taut band to the bones also should be needled and infiltrated, using a similar technique. In comparison the PIB coating technique requires a larger deposit of 0.5–1 ml of 1% lidocaine at each needle stop. After proper N and I the fibrotic core of the taut band and tender spots or trigger point also disappears, as confirmed by palpation.

The PIB has several beneficial effects.[7] It frequently makes trigger point injection pain-free. Even when complete anesthesia is not achieved, PIB reduces substantially the pain caused by penetration of tender and painful tissues. In addition, PIB prevents the sensitization that would be caused by local tissue injury during N and I. The nociceptive impulses generated by needling are blocked from reaching the central nervous system, and pain fails to enter the memory in the brain. Relaxation of the neurogenic component within the taut band facilitates substantially the second step of the trigger point injection, which consists of N and I. The relaxation of the neurogenic component exposes the remaining fibrotic core and allows the practitioner to concentrate the needling on this structure. The needling seems to be the most effective modality to break up the fibrotic tissue, when conservative therapy for relaxation of taut band may not be effective.

PIBs themselves are effective in relieving pain and may be used for treatment without subsequent N and I. However, once a fibrotic core is palpated, N and I is the only modality, in the author's experience, that brings long-term results and prevents recurrence by eliminating the underlying pathology.[7–10] It should be noted, however, that the PIB, which induces local anesthesia for about 45 minutes, actually relieves the pain and tightness for a longer period, sometimes weeks or even longer. The long-term relief and improvement of function are enhanced and maintained by follow-up physical therapy, particularly electric stimulation and relaxation exercises as described in the section on physical therapy.

Local infiltration is effective also for desensitization of sensitized (inflamed, damaged, overused) tissues that are tender and painful.[7–10] Infiltration normalizes the tenderness and pain by interrupting the continuous activity (after discharges) characteristic of sensitized nerves. As a result of normalization of nerve function, the effect of infiltration outlasts by a long period the action of anesthetic, which is usually limited to 45 minutes if 1% lidocaine is used. Desensitization may last weeks or longer. The anesthetic of choice for N and I and other blocks is 1% lidocaine.

### Preinjection Blocks Prevent Pain on Penetration of Tender Areas

PIBs are a new approach that prevent pain caused by needle penetration of tender and painful areas. The technique of PIB requires some knowledge of regional anatomy, but essentially it is quite simple. The goal is to block the sensory input going to the central nervous system from the tender, painful area to be injected. The simplest technique, called "coating block," consists of diffuse spreading of 1% lidocaine into the sensory supply of the area to be injected (see Fig. 2). In the extremities this area is located proximally to the injected spot.

Over the trunk the medial corresponding (paraspinal) areas are infiltrated diffusely (Fig. 3). In a few minutes the pain and tenderness disappear or are substantially reduced. The N and I can then be performed with no pain or only minimal discomfort. For injection of the teres minor muscle, PIB is administered to the lateral aspect of the muscle, where the axillary nerve enters (Fig. 3).

Paraspinous PIB is useful before N and I of paraspinal structures (Fig. 4). Paraspinous PIB frequently alleviates pain in radiculopathy and supraspinous ligament sprain.[7–10] N and I of supraspinous ligament sprain, which is a frequent irritative focus that causes segmental (radicular) sensitization,[7] can be performed without pain after paraspinous PIB. Peripheral nerve blocks are also effective for PIB, particularly for N and I in traumatic dystrophies. In addition to preventing pain, PIBs also desensitize (i.e., stop sensitization) the painful area and allow early resumption of activities.

### CASE STUDIES

**Patient 1: A 45-year-old Female Recreational Tennis Player.**    Sports injuries, motor vehicle accidents, and work injuries respond particularly well to N and I in the early stage after acute injury. The patient was a real estate agent and sustained **a tear in her right gastrocnemius muscle during a tennis game** on Friday morning at 10 AM.

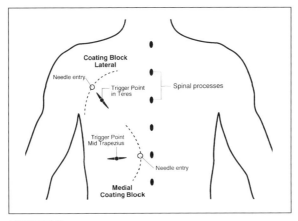

**FIGURE 3.**
The PIB technique called "coating" block anesthetizes the sensory input from the tender area to be injected. The coating block for the paraspinal and back muscles is performed medially from the injected trigger point. The PIB of teres minor muscles is administered over the lateral aspect of the trigger point, where the axillary nerve enters the muscle.

She called my office immediately and was given an emergency appointment as soon as she was able to come. After obtaining the necessary approval from the primary care physician, she arrived in the office at 2 PM, limping and able to put only minimal weight on the injured limb. Figure 5 shows the pressure threshold findings by algometer. The maximal tender spot (MTS) was 1.9 kg/cm². Other tender spots over the sprain across the gastrocnemius muscle also showed decreased pressure threshold, indicating high sensitivity relative to the opposite normal side, which showed a pressure pain threshold of 5.3 kg/cm². Ankle dorsiflexion with extended knee was decreased by 30° due to tightness of the injured gastrocnemius muscle. PIB was performed proximally to the

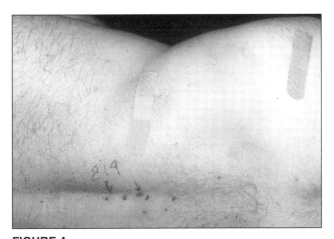

**FIGURE 4.**
Paraspinous preinjection block at lumbar level prevented pain from trigger point injection (N and I) of the quadratus lumborum muscle. In the same session injection of the trigger point in the gluteus medius was very painful.

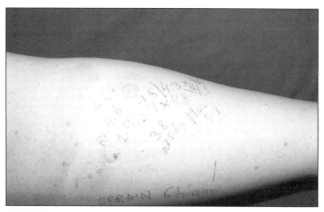

**FIGURE 5.**
Gastrocnemius tear with indication of pressure pain threshold for patient 1. The most tender spot over the sprained gastrocnemius muscle was 1.9 kg/cm² as compared with 5.3 kg over the opposite normal control side. After PIB, which was administered in a V shape proximally to the sprain, the pressure threshold increased to 3.7 kg. After needling and infiltration (N and I) of the most tender areas within the sprain, the pressure threshold further increased to 4.8 kg. Pain during PIB was minimal, and no pain was experienced during N and I. If performed without PIB, N and I is extremely painful in acute injuries.

sprain, reaching deeply into the muscle, with a 3½-inch, 25-gauge needle. Lidocaine 1% was infiltrated in a V shape (see Figure 2). During the PIB the patient felt no pain except when the needle penetrated the end of the taut band, which extended from the injury proximally and reached the insertion of the muscle. The second set of numbers in Fig. 5 indicates how, after PIB, the pressure threshold increased over the point of maximal tenderness from 1.9 to 3.7 kg. There was a similar increase in pressure threshold over the other measured tender spots. A few minutes after PIB, when pain sensitivity to finger pressure had decreased, N and I of the sprained areas was performed with 1% lidocaine. Such a procedure is extremely painful without PIB. Thanks to the PIB, the N and I was tolerated by the patient without pain. The pressure threshold increased further after N and I, as shown by the third set of numbers in Figure 5. The pressure threshold over the maximal tender spot increased to 4.8 kg, which almost corresponded to normal control levels. After N and I the patient was able to walk with minimal limp and only some pain, which was located in the taut band but proximally to the site of PIB. Spraying of the tight and tender muscle fibers with ethyl chloride was combined with reciprocal inhibition by activation of the antagonists (i.e., ankle dorsiflexors). The tightness and pain were relieved, enabling the patient to walk without limping and without discomfort.

Although functional recovery was complete after PIB and N and I, the patient was advised to use crutches to avoid weight-bearing on the injured limb. She was instructed to apply ice or to massage the area with ice for 10 minutes, to elevate the limb, and to perform active movements, particularly reciprocal inhibition (active ankle dorsiflexion) to maintain range of motion. The exercises also prevented edema formation and increased circulation, thus cleansing away algogenic and inflammatory substances that may accumulate in tissues injured by sprain or N and I and cause inflammation and edema. She returned on Monday (the fourth day after injury). She reported that on Saturday, the day after the injury, she attended two social events, at one of which she danced "a little bit." She had no pain after the PIB. She needed another session of N and

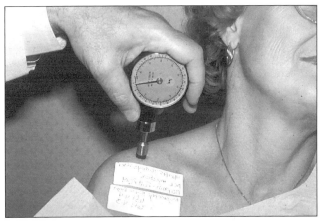

**FIGURE 6.**
Effect of needling and infiltration after preinjection block applied to the sprained ligaments of the acromial clavicular joint secondary to a ski injury.

I to patch up the damaged area that had not been attended to previously. She was receiving physical therapy, which consisted of hot packs for 20 minutes, followed by 15 minutes of high-frequency sinusoid surging current with deep penetration. The maximal volume of current as tolerated was selected to induce strong muscle contractions. The third component of physical therapy consisted of range of motion and relaxation exercises by reciprocal inhibition.

This case demonstrates two noteworthy points:

1. N and I in the acute stage immediately after injury achieved three major goals: (1) immediate and complete relief of pain; (2) restoration of function in terms of almost complete range of ankle dorsiflexion, which had been limited by the tight gastrocnemius muscle; and (3) prevention of inflammatory reaction and sensitization of nerve endings, both of which cause pain. The weight-bearing function of the extremity was restored, and the patient experienced no limitation in this respect.

2. Rapid and excellent recovery was achieved with minimal or no pain experienced by the patient during N and I because of the preinjection block. A similar case involved a 45-year-old male tennis player who had sustained an identical tear in the gastrocnemius muscle and was treated by N and I before the introduction of PIBs. The patient was examined about 6 months later and stated that after the N and I, which took place within 1 hour of injury, he experienced no pain. However, the N and I procedure itself, without PIB, was quite painful. Functional recovery is accelerated substantially by PIB. Other clinicians also have observed that PIB seems to prevent bleeding secondary to the N and I.

**Patient 2: A 26-year-old Manual Worker.** A 26-year-old manual worker sprained the quadratus lumborum muscle while lifting a heavy object and experienced acute low back pain. He called the office and was told to come in immediately. **Sprain of the quadratus lumborum** was diagnosed. The patient had severe pain at rest and was unable to move his trunk. N and I alleviated the pain instantaneously and restored complete mobility. He received one more injection and had follow-up physical therapy sessions daily.[7] On reevaluation in 2 weeks he reported no spontaneous pain or tenderness after N and I and returned to work 3 weeks after injury in good shape. This case illustrates the efficacy of N and I in the early stage of injury sustained at work. N and I accelerated recovery and made possible his return even to manual work shortly after the accident.

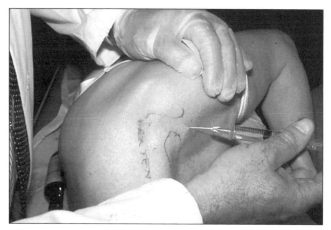

**FIGURE 7.**
Preinjection block technique for the acromial clavicular joint sprain (same patient as Figure 6).

**Patient 3: A 59-year-old Female Psychiatrist.**    A 59-year-old female psychiatrist presented with **acute acromioclavicular joint sprain** and dislocation of bones (Figs. 6 and 7). After PIB, N and I of the sprained ligaments was performed (Fig. 7). The patient reported immediate relief of pain. Follow-up 10 days after N and I showed normal pressure thresholds practically identical with the opposite control side. Follow-up 2 years after the accident showed complete healing, no tenderness whatsoever, and full function of the shoulder.

**Patient 4: A 66-year-old Woman.**    A 66-year-old woman developed **chest pain**, dizziness, and spells of weakness **after open heart surgery** for valve replacement. Cardiologic work-up failed to identify the cause of pain. About 9 months after surgery the patient still could not lead a normal life. Figure 8 shows how the patient pointed

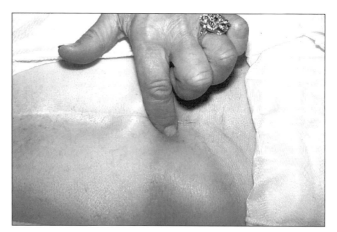

**FIGURE 8.**
Patient complaining of severe pain causing dizziness and inability to function after open heart surgery (valvular replacement). Several cardiologists were unable to establish the cause of pain. About 9 months after the operation tender spots were detected within the scar tissue, as indicated above by the patient.

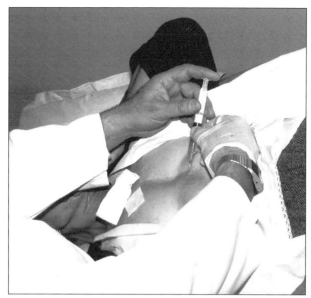

**FIGURE 9.**
Same patient as Figure 8. Needling and infiltration of the tender spots within the surgical scar brought gradual but substantial improvement.

with one finger to the point of maximal pain. N and I gradually relieved her complaints. PIB was administered as feasible. A total of 10 injections was given, one weekly. A different tender spot, which the patient identified as the site of pain within the operation scar, was needled and infiltrated at each session (Fig. 9). The patient stated that the injections "gave back her life". Her pain and other complaints improved so much that she was able to resume a normal lifestyle.

## MANAGEMENT OF MUSCLE SPASMS

The most important goals in management of muscle spasms are to identify and eliminate the irritative focus (trigger area) that caused the spasm. Ask the patient where the pain or injury started and where the pain originates. Usually the patient can point with one finger to an area or to a point that is sensitive to pressure. If pressure on the point reproduces the patient's complaints or aggravates the muscle spasm, as monitored by palpation, the point should be treated as the **irritative focus responsible for the spasm**. Muscle spasm and tightness can be documented objectively by a tissue compliance meter.[5] This mechanical, handheld instrument measures muscle tone objectively.

PIBs administered to the irritative focus (coating or paraspinous) are usually effective in relieving pain and spasm. After the spasm has been relieved, taut bands, tender spots, and trigger points can be easily palpated. They should be needled and infiltrated for complete and long-term relief of pain and to prevent recurrence. If the irritative focus that triggered the muscle spasm cannot be identified, diffuse infiltration of the spasmodic muscle brings prompt relief. This is again done best after PIB.

After N and I, PIB, or diffuse infiltration, a course of physical therapy is administered 3 times/week. Hot packs (20 minutes) are followed by electric stimulation (10 minutes of tetanizing current), which breaks up the spasm. Tetanizing current is followed by 10 minutes of sinusoid surging currents, which relax the muscle, squeeze out the edema, and increase blood flow. The patient is instructed to perform relaxation (limbering) exercises, particularly reciprocal inhibition of the treated muscle. The exercises are performed on the hour in the acute stage and every 2 hours later. The maintenance regimen consists of 3 exercise sessions per day.

Muscle relaxants may help to prevent recurrences of muscle spasms, but injections, as described above, are incomparably more effective in breaking up the vicious cycle of pain–spasm–pain. Only N and I can remove completely the irritative focus that caused the spasm. Only injections bring instantaneous relief, which usually is dramatic.

## PHYSICAL THERAPY FOR MUSCLE PAIN SYNDROMES

### General Relaxation Exercises—Patient Instructions

Relaxation by eye movement and deep breathing is part of every treatment of pain.

1. Lie or sit comfortably; head, trunk, and all limbs should be supported.
2. Look up to your eyebrows without moving your head. Breathe in as deeply as you can, and expand your chest. Hold your breath for 2 seconds.
3. Look down to your chin again without moving your head. Breathe out very slowly but completely between your teeth, producing a hissing sound. At the end of exhalation, pull in your belly to force all of the air from your lungs. Feel how the tension reflexly melts away in your muscles during exhalation. The longer you exhale, the more you relax. Repeat the above sequence 4–5 times for basic relaxation and also at the end of each session.

This basic exercise is followed by stretching or postisometric relaxation exercises specifically aimed at the treated trigger point or muscles. The patient should stretch only during exhalation when muscles relax.

### Spray and Stretch Technique[35,36]

One-directional parallel sweeps of Fluori-Methane are sprayed slowly (10 cm/sec) over the 45-cm area surrounding the trigger point and over the entire referred pain zone. Frosting should be avoided. After cooling, a moist electric heating pad is applied for 5–15 minutes to warm the muscle. The injected muscle is stretched slowly for about 30 seconds. Full active range-of-motion exercise is performed 5 times.

### Spray and Active Limbering[20-22]

1. Ask the patient to point with one finger to the spot of maximal pain.
2. Spray ethyl chloride over the area, concentrating on the maximal tender point.
3. The patient moves through full range of joint exercises, using the sprayed muscles, 3–5 times. This step can be combined with breathing and eye movement. Movement in the direction of stretching (for example, backward to limber the pectoralis muscles) is synchronized with exhalation and the look-down phase. Ask again whether any pain remains. If pain is still present, it shifts to another location. Spray the painful area, and follow with limbering movement to full active range of motion.
4. Repeat the above procedure until pain is relieved completely or no more progress can be achieved.

Active limbering exercises are characterized by slow full range-of-motion exercises with minimal effort. Therefore, elimination of gravity helps. With shoulder movements, gravity is eliminated by dragging the arm over the table. In hip-knee flexion and extension, the heel is dragged over the table.

### Relaxation by Activation of Antagonists

Relaxation by activation of antagonist muscles, also called the reciprocal inhibition technique, is most effective, in the author's experience, for relaxation of tight muscles, spasms, trigger points or tender spots, and taut bands.[10] Resistance to the antagonist is mild.

## Isometric Contraction–Reciprocal Inhibition Stretch[10]

Isometric contraction–reciprocal inhibition stretch is a combination of three effective relaxation techniques described earlier.[10]

## Physical Therapy for the Injured Muscle after Needling and Infiltration[7–10]

Patients should have follow-up physical therapy after N and I daily during the first week. The frequency is reduced later to 3 times per week. Therapy consists of hot packs for 20 minutes to relax the muscle and to increase circulation. Hot packs are followed by electrical stimulation with sinusoid surging current to induce strong, slow physiologic contractions of the injured muscle. The degree of contraction increases gradually and then slowly decreases. The current should be of the highest available frequency to achieve deep penetration, whereas the frequency of contractions should be as slow as possible to allow maximal time for relaxation. The duration of contractions is as long as the patient tolerates. After 15 minutes of such contractions the edema caused by the injury as well as by the needling usually disappears. The high degree of tenderness also improves, essentially reaching levels close to normal. The explanation of this positive result lies in removal of edema by contractions, which in turn allows the augmented circulation to remove the algogenic inflammatory substances that sensitize nerve endings.

The third component of physical therapy consists of relaxation exercises,[2,10,20,21,25] including reciprocal inhibition, or relaxation of muscle tightness, spasm, and tension by mild contraction of the antagonist. In the experience of the author and his coworkers, this approach seems to be the most effective in relieving spasm, tension, tightness, and taut bands of myofascial trigger points. Such taut bands are invariably formed by any injured muscle fibers and extend usually to the myotendinal junction as well as over the attachment of the tendons to the bone (enthesopathy). The other type of exercises consists of slow full range of motion, contracting and relaxing the injured muscle. Such dynamic exercises prevent sensitization from immobilization, maintain the restored range of motion, enhance local circulation, and prevent consequences of disuse. The specific exercises for each muscle group are repeated 5 or 6 times and performed on the hour in the acute stage. During the subacute period of recovery exercises are performed 4 or 5 times/day and later 3 times/day. Twice daily is the minimal amount of exercise needed to maintain function and to prevent the muscle from becoming sensitized and tight.

The relaxation exercises are performed on the day after the injury, using mild active contractions without resistance. Relaxation of the injured muscle by reciprocal inhibition (i.e., relaxation by activation of the antagonist muscle) is safe and highly effective. Passive stretching, on the other hand, should be avoided until the sprain heals (about 4 weeks). Passive stretching may cause reinjury, particularly if it is performed by the therapist and not by the patient. Range-of-motion exercises, particularly with relaxation by activation of the antagonist muscle, are also encouraged, but strengthening exercises are deferred until healing is complete. Until such time, low-resistance, high-repetition exercises are used to develop endurance.

## REFERENCES

1. Bonica JJ: The Management of Pain. Philadelphia, Lea & Febiger, 1990.
2. Deyo RA: A controlled trial of transcutaneous electrical nerve stimulation (TENS) and exercise for chronic low back pain. N Engl J Med 322:1627–1634, 1990.
3. Fields HL: Pain. New York, McGraw-Hill, 1987.
4. Fischer AA: Pressure algometry (dolorimetry) in the differential diagnosis of muscle pain. In Rachlin ES (ed): Myofascial Pain and Fibromyalgia: Trigger Point Management. St. Louis, Mosby, 1994, pp 121–141.

5. Fischer AA: Clinical use of tissue compliance meter for documentation of soft tissue pathology. Clin J Pain 3:23–30, 1987.

6. Fischer AA: New developments in diagnosis of myofascial pain and fibromyalgia. Phys Med Rehabil Clin North Am 8:1–21, 1997.

7. Fischer AA: New approaches in treatment of myofascial pain. Phys Med Rehabil Clin North Am 8:153–169, 1997.

8. Fischer AA: Injection techniques in the management of local pain. J Back Musculoskel Rehabil 7:107–117, 1996.

9. Fischer AA: Trigger point injection. In Lennard TA (ed): Physiatric Procedures in Clinical Practice. Philadelphia, Hanley & Belfus, 1995, pp 28–35.

10. Fischer AA: Local injections in pain management: Trigger point needling with infiltration and somatic blocks. Phys Med Rehabil Clin North Am 6:851–870, 1995.

11. Fishbain DA, Goldberg M, Meagher BR, et al: Male and female chronic pain patients categorized by DSM-III psychiatric diagnostic criteria. Pain 26:181–197, 1986.

12. Fricton JR, Kroening R, Haley D, Siegert R: Myofascial pain syndrome of the head and neck: A review of clinical characteristics of 164 patients. Oral Surg 60:615–623, 1985.

13. Frost FA, Jessen B, Siggaard-Andersen J: A controlled, double-blind comparison of mepivacaine injection versus saline injection for myofascial pain. Lancet i:499–500, 1980.

14. Garvey TA, Marks MR, Wiesel SW: A prospective, randomized, double-blind evaluation of trigger-point injection therapy for low-back pain. Spine 14:962–964, 1989.

15. Gerwin RD: Neurobiology of the myofascial trigger point. In Massi AT (ed): Fibromyalgia and Myofascial Pain Syndromes. Bailliere's Clinical Rheumatology. London, Bailliere-Tindall, 1994, pp 747–762.

16. Hackett GS: Ligament and tendon relaxation treated by prolotherapy, 3rd ed. Springfield, IL, Charles C Thomas, 1958, pp 27–36, 70.

17. Hong C-Z: Lidocaine injection versus dry needling to myofascial trigger point. Am J Phys Med Rehabil 73:256–263, 1994.

18. Jaeger B: Are "cervicogenic" headaches due to myofascial pain and cervical spine dysfunction? Cephalalgia 3(9):157–164, 1989.

19. Jaeger B, Skootsky SA: Double-blind, controlled study of different myofascial trigger point injection techniques. Pain 4(suppl):S292, 1987.

20. Kraus H: Clinical Treatment of Back and Neck Pain. New York, McGraw-Hill, 1970.

21. Kraus H: Diagnosis and Treatment of Muscle Pain. Chicago, Quintessence, 1988.

22. Kraus H, Fischer AA: Diagnosis and treatment of myofascial pain. Mt Sinai J Med 58:235–239, 1991.

23. Mense S: Nociception from skeletal muscle in relation to clinical muscle pain. Pain 54:241–289, 1993.

24. Njoo KH: The occurrence and inter-rater reliability of myofascial trigger points in the quadratus lumborum and gluteus medius: A prospective study in non-specific low back pain patients and controls in general practice. Pain 58:317–323, 1994.

25. Rachlin ES: Trigger points. In Rachlin ES (ed): Myofascial Pain and Fibromyalgia. St. Louis, Mosby, 1994.

26. Rosen NB: Myofascial pain: The great mimicker and potentiator of other diseases in the performing artist. Md Med J 42(3):261–266, 1993.

27. Simons DG: Myofascial pain syndromes due to trigger points. In Goodgold J (ed): Rehabilitation Medicine. St. Louis, Mosby, 1988, pp 686–723.

28. Simons DG: Referred phenomena of myofascial trigger points. In Vecchiet L, Albe-Fessard D, Lindblom U, Giamberardino MA (eds): New Trends in Referred Pain and Hyperalgesia. Amsterdam, Elsevier, 1993, pp 341–357.

29. Simons DG, Fischer AA: Myofascial pain. In Fields HL (ed): Core Curriculum for Professional Education in Pain, 2nd ed. Seattle, IASP Press, 1995, pp 79–81.

30. Simons DG: Clinical and etiological update of myofascial pain from trigger point. J Musculoskel Pain 4:93–121, 1996.

31. Simons DG, Travell JG: Myofascial origins of low back pain. Parts 1, 2, and 3. Postgrad Med 73:66–108, 1983.

32. Sola AE, Rodenberger ML, Gettys BB: Incidence of hypersensitive areas in posterior shoulder muscles. Am J Phys Med 34:585–590, 1955.

33. Sola AE, Bonica JJ: Myofascial pain syndromes. In Bonica JJ, Loeser JD, Chapman CR, Fordyce WE (eds): The Management of Pain, 2nd ed, vol 1. Philadelphia, Lea & Febiger, 1990, pp 352–367.

34. Skootsky SA, Jaeger B, Oye RK: Prevalence of myofascial pain in general internal medicine practice. West J Med 151:157–160, 1989.

35. Travell JG Simons DG: Myofascial Pain and Dysfunction: The Trigger Point Manual, vol I. Baltimore, Williams & Wilkins, 1983.

36. Travell JG, Simons DG: Myofascial Pain and Dysfunction: The Trigger Point Manual. The Lower Extremities, vol II. Baltimore, Williams & Wilkins, 1992.

37. Wolfe F, et al: The American College of Rheumatology 1990 criteria for the classification of fibromyalgia. Report of the Multicenter Criteria Committee. Arthritis Rheum 133, 1990.

# 7

# Fibromyalgia

## DENNIS M. LOX, MD

Muscular pain has been present for as long as medicine has been an art and science. Diverse terms, such as lumbago and rheumatism, have long been used. In 1904, Gowers[4] adopted the term *fibrositis* because he believed that widespread and diffuse pain was due to pathologic process in the fibrous tissue. Stockton[13] noted "patchy, inflammatory changes in white fibrous tissue." Yunnis[19] adopted the term *fibromyalgia*, which replaced fibrositis in the late 1980s after numerous studies failed to reveal inflammatory changes in the muscle, which were the basis for the term *fibrositis*.[13,18]

Associated symptoms are varied and not uniformly accepted. Some, such as sleep disturbances, irritable bowel, stiffness, fatigue, and symptom changes with the weather, also may be seen in other chronic pain syndromes or associated with stress. Sleep disturbances, including stage IV rapid-eye-movement sleep, are found frequently in the general population and are not endemic to fibromyalgia, and the classic alpha intrusions were not found consistently in patients with fibromyalgia.[6]

In 1990, a 24-member committee of the American College of Rheumatology, chaired by Frederick Wolfe, M.D., published Criteria for the Classification of Fibromyalgia[16] (Table 1). The intention was to create easy-to-follow guidelines for research criteria and to develop useful dialogue among numerous practitioners. An easy, usable framework was necessary for researchers to communicate and gather data. Two elements resulted. First, widespread pain was a feature, and second, 11 or more tender points at 18 predetermined sites were necessary to fulfill the research criteria (Fig. 1). There was no criterion for objective findings—only subjective responses of widespread pain and 11 tender points. A widespread explosion in the diagnostic frequency of fibromyalgia quickly resulted, and the research criteria shifted to a highly subjective, two-pronged approach to diagnosis. Of interest, what had previously been an obscure diagnosis in motor vehicle collisions and industrial injuries was now becoming suddenly prevalent. Unfortunately, many patients with chronic pain were labeled with the diagnosis of fibromyalgia because its diagnosis implied diffuse widespread pain.

No current objective test, serum blood studies, muscle biopsy, or demonstrable abnormality can account for the symptoms. Researchers have attempted to draw conclusions from indirect data that are nonspecific.[1,12] Such findings may be noted in multiple processes such as depression, loss of sleep, or chronic stress. The relationship with psychologic and personality factors has been questioned,[2,8,15] and, as in many chronic pain syndromes, authors have pointed to fibromyalgia as a product of failure to handle

**TABLE 1.**
The American College of Rheumatology 1990 Criteria for the Classification of Fibromyalgia

1. History of widespread pain, which includes the upper and lower extremities and pain above and below the waist.
2. Tender points in 11 of 18 predetermined sites. A tender point is considered present if, to manual palpation, the patient reports that the palpation was painful.

First Region—Head and Neck
1. Suboccipital muscles, insertions left and right.
2. Cervical paraspinalis muscles between the inner transverse process spaces at C5 through 7.
3. Trapezius muscles, left and right, at the upper midpoint.
4. Supraspinatus muscles, left and right, at the origins at the medial border above the scapula.

Second Region—Trunk
4. At the second rib, left and right, at the second costochrondral junctions lateral to the upper surfaces.

Third Region—Upper Extremity
6. The lateral epicondyles, left and right, 2 cm distal to the epicondyle.

Fourth Region—Lower Extremity
7. Gluteal musculatures, left and right, in the upper outer quadrants.
8. Greater trochanter, left and right, just posterior to the trochanteric prominence.
9. Left and right knee, proximal to the joint line at the medial fat pad.

The 9 anatomic regions with bilateral sites equate to 18 tender points, and the diagnosis requires 11 tender points to palpation at 18 of the predetermined sites.

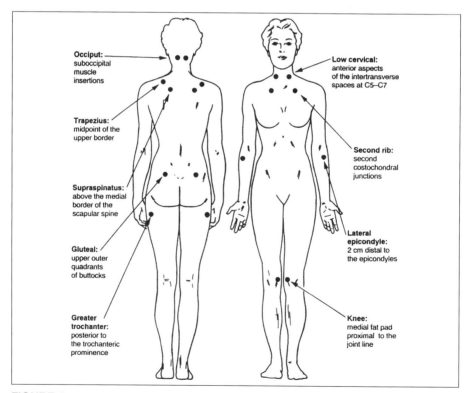

**FIGURE 1.**
Location of specific tender points in fibromyalgia. (From Freundlich B, Leventhal L: The fibromyalgia syndrome. In Schumacher HR Jr, Klippel JH, Koopman WJ (eds): Primer on the Rheumatic Diseases, 10th ed. Atlanta, Arthritis Foundation, 1993, pp 247–249, with permission.)

stress effectively and the medical system's inability to deal with such patients.[7,9] Fibromyalgia is reported 5–10 times more frequently in women than in men.[1]

Recently, fibromyalgia has been accepted by some authorities as a disabling condition. However, the literature fails to support this position. Indeed, in 2-year followup studies of patients diagnosed with fibromyalgia, Granges[5] found that some no longer had symptoms or met the criteria for fibromyalgia and that in some patients the symptoms waxed and waned. Like many conditions, fibromyalgia may have a natural course of exacerbations influenced by multifactorial associations, including stress.[7,10] Unfortunately, patients often receive inappropriate education and misinformation in the form of pamphlets or support groups, which reflect the condition as disabling and progressive, although research does not support this conclusion. One of the author's patients recalled being told that she might as well go on Social Security and probably would end up in a wheelchair. This misinformation is a disservice to the patient. It is the physician's responsibility to provide accurate and informative information.

The American College of Rheumatology encourages patients to work, does not promote disability, and indeed encourages active exercises.[17] Exercise, in essence, is the only treatment. Frequently, patients complain that exercise causes too much pain, which perpetuates a vicious cycle of immobility and promotes loss of functional ability and decreased aerobic capacity. At this point, the physician must act not only as a medical advisor but also as supportive coach and counselor to encourage the patient to continue. The old adage—no pain, no gain—is extremely appropriate in this case. As in any condition, however, a thorough examination is necessary to rule out occult pathology that may account for symptoms. If sleep disturbances are present, they should be tested. Various authors have looked at numerous medications; low-dose tricyclic antidepressants may have a value. Antiinflammatories and steroids have no effect on the outcome, unlike myofascial pain syndrome, which has a discrete palpable taut band. The hallmark of fibromyalgia is a tender point, and no controlled studies suggest that infiltration and injection of tender points promotes lasting relief.

Hidding[9] found a great disparity between self-report questionnaires about functional ability in patients with fibromyalgia and what was observed in functional levels. A team approach with a compassionate, educated physician and a rehabilitation team with a behavioral and functional approach appears to be the best measure to prevent progressive deconditioning and disability.

In 1994, the American College of Rheumatology committee discussed the consequences of the 1990 consensus report. Their recommendations, recently published by Wolfe,[17] were to eliminate the term posttraumatic fibromyalgia or reactive fibromyalgia, because no specific research suggests that trauma induces fibromyalgia. The concept of trauma-induced fibromyalgia had been advocated by proponents who reviewed case studies and concluded that fibromyalgia occurred after trauma; therefore, it was post-traumatic in origin.[11,14] The American College of Rheumatology also calls for more research to help address and discern the problems associated with fibromyalgia.

In summary, there is no known cause, diagnostic test, or state-of-the-art treatment, except to encourage mobility, prevent deconditioning, restore normal sleep, encourage the patient to remain at a functionally active level, and not to promote disability. The physician has the responsibility of providing the patient with accurate information.

## REFERENCES

1. Bennet RM, Clark SR, Campbell SM, Burckhardt CS: Low levels of somatomedin C in patients with the fibromyalgia syndrome—A possible link between sleep and muscle pain. Arthritis Rheum 35:1113–1116, 1992.
2. Buckelew SP: Fibromyalgia: A rehabilitation approach—A review. Am J Phys Med Rehabil 68:37–41, 1989.

3. Drewes AM, Andreasen A: Pathology of skeletal muscle and fibromyalgia: A histo/immuno/chemical and ultrastructural study. Br J Rheumatol 32:479–483, 1993.

4. Gowers W: Lumbago—Its lessons and analogs. BMJ 1:117, 1904.

5. Granges G, et al: Fibromyalgia syndrome: Assessment of the severity of the condition 2 years after diagnosis. J Rheum 21:283, 1994.

6. Farney RJ, Walker JM: Office management of common sleep/wake disorders. Med Clin North Am 79(2):391–414, 1995.

7. Hadler NM: Occupational Musculoskeletal Disorders. New York, Raven Press, 1993.

8. Hartfo: Fibromyalgia—A common non-entity? Drugs 35:320–337, 1988.

9. Hidding A, et al: Comparison between self-report measures and clinical observations of functional disability in ankylosing spondylitis, rheumatoid arthritis and fibromyalgia. J Rheum 21:818, 1994.

10. Lorenzen J: Fibromyalgia: A clinical challenge. J Intern Med 235:191–203, 1994.

11. Romano TJ: Clinical experiences with post-traumatic fibromyalgia syndrome. W Va Med J 86:198–202, 1990.

12. Russell IJ, et al: Elevated cerebrospinal fluid levels of substance P in patients with the fibromyalgia syndrome. Arthritis Rheum 37:593–601, 1994.

13. Stockman R: The causes, pathology and treatment of chronic rheumatism. Edin Med J 15:107–116, 223–235, 1904.

14. Waylonis GW, Perkins RH: Post-traumatic fibromyalgia: A long-term follow-up. Am J Med Rehabil 73:403–412, 1994.

15. Wolfe F, Cathey MA, Kleninheksel SM: Psychological status in primary fibrositis and fibrositis associated with rheumatoid arthritis. J Rheumatol 11:500–506, 1984.

16. Wolfe F, et al: The American College of Rheumatology 1990 Criteria for the Classification of Fibromyalgia. Arthritis Rheum 33:160, 1996.

17. Wolfe F: The fibromyalgia syndrome: A consensus report on fibromyalgia and disability. J Rheumatol 23:534–537, 1996.

18. Yunnus M, et al: Primary fibromyalgia (fibrositis): Clinical studies of fifty patients with matched normal controls. Semin Arthritis Rheum 11:151–171, 1981.

19. Yunnus MB, Kalyan-Raman UP, Masi AT: Electron-microscope studies of muscle biopsy in primary fibromyalgia syndrome: A controlled and blinded study. J Rheum 16:97–101, 1989.

# 8

# Soft Tissue Injuries of the Lower Limbs

FRANCIS P. LAGATTUTA, MD
TERRY L. NICOLA, MD, MS
LAWRENCE W. FRANK, MD

## HIP

The hip as a joint of the lower extremity refers specifically to the spheroid femoral acetabular joint or femoral articulation with the fused coxal bone of the pelvis. This articulation is highly stable; subluxation and dislocation are rare, in part because of the acetabular lip and labrum around the femoral head in the acetabular fossa.[47] The severe loss of function from hip fractures and avascular necrosis is well known; however, pain and loss of function from soft tissue injuries in relation to the hip are also significant. Sources of local hip pain include the fibrous capsule, ligaments, synovial lining, periosteum, and muscles.[14,92,101] Soft tissue injuries of the hip can be divided into four basic categories: (1) injury to the hip capsule, (2) direct trauma, (3) musculotendinous strains, and (4) nerve entrapments. Hernias and pain referred from thoracolumbar and pelvic joints also may be implicated.

### Injury to the Hip Capsule

Sprains to the hip capsule from sudden and accidental extremes of extension and rotation can be diagnosed by isolated testing of the hip in flexed position, under stress in internal or external rotation, or in full extension in the prone position.[14,34,89] The Thomas test in the supine position stresses the iliopsoas muscle and possibly the anterior capsule of the hip. The iliofemoral or Y ligament of Bigalow is a key restraint of hip extension, whereas the ischiofemoral and pubicofemoral ligaments provide rotatory restraints.[47]

A review of joint innervation also provides insight into pain patterns referred from the hip.[14,28,47,83,92,101] The femoral nerve innervates the iliofemoral ligament and may explain pain referred to the knee from injury to this ligament. The accessory obturator nerve also provides innervation to the ligament. The capsule is innervated on the medial side from the obturator nerve, on the superolateral side by the superior gluteal nerve, and on the posterior side by the sciatic nerve. Sensory patterns from these nerves and guarding of their respectively innervated muscles may be correlated with referred pain or cramping. Shared innervation of the hip capsule with other S1- and S2-innervated muscles may explain weakness of the external rotation muscles; guarding of the gemellus and quadratus femoris muscles may be associated with injuries to the capsule. Stress applied by the examiner to the hip joint in the supine or side-lying position and passive joint stress in the extremes of the respective range of motion help to differentiate capsule injury from musculotendinous injuries in difficult cases with significant contractures. Fluoroscopic injection of the hip joint helps to differentiate hip capsule and ligament injuries from musculotendinous injuries in difficult cases.[92]

Treatment for hip capsule sprains generally involves crutch assistance, partial or toe-touch weight-bearing, and avoidance of flexion contracture by frequent supine stretches with one leg suspended over the edge of a bed and the other leg in a hip-and-knee tuck position. Sleeping prone also may be advised. All stretches are actively assisted by the patient to protect against excessive potential stress to the hip in examiner-applied passive stretches. In approximately 4 weeks muscle contraction exercises are followed by resistance exercises, with use of standard free weights at approximately 8 weeks. Axial-directed traction is another safe stretch applied to capsule and ligaments.[65] Recovery varies from 6–12 weeks. In certain refractory cases, intraarticular injection of combined corticosteroid and local anesthetic solution may be tried. Successful treatment assumes that stress fractures, avascular necrosis, and congenital hip or epiphyseal subluxation have been ruled out.

### Direct Trauma

Direct trauma to the surrounding pelvis and thigh tends to involve bony prominences with secondary bursal inflammation, muscular hemorrhage, or periosteal hematoma. Soft tissue contusions are among the most common pelvis and hip injuries in athletes.[103] Muscle hemorrhage results in significant loss of function. If bleeding is prolonged, pain, tenderness, and guarding may progress on the day after injury. Areas most susceptible to bursa, muscle, or periosteal contusions include the greater trochanter, ischial tuberosity, and pubic rami.

Direct contusion of the iliac crest with periosteal hematoma is called a hip pointer. The initial goal of treatment is to control the local bleeding with ice, compression, and padding or brace. Radiographs are recommended to rule out fracture. Heat, massage, and vigorous activity should be avoided for 48 hours. Attempts at aspiration of the area and nonsteroidal antiinflammatory drugs (NSAIDs) should be avoided initially to minimize bleeding.

Contusion of the sciatic nerve with blows to the buttock area may be a surgical emergency because of gluteal compartment syndrome, which is heralded by progressive referred symptoms over hours rather than a more immediate onset. Immediate and transient referred pain are unlikely signs of severe injury.

Myositis ossificans is a difficult posthemorrhage muscular complication.[34] Pain and tenderness with decreased range of motion and a local palpable mass are the first indications of local heterotopic calcification, usually near a bony surface. Radiographs do not show calcification for weeks. Range of motion should be actively assisted by the patient, without passive force through painful barriers, to avoid inciting more bleeding. Crutches are often necessary because hip splinting is difficult. Passive stretching in general should be avoided for 4–6 months. Radiographic evidence that heterotopic calcification has resolved is not necessary for final determination of clinical recovery. Surgical treatment is not necessary unless problems with pain and range of motion persist at 9–12 months.

### Musculotendinous Strains

Musculotendinous strains of the hip occur in conjunction with bursal inflammation in the areas of the ischial tuberosity, iliopectineal bursa and prominence, and greater trochanter.[34] Inflammation is related typically to cumulative friction involving the tendon over the bursa. Chronic bursitis may be accompanied by an audible snap.

Ischial bursitis occurs in conjunction with the hamstring aponeurosis and possibly in conjunction with injury to this muscle group.[78] Pain is persistent throughout the day. Treatment consists of pressure relief, aspiration of the bursa, and cryotherapy. Massage and actively assisted range of motion exercises involving the hamstring may be added to the regimen, along with corticosteroid injection for refractory cases.

Iliopectineal bursitis occurs in conjunction with strains and overuse of the iliopsoas tendon.[23,44] Snapping of the iliopsoas tendon may occur at the pectineal eminence and is quite audible with extension of the hip joint. The pain may be severe over the anterior aspect of the hip and disrupt normal gait. Patients may assume resting postures of flexion and external rotation for relief. Partial rupture of the iliopsoas tendon at its insertion is also possible. Treatment should limit the ranges of motion and exercises that reproduce painful snapping of the iliopsoas; a spica splint may be used during ambulation. Contract-and-relax exercises and eventual stretching and strengthening of the iliopsoas mechanism are recommended.

Trochanteric bursitis is familiar to most medical practitioners in association with overuse and trauma to the iliotibial tract (ITT). Pain localized to the greater trochanter increases with external rotation and adduction of the hip.[14,34] Contributing factors include a broad female pelvis, leg length discrepancy, and excessive foot pronation. The combined attachments of the gluteus maximus and tensor fascia lata require a thorough flexibility program for the ITT, with the hip in both extension and flexion positions to apply adduction stretch to both muscle groups. Strengthening of the gluteus medius and minimus abductors is important to control pelvic tilt. Occasionally corticosteroid injection into the bursa is necessary.

The term *snapping hip* requires separate mention. Like iliopectineal bursitis, snapping hip syndrome may occur within the ITT over the greater trochanter.[34] The long head of the biceps femoris off the hamstring group may cause a snapping sound over the ischial bursa and tuberosity. Iliofemoral ligaments over the femoral head, even in the absence of a bursa, may cause a snapping sound. On rare occasions, the snapping sound comes from synovial chondromatosis, osteochondral exostoses, or subluxation of the hip.

The symphysis pubis may receive asymmetrical shear forces from overuse of the gracilis and adductor muscle groups. Myofascial restrictions should be treated with a flexibility program in conjunction with relative rest, ice, and elastic trousers compression. Response to treatment is expected in 2–3 months.

The sacroiliac joint is the local source of pain in the posterior base of the spine between the two iliac extensions, although nonspecific aching pain may involve the lower extremities. Although the joint is well supported by a thick ligament complex and wedge-shaped articulation between the two iliac bones, sprains may result from sudden torsion and direct blows or falls on the buttock. On physical examination local tenderness may be present, with positive provocation tests and the March sign. Radiologic evaluation should be done if loss of mobility is noted. Although sacral fractures are rare, coccyx fractures are not, and coccydynia is a painful disorder. Initial treatment consists of bracing to maintain the lumbar lordosis, relative rest from near-maximal loads to the spine, NSAIDs, and cold packs for 1–2 weeks, followed by ultrasound and isometric hip exercises. A program for full neutral spine posture control, known as dynamic lumbar stabilization, should be in place within 4 weeks, along with back-bridging, lunges, control of the lower abdominal oblique muscles, and aerobic activity. Occasionally corticosteroid injection is necessary. Resolution of pain or at least return to full function should occur in less than 4 months.

Treatment of specific strains to supporting muscles of the hip and pelvis can be considered in five phases:

1. For the first 48–72 hours, rest, ice, compression, and elevation (RICE) are used to control bleeding and swelling. The ice pack should be applied for 20 minutes, then

removed for 1 hour. Crutch-protected ambulation, spica elastic wrap or compression trousers, and abdominal corset also may be used. NSAIDs are not recommended, at least in the initial healing phase.

2. Active and actively assisted range of motion exercises may begin within limits of pain to prevent contractures; nonresisted muscle contractions without external weight limit atrophy. Heat, ultrasound, and electrical modalities may begin, along with use of NSAIDs, after 72 hours.

3. When range of motion is pain-free and no muscle-guarding is noted, isometric resistance exercises may begin, along with bicycling. Passive stretching is part of this phase.

4. Resistance strengthening begins. Cryotherapy is still part of the treatment plan.

5. After at least 70% return of strength, hopefully within 8–10 weeks, specific co-ordination and proprioception drills are the final assignments before return to full activities of daily living, sports, and heavy labor. These drills are typically simulations of the patient's desired skills or lifting activity.

Specific strain to the external oblique muscle is common in sports, such as hockey and football, that involve tackle or checking moves. The site of tear is off the aponeurosis and its insertion into the anterior and inner iliac crest. The patient may be unable to regain full upright posture, with local tenderness at the iliac crest. A muscle defect is palpable, and gluteal injury must be ruled out. The side-lying abduction test against manual resistance of the examiner is one method.

The mechanism of strain to the iliopsoas muscle may involve collision with a ground-fixed or hip-extended lower extremity, as with a blocked kick or soccer play. Occasionally injury may occur from overuse, as in long-distance running and overtraining (Fig. 1). A stabbing pain in the groin may increase with resisted hip flexion. Recovery may require up to 4 months.

Adductor muscles that cross two joints, such as the gracilis, are especially susceptible to injury. A typical mechanism for adductor strains is forced external rotation or abduction of the hip. Pain is immediate and localized in the area of the symphysis pubis or pubic ramus. An inguinal hernia must be ruled out. This possibility should be considered even in the absence of a canal protrusion in patients with significant inguinal ligament tenderness and symptoms induced by the Valsalva maneuver. A herniagram may be necessary in difficult cases. For most adductor strains resistance exercises may begin in 3–6 weeks, with gradual return to high-level physical activity over the next 3–6 weeks. Coordination drills may be used for lifting, climbing stairs, pivot maneuvers, and running start–stop trials, if necessary.

### Nerve Entrapments

Nerve entrapment syndromes occur in close relation to myofascial syndromes and muscle strains when the margin for nerve passage is narrow or the nerve is subject to blunt trauma.[34,83]

Iliacus muscle syndrome is a surgical complication with femoral nerve entrapment within the pelvic basin. Other causes include retroperitoneal hemorrhage, hernias, and iliopsoas hemorrhage. The entrapment is associated with loss of knee extension and possibly of hip flexion if the iliopsoas is involved. Loss of the patellar tendon reflex and sensory loss in the distribution of the femoral nerve in the thigh and possibly of the saphenous nerve in the medial calf may be present. Treatment of the underlying cause should be accompanied by crutch-assisted walking (when necessary), actively assisted range of motion of the hip flexors and knee extensors, and gluteal sets with exercises for maintenance of neutral spine.

Obturator tunnel syndrome involves trauma to the obturator nerve along its course across the sacroiliac joint, psoas major muscle, and obturator foramen. The

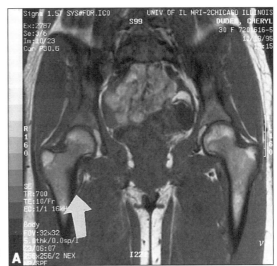

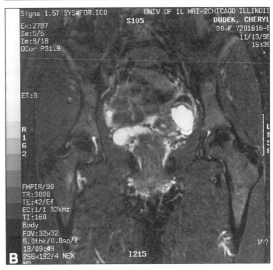

**FIGURE 1.**
T1-weighted *(A)* and T2-weighted *(B)* MRI scans of a 31-year-old female runner with right anterior hip and groin pain. Note the insertion of the distal iliopsoas tendon into the lesser trochanter of the femur *(arrows).* Decreased T1 and increased T2 signals verify a strain of the tendon at its insertion.

many possible causes include genitourologic procedures, hip arthroplasty, herniorrhaphic surgery, pelvic fractures, obstetric procedures, tumors, and osteitis pubis. Pain from the symphysis may be referred to the medial knee.[14,28] Adductor paresis and circumducted gait pattern should raise suspicion of an obturator neuropathy. Adductor paresis may not be obvious because of dual innervation by the femoral nerve for the adductor longus and the sciatic nerve for the adductor magnus. Avoidance of single-leg stance with crutches for the symptomatic side prevents symphysis pubis shear. A supportive inguinal or girdle-like garment may be helpful.

Piriformis syndrome may be diagnosed if entrapment of the sciatic nerve is suspected. The entrapment may involve the entire sciatic nerve (whole) or only the peroneal division crossing through the piriformis muscle (partial). This syndrome has been attributed to direct buttock trauma, such as a fall. Other causes include piriformis muscle-guarding due to another disorder of the sacroiliac joint, muscle strain or inflammation, or inflammation of the synovial bursa between the sacrum and piriformis muscle. This syndrome should not be confused with lumbosacral radiculopathies. The more specific features of piriformis syndrome include decreased pain with external rotation of the hip, increased pain with internal rotation of the hip and extended knee, local tenderness, and sometimes a palpable piriformis mass. Weakness in the peroneal division for the ankle-supporting muscles may require an ankle-foot orthosis. Local cold modalities to the buttock region, gluteal squeezes with hips externally rotated, and actively assisted hip rotation exercises that avoid extremes of internal rotation may be successful. Local corticosteroid injection may be helpful, although care must be taken to avoid injection directly into the nerve itself and the possible complication of nerve compartment pressure necrosis.[92] The patient may be placed in the contralateral decubitus position. A landmark connecting line is drawn between the greater femoral trochanter and posterior superior iliac spine. Needle entry is 3 cm below the midpoint of the line. If conservative measures are not effective, surgical release may be necessary.

Meralgia paresthetica, or inguinal entrapment of the lateral femoral cutaneous nerve, is more an annoyance than a truly disabling problem. The causes of entrapment include retroperitoneal hematoma, tumors, tight clothing, or sudden hip hyperextension injury. Exercises involving active hip flexion followed by extension, local cold therapy, and strengthening of the lower abdominal muscles, along with treatment of the underlying causes, usually result in cure.[34]

Ilioinguinal syndrome results from local injury of the ilioinguinal nerve. The nerve begins its pathway through the transversus abdominis and external oblique muscles, accompanying the spermatic cord (in men) or the round ligament (in women), and innervates the labia majora or scrotum. Causes other than local muscle damage include entrapment with the spermatic cord in an inguinal hernia or renal or retroperitoneal pathology. Pain may be evoked with pressure immediately distal and medial to the anterior superior iliac spine, with referral to the inguinal ligament. The patient may describe difficulty with lumbopelvic extension maneuvers. Arising from a supine position is difficult. A crooked gait is noted because of loss of the pelvic gait component. Crutch-assisted walking may be necessary for antalgic gait, along with treatment of the hernia or other cause. An abdominal and hip flexor isometric program may be considered as part of a general lumbar dynamic stabilization program. If corticosteroid injection is used, landmark identification of the nerve is 1 inch medial to the anterior superior iliac spine and inferior to the inguinal ligament. The needle is inserted to a depth of 1 inch,[92] and injection of 5–10 cc of local anesthetic with the corticosteroid is recommended for adequate perfusion and identification of the nerve. Much less is needed when an electroinjection needle is used.

With all injuries to the hip and pelvis, the goal is symmetrical motor control of the hip and back during periods of sedentary activity and the extremes of lifting and rotation maneuvers at work or sports and fitness events.

## KNEE

The knee is one of the most commonly injured joints in the body. Numerous pain-sensitive structures may produce clinical symptoms about the knee. This section discusses basic anatomy and the differential diagnosis of midarticular, anterior, posterior, medial, and lateral pain. Narrowing the focus of the patient's symptoms in a regional fashion leads to specific evaluation and accurate diagnosis.

### Anatomy

#### Bones
Knowledge of the anatomy of the knee is crucial to diagnosis and accurate treatment. The bony articulations are the patellofemoral joint and the tibiofemoral joint. The

proximal fibula and tibiofibular joint are not part of the knee joint per se but may be injured with the knee.

The femur is the longest bone in the body. The femoral condyles articulate with the tibia, and hyaline cartilage covers the articular surfaces. The articular surface of the medial condyle is longer than the lateral condyle, causing axial rotation around the knee during flexion and extension.[72] The intercondylar fossa contains attachments of the anterior and posterior cruciate ligaments. The femoral surface of articulation with the patella is the trochlear groove, which is bordered by anterior prominences of the medial and lateral femoral condyles. The lateral femoral condyle extends more anteriorly than the medial condyle, protecting against lateral patellar subluxation.

The proximal tibia is a flat bony surface consisting of the medial and lateral condyles and the intercondylar eminence. The tibial condyles articulate with their respective femoral condyles through the intervening menisci. The anterior intercondylar area is the site of tibial attachment of the anterior cruciate ligament. The tibial tuberosity is the distal attachment of the quadriceps mechanism and patellar tendon. The pes anserinus area is just medial to the insertion of the patellar tendon. The tendons of the sartorius and gracilis muscles and the semitendinous tendons insert at this point. The lateral tibial or Gerdy's tubercle is the site of attachment of the iliotibial band (ITB), which originates from the tensor fascia lata, gluteus maximus, and gluteus medius muscles at the pelvis.

The knee articulation is not a strictly hinged joint. The bony anatomy and cruciate ligaments determine multiple axes of rotation.[70] In flexion and extension, a rolling-gliding motion allows constant contact of the femoral and tibial condyles despite their asymmetrical shape.[54] As a result, physiologic compression and shear forces are applied to the menisci with knee motion. The anterior cruciate ligament and medial collateral ligament passively control axial rotation about the knee. The popliteus and hamstring groups provide dynamic rotational control.

### Muscles

The hamstring muscle group exerts muscular control of flexion and consists of the biceps femoris laterally and the semimembranosus and semitendinosus medially. Because of their insertion on the proximal tibia, the hamstrings also pull the tibia posteriorly on the femur, a property that is emphasized in anterior cruciate ligament rehabilitation.[94] The gastrocnemius flexes the knee when the foot is planted on the ground. The plantaris, gracilis, and sartorius muscles also may play minimal roles.

The quadriceps muscles control knee extension via their common tendinous insertion into the tibial tuberosity. The presence of the patella in the common extensor tendon enhances the mechanical lever arm of the quadriceps[39] and increases knee power during terminal extension. The quadriceps group consists of the vastus lateralis, intermedius, medialis, and rectus femoris muscles. The rectus femoris is a two-joint muscle that crosses the hip joint anteriorly; contracture of the rectus femoris may alter the biomechanics of both hip and knee. The vastus medialis obliquus (VMO) controls patellar tracking by pulling medially on the patella. Its fibers are oriented 50–55° medially in the frontal plane, originate from the adductor tubercle[60] and the tendon of the adductor magnus,[10] and insert at the medial patella.

Muscular control of axial rotation about the knee may be used to substitute for injuries to the static rotatory stabilizers, such as the anterior cruciate and medial collateral ligaments. The semitendinosus, gracilis, and sartorius muscles control internal tibial rotation and insert at the pes anserinus. The biceps femoris controls external tibial rotation.

### Menisci

The menisci are cantaloupe-shaped cartilaginous structures attached to the tibial condyles. They form a cuplike articulation with the rounded femoral condyles. The menisci protect the articular cartilage by providing shock absorption,[102] enhance joint stability by deepening the femoral articulation,[41] and distribute joint lubrication and nutrients. The medial geniculate arteries supply blood to the outer one-third of the menisci.[4] The inner two-thirds are avascular. Symptomatic tears of the outer third are thus more amenable to spontaneous healing or surgical repair than the inner areas, which are often surgically excised.

### Ligaments

Ligaments are static stabilizers of the knee. The major ligaments are the anterior cruciate ligament (ACL), posterior cruciate ligament (PCL), medial collateral ligament (MCL), and lateral collateral ligament (LCL). In combination, these ligaments control rotation, anterior and posterior translation, and mediolateral stability of the knee. They are generally strong, thick ligaments, but they are frequently injured. They suffer a biomechanical disadvantage because they are often unable to withstand the large varus–valgus and rotational forces applied over the long lever arms of the limbs.

Ligament injury has been classified in the following manner:

Grade I lesion   Localized tenderness without joint laxity.
Grade II lesion   Tenderness without laxity, but functional loss and effusion are present.
Grade III lesion   Joint laxity.[1]

**Anterior Cruciate Ligament.**   The ACL travels from the inner aspect of the lateral femoral condyle anteriorly, medially, and inferiorly to the anterior tibial intercondylar area.[5] It contains two fiber bundles, the anteromedial and posterolateral bands.[19,21] The anterolateral band tightens in flexion, whereas the posterolateral band tightness in extension. The ACL prevents excessive internal rotation of the tibia on the femur, anterior translation of the tibia on the femur, and knee hyperextension. The ACL is innervated by branches of the tibial nerve[5] that may transmit afferent information for proprioception of the knee.[94] Prolonged ACL laxity and resultant knee instability may lead to meniscal degeneration and degenerative joint disease.[74] There is debate as to whether partial ACL tears are detectable by physical examination;[90] however, such tears respond well to nonoperative treatment.[52]

The astute patient may recall that the injury occurred with a combination of internal rotational and valgus stress on the knee. In football, the classic injury mechanism is the clip, a lateral blow to the knee with a planted foot while the athlete makes a directional change. Hyperextension is another mechanism of injury.[73] Symptoms may include giving way or involuntary buckling of the knee. There may have been an initial "pop" with rapidly progressive swelling of the knee. Examination in the acute phase is difficult because the pain includes local muscle spasm that invalidates many of the physical examination signs. Arthrocentesis is necessary only for severe effusions, but a blood-tinged aspirate is almost diagnostic. Full knee flexion is not possible because of effusion and pain. Knee effusions may inhibit quadriceps contraction by reflex mechanisms,[2] and the quadriceps muscles often atrophy with ACL injury. Once pain is somewhat decreased, the Lachman test[100] is most sensitive to ACL rupture. The pivot shift[27] also may be positive, especially under anesthesia. The anterior drawer sign is less sensitive because tautness of the collateral ligaments at 90° may obscure anteroposterior laxity of the ACL. There may be concomitant disruption of the medial collateral ligament and medial meniscus in the classic triad of O'Donoghue. Lateral meniscal tears also may occur with ACL tears.

Anteroposterior and lateral plain films may show an avulsion fracture of the lateral tibial plateau (Segond's sign), which is associated with ACL or meniscal damage in more than 70% of cases.[32] A notch view may show avulsion of the tibial intercondylar eminence; however, this is rare. MRI may show disruption of the ACL in the axial and sagittal planes, and bone contusion of the lateral tibial or femoral condyles is a strong secondary sign for ACL disruption.

**TABLE 1.**
Modalities for Treatment of Soft Tissue Injuries

| Before 48 Hours | After 48 Hours | Soft Tissue Extensibility |
| --- | --- | --- |
| Ice | Hot packs | Neuromuscular massage |
| Electrical stimulation | Ultrasound | Massage |
| Elevation | Iontophoresis | Joint mobilization |
| Wrap | Contrast bath | |
| Protective gear | Hydrotherapy | |
| | Acupuncture | |

Successful conservative treatment is predicated on patient compliance with a rigorous physical rehabilitation program. Initial treatment consists of joint rest, ice, compression, and elevation (RICE) as well as NSAIDs to reduce inflammation and edema (Table 1). Muscle spasm may be treated with interferential electrical stimulation, ice, muscle stretching, reciprocal inhibition techniques, and contract–relax techniques. Gastrocnemius stretching is necessary to diminish its pull of the femur posteriorly on the tibia. Hamstring strengthening is emphasized to pull the tibia posteriorly on the femur. Quadriceps strengthening is required to restore strength lost with effusion. Short arc squat exercises are ideal because they promote closed kinetic chain cocontraction of the hamstrings and quadriceps (Tables 2–4). Anterolateral rotational instability is treated with selective strengthening of the lateral hamstrings. Gait abnormalities such as decreased weight-bearing on the injured leg are corrected. Once weight-bearing and walking are relatively stable and pain-free, proprioceptive rehabilitation may begin with a wobble board and trampoline and advance to jumping and slideboards. In athletes, upper body aerobic conditioning and sport-specific rehabilitation are necessary. Reports of rehabilitation time for ACL injuries are variable.

The effectiveness of bracing is under debate. Prophylactic bracing has been shown to be ineffective in college football players.[99] Functional braces, such as the Lenox-Hill brace, may be useful in the initial stages of rehabilitation but may not control anterior

**TABLE 2.**
Stretching Protocol*

| Thoracic lumbar fascia | Iliotibial band |
| --- | --- |
| Hips | Hamstrings |
| External rotation | Knee flexion |
| Internal rotation | Ankle |
| Flexion | Heel cords |
| Extension | |

* Stretching the entire lower limbs as well as the thoracolumbar fascia is required to facilitate healing and prevent future injuries.

**TABLE 3.**
Closed Kinetic Chain/Plyometric Exercises*

| | |
| --- | --- |
| Jump/shuttle | Split squat |
| Inverted leg press | Lunge series |
| Leg press | Rubber tubing |
| Squat | Step-ups/downs |

* Allow safe and functional return of strength to the lower limbs with an emphasis on proprioception.

**TABLE 4.**
Advanced Closed Kinetic Chain Exercises*

| |
| --- |
| Medicine ball |
| Side-step cut |
| Cross-over cut |
| Sport-specific activities |

* Minimize sport-neglected activity and lead to participation in specific sport.

translation or rotational instability sufficiently during high-demand activity.[50] Neoprene sleeves may add to proprioceptive input to the knee via the skin but offer little mechanical support.

The details and outcomes of ACL repair are beyond the scope of this chapter; however, patients with severe rotational instability or concomitant injury of the meniscus or MCL may be surgical candidates. Other candidates may include athletes placing high demands on the knee and patients who have failed a supervised, ACL-specific rehabilitation program.

**Posterior Cruciate Ligament.** The PCL travels in the intercondylar notch from the medial surface of the medial femoral condyle posteriorly, laterally, and inferiorly to the posterior tibia. Again there are two bundles: an anterior bundle that tightens in knee flexion and a posterior bundle that tightens in extension. The PCL controls primarily posterior translation of the tibia on the femur, providing 95% of the resistance in this direction.[13]

Isolated PCL injury is less common than ACL injury and may have a 9–23% incidence.[9,17,20,77] The PCL is injured most commonly with posteriorly directed forces to the tibia with the knee in flexion, as may occur in a car accident, with the knee hitting the dashboard, or in falling on a flexed knee. Knee hyperextension injury or stepping inadvertently into a hole also may cause PCL injury. Patients may report effusion and muscle spasm, as in ACL injury, but knee instability is not generally a hallmark of PCL injury. Physical examination may show joint effusion, positive sag sign, positive reverse Lachman's sign,[98] and positive posterior drawer sign. Anterior translation of the tibia on the femur may be increased with PCL injury because of reduction of the posterior displacement of the tibia on the femur. This finding may be confused with a positive anterior drawer sign, and ACL laxity may be misdiagnosed if it is misinterpreted.

Plain films should be done with notch views to rule out bony avulsion of the tibial or femoral insertions. The PCL has an "upside-down hockey stick" appearance on sagittal MRI cuts. Absence of this signal indicates PCL disruption.

Initial conservative measures are aimed at reducing edema and inflammation. Therapeutic exercise includes reduction of muscle spasm and attainment of proper muscle length. It is especially important to stretch the hamstrings to prevent excessive posterior pulling of the tibia over the femur. Closed kinetic chain and multiangle isometric quadriceps strengthening are then initiated to promote anterior translation of the tibia over the femur. Gait abnormalities, such as decreased weight-bearing on the injured leg, are corrected. Proprioceptive rehabilitation, aerobic conditioning, and sport-specific rehabilitation are necessary for athletes and patients who place high demands on their knees. Outcomes for nonoperative PCL management and rehabilitation are encouraging.[82]

## Anterior Knee Pain

### Patellofemoral Tracking

Abnormal patellofemoral tracking is the most common cause of anterior knee pain, and patellofemoral anatomy deserves special attention. The patella is a sesamoid bone formed within the common tendon of the quadriceps during fetal development. It has a number of facets that articulate with the distal femur at different knee flexion angles. Wearing of the facets may cause knee flexion pain at specific angles. The patella tracks within the confines of the femoral trochlear groove. Wiberg[104] has proposed an anatomic classification system to describe patellar anatomy and susceptibility to tracking abnormalities.

The patella normally travels within the femoral trochlea when the knee is flexed from 20–135°. From 0–20° there is no contact between the patella and femur. The greatest patellofemoral forces occur at midflexion. Medially and laterally, the patella has static and dynamic stabilizers that control tracking. Abnormal patellar tracking is most often laterally directed because of the predisposition to genu valgum, lateral stabilizer strength and tightness, and medial stabilizer weakness and laxity.

The medial static stabilizers are the medial retinaculum and medial patellofemoral ligament. The vastus medialis obliquus (VMO) muscle is the only dynamic stabilizer medially. The lateral static stabilizers are the lateral femoral condyle, lateral retinaculum, lateral patellofemoral ligament, and ITB. The vastus lateralis obliquus muscle,[35] the lateral component of the VMO, may be lateral dynamic stabilizer of the knee.

Excessive femoral anteversion,[38] external tibial torsion,[39] genu valgum,[66] and foot pronation[40] also may predispose to abnormal patellofemoral tracking. The Q angle and Insall ratio are anatomic indices of susceptibility to abnormal patellofemoral tracking. The Q angle grossly measures the amount of valgus and axial rotation between the tibia and femur. It is the angle formed by the intersection of lines drawn from the anterior superior iliac spine and the tibial tuberosity through the midpoint of the patella when viewed in the coronal plane. The average Q angle is about 10°, and angles greater than 14° may predispose to abnormal patellofemoral tracking. The Insall ratio is defined as the ratio of patellar tendon length to patellar height and may be calculated from plain film lateral views. An Insall ratio greater than 1.2 (patella alta) may cause the patella to engage the trochlea later in flexion than normal, predisposing to lateral patellar displacement in the early stage of flexion. Patella baja is associated with an Insall ratio less than 0.8.

Patients with patellofemoral pain have symptoms of anterior knee pain with repetitive knee motion or prolonged static knee flexion. Pain is usually worst in the mid-flexion position when the patellofemoral forces are greatest. Examples of aggravating activities including walking stairs or prolonged sitting, often described as "theater knee." A history of recurrent patellar subluxation may accompany patellofemoral pain. Patients may notice crepitus with knee motion or knee swelling. Inspection of the knee may reveal "grasshopper eye"[37] patellae, which face laterally and superiorly. Muscle bulk of the medial quadriceps, especially the VMO, may be decreased. Palpation may reveal diffuse knee tenderness and mild effusion. The patella may not translate well medially because of a tight lateral retinaculum. Pain may be reproduced with passive knee range of motion, active squatting, or Clarke's patellar grind test.[84] Ober's test may identify ITB tightness.[76] Rectus femoris tightness also may contribute to increased patellofemoral forces.

Plain films with sunrise views may show lateral patellar tilting, frank subluxation, or narrowed joint space. Eburnation, erosion, or osteophyte formation of the patella may be seen in severe cases. MRI may show secondary osteochondritis dessicans or chrondromalacia patella on axial cuts. Although currently investigational, cine-MRI may provide useful dynamic patellofemoral tracking information in the future.

Initial treatment consists of reducing edema and inflammation. Exercise treatment may begin immediately, focusing at first on ITB, gastrocnemius, and hamstring stretching to help decrease factors contributing to lateral tracking and abnormally high patellofemoral joint forces. If the feet are pronated, corrective orthotics may be necessary to reduce the resulting valgus stress on the knee. Initial strengthening should consist of isotonic, closed kinetic chain, short-arc VMO strengthening in a pain-free range of motion. The VMO is thought to be selectively isolated with combinations of hip adduction and knee extension. Multiarc isometric VMO strengthening also may be useful. With improvement in pain, isotonic VMO strengthening may be upgraded to greater flexion angles. Ice is helpful for inflammation after exercise sessions. Eventually, proprioceptive and plyometric knee exercises may be necessary for athletes and other patients who place high demands on their knees. Patellar taping may be useful, and patients may find bracing or neoprene sleeves helpful as proprioceptive aids, although these interventions have not been proved to help with tracking.

The differential diagnosis for anterior knee pain related to abnormal patellar tracking includes recurrent patellar subluxation, chondromalacia patellae, osteochondritis dessicans, plica inflammation, and retinacular pain.[25,26] Recurrent patellar subluxation is obvious from the history and may be caused by abnormal lateral patellar tracking and shallow patellar anatomy in combination with tight quadriceps or hamstrings. Chondromalacia patella is defined as softening of the patellar cartilage and is reliably diagnosed only by radiographs and arthroscopy. Although there are various stages of cartilaginous damage,[8] damage does not correlate with symptoms. Osteochondritis dessicans (OCD) is an osteochondral surface deficit of unclear origin. The incidence of OCD on the lateral wall of the medial femoral condyle is 70%. Free fragment production from an osteochondral deficit may cause symptoms of knee locking. The retinacula are innervated and may be a source of pain with direct trauma or excessive tension with abnormal patellar tracking.

The plica is a horseshoe-shaped, extraarticular, embryologic vestige of synovium. It extends from the fat pad over the medial femoral condyle and under the quadriceps tendon, then wraps over the lateral femoral condyle to the lateral retinaculum.[43] Abnormal patellofemoral tracking may cause repetitive friction over the plica, resulting in inflammation. The plica may be palpated over the medial femoral condyle as a discrete, tender, fibrous band. The lateral plica is less commonly symptomatic. An inflamed plica may be seen on MRI. Treatment begins with rest, ice, and NSAIDs, which are followed by treatment of abnormal patellofemoral tracking. Corticosteroid injection may be useful in resistant cases.

### Other Causes of Anterior Knee Pain

Bony causes of anterior knee pain include patellar contusion and fracture. Osgood-Schlatter disease (tibial tuberosity epiphysitis) should be considered in adolescents with complaints of tibial tuberosity pain after growth spurts.

Patellar tendinitis or "jumper's knee" is common in basketball players. Tenderness is usually localized near the tendon's proximal insertion into the patella. This area is most susceptible to injury because of its tenuous blood supply. Patellar tendon rehabilitation requires initial pain relief and NSAIDs followed by stretching of the hamstring and gastrocnemius muscles to allow pain-free and resistance-free normal knee extension. Stretching of tight quadriceps muscles also may decrease tension on the patellar tendon. Eccentric strengthening is recommended for tendon rehabilitation.[97] Closed chain, isotonic, eccentric exercise mimics the maximal natural stresses incurred by the extensor tendon during ambulation. Open chain exercises may be added if they are task- or sport-specific for the patient's activities after rehabilitation (e.g., kicking a soccer ball).

Commonly confused with patellar tendinitis, fat pad inflammation or necrosis may cause subpatellar pain.[38] Fat pad pain may be caused by direct trauma or surgery-induced scarring of the infrapatellar bursa. With patella baja, the patella may impinge on the fat pad during knee extension. On examination, the fat pad is tender to palpation on either side of the patellar tendon. Treatment consists of NSAIDs, ice, and relative rest. Excision may be considered for disabling cases refractory to conservative treatment.

Synovial inflammation of the knee usually manifests as exquisitely painful range of motion and effusion. Common causes include infection (e.g., gonorrhea, staphylococci), autoimmune disease (e.g., rheumatoid arthritis, systemic lupus erythematosus), or crystalline arthropathy (e.g., gout, calcium pyrophosphate deposition disease). Diagnosis may require arthrocentesis and joint fluid analysis, complete blood count with differential, sedimentation rate, and other autoimmune test batteries as guided by the history. Initial treatment is directed at the cause of inflammation. Once inflammation, effusion, and pain are adequately controlled, rehabilitation goals include maintenance of knee range of motion and appropriate strengthening of the hamstrings and quadriceps, which may have been weakened by disuse atrophy.

A number of bursae are located about the knee. Common bursal sources of anterior knee pain include the prepatellar, infrapatellar, and suprapatellar bursae. Rest, ice, compression, and NSAIDs are the treatments of choice. Prepatellar bursitis or "housemaid's knee" may be caused by irritation due to prolonged kneeling. There may be crepitus over the patella. The prepatellar bursa does not respond well to aspiration and corticosteroid injection, which may cause cutaneous fistula formation. Compression, knee cushioning, and decreased kneeling are often helpful. Infrapatellar bursitis may be differentiated from patellar tendinitis and fat pad syndrome by the finding of tenderness directly over the mid-substance of the patellar tendon. The suprapatellar bursa may communicate with the knee joint synovium and be irritated by intraarticular processes. Aspiration and fluid analysis may be helpful in decreasing pain and obtaining a diagnosis. Corticosteroid injection may be helpful for noninfectious effusions.

### Posterior Knee Pain

Posterior knee pain is much less common than anterior knee pain. A detailed knowledge of posterior anatomy is necessary for accurate diagnosis.

The posterior capsule is a pain-sensitive structure that may be injured with extreme knee hyperextension. The oblique popliteal ligament is a continuation of the semimembranosus tendon that runs superolaterally across the posterior capsule, eventually blending into the substance of the capsule. Tight hamstrings or repetitive overload of the hamstrings may result in secondary irritation of the oblique popliteal ligament. Semimembranosus tendinitis[85] may result from repetitive eccentric overload in the deceleration phase of gait. Tenderness is maximal over the posteromedial corner of the knee. Treatment consists of adequate lengthening and eventual eccentric strengthening of the hamstrings. The Slocum test[93] is useful to assess the integrity of the posteromedial or posterolateral capsule.

Vascular disease of the popliteal artery or vein may be responsible for posterior knee pain. Generally pain radiates into the calf. Venous and arterial blood flows may be necessary for diagnosis. Older patients are most susceptible to vascular problems.

The tibial nerve is relatively protected; however, direct trauma or rotational instability[88] may predispose to injury. Plantarflexion weakness or plantar sensory loss may be apparent. Electromyography (EMG) may be useful if the differential diagnosis includes sciatic nerve or radicular lesions. Microsurgical reconstruction may be necessary for nerve transection; however, the anatomically intact nerve is allowed to regenerate. Medications such as tricyclic antidepressants or carbamazepine may be helpful for neuropathic pain. Splinting and bracing for functionally limiting weakness also may be indicated.

The gastrocnemius bursa may be a source of posterior knee and calf pain. The bursa may communicate with the knee joint space and become quite enlarged to form a Baker's cyst. Knee effusions secondary to intraarticular pathology are usually the cause and should be diagnosed and treated appropriately. Duplex ultrasound may confirm the diagnosis. Recurrences after aspiration and treatment of effusion may necessitate surgical resection.

### Medial Knee Pain

Although management of bone injury is beyond the scope of this chapter, contusion or fracture of the medial tibial plateau of the medial femoral condyle must be recognized as possible causes of medial knee pain.

#### Medial Collateral Ligament

The MCL is a broad band of connective tissue passing from the medial epicondyle of the femur to the proximal tibia. It has superficial and deep portions with an intervening bursa. The deep portion is incorporated into the medial knee capsule and is also attached directly to the medial meniscus. The MCL is a broad band that confers a large degree of valgus and rotational stability to the knee; however, excessive forces in these directions lead to injury. Because of its attachments, the MCL is commonly injured together with the medial capsule.

Examination may reveal mild localized edema, and palpation reveals tenderness above and below the joint space over the ligament. Grade III tears may be associated with gapping of the medial joint space with valgus stress. The MCL is best tested with valgus stress at 20° of flexion. The knee also should be valgus-stressed in full extension to test the integrity of the posteromedial capsule. Plain films may be unremarkable; however, valgus stress views may reveal joint gapping. MRI is excellent for imaging the MCL. Ligamentous disruption is best seen on T2-weighted coronal views of the knee.

Treatment depends on the patient's demands on the knee. Elite athletes in sports that require cutting and directional change during running may require reconstruction of grade III tears, but an initial trial of bracing and rehabilitation may suffice. Sedentary patients and patients with grade I or II tears may do well with nonoperative treatment alone. RICE and NSAIDs are used initially. Protective bracing or casting with the knee in extension may be protective in initial stages of healing. Bracing may be removed when range of motion is 75–80% of normal. Exercise treatment usually consists of maintaining normal knee joint range of motion and strength while the ligament heals.

### Medial Meniscus

The medial meniscus is commonly injured in valgus and rotational knee trauma. Its medial margin attaches to the joint capsule and MCL. A sharp valgus stress may tear the MCL and pull a piece of the meniscus with it. Crush injury to the meniscus may occur with a strong varus injury, but this mechanism is less common than valgus injury. The ACL and MCL may be injured with the meniscus in the triad of O'Donoghue. Patients complain of knee locking or catching with medial knee pain. In older patients a degenerative meniscus may present with insidious onset of medial knee pain.

Examination may reveal medial joint line tenderness due to synovial and capsular inflammation. McMurray's test is positive, particularly with valgus and external tibial rotation.[68] The Apley grinding test[3] is less specific for meniscal injury. The distraction test may relieve pressure on the injured meniscus. Meniscal tears may be imaged with plain arthrography, CT-arthrography, and MRI. On MRI, complete and partial tears are best seen on T2-weighted images. Complete tears extend through the entire meniscus to the articular surface, whereas partial tears do not; meniscocapsular dissociation is a secondary sign of a medial meniscal tear. Tears may be radial or vertical in orientation. "Bucket-handle" tears may cause the greatest symptoms of locking. Chronic meniscal degeneration is clearly identified with MRI.

Symptomatic meniscal tears are often surgically repaired or resected. Subtotal meniscectomy avoids the development of degenerative arthritis associated with total meniscectomy. Meniscal tears without major pain and locking may be treated conservatively but may evolve into symptomatic tears. Physical therapy focuses on normal joint range of motion and muscle length and strength. Deep heat prior to soft tissue stretching helps to improve soft tissue elasticity. Residual gait abnormalities from acute injury are also addressed. Proprioceptive, plyometric, and task-specific exercise complete the rehabilitation program. NSAIDs may be used to decrease swelling and pain due to inflammation during rehabilitation.

### Bursae

The pes anserinus bursa is located medial to the tibial tubercle and underlies the insertions of the sartorius, gracilis, and semitendinosus tendons. Local trauma or tendon tightness may predispose to inflammation. RICE, NSAIDs, and possibly steroid injection may be useful. Stretching of the pes anserinus muscles may lessen tension over the bursa. The medial collateral ligament bursa may be inflamed and is distinguished from MCL injury by tenderness inferior but not superior to the joint space.[55]

### Nerves

Nerve injury may be an easily overlooked cause of medial knee pain. The saphenous nerve may be injured by traumatic laceration or inadvertent transection during knee surgery, especially arthroscopy. Reproduction of pain with palpation or Tinel's sign over the saphenous nerve is diagnostic. If knee pain is associated with low back pain, the differential diagnosis includes L3 or L4 radiculopathy. EMG may be useful if the history and physical examination do not lead to an obvious diagnosis.

## Lateral Knee Pain

Although management of bone problems is beyond the scope of this chapter, contusion or fracture must be recognized as possible causes of lateral knee pain. The Maisonneuve fracture is a fracture of the proximal fibula associated with medial ankle injury. Fibular dislocation may occur with lateral blows to the knee.

### Posterolateral Corner

Injuries of the posterolateral corner have been mentioned as a discrete group in the literature. The entities that make up this complex are the posterior horn of the lateral meniscus, lateral collateral ligament, popliteus tendon, and arcuate ligament. Differentiation among these structures is difficult both clinically and radiographically because of their proximity. The posterolateral corner is tested most reliably by the reverse pivot shift test.[45]

The popliteus muscle deserves special attention. In full extension during weight-bearing, the femur is locked in internal rotation relative to the tibia. This so-called "screw home" mechanism allows the knee to remain in extension in static standing without muscular support. Before initial flexion the femur must rotate externally with respect to the tibia to "unlock" the knee. The popliteus performs this function. It originates at the posterior tibia, passes through the capsule under the arcuate ligament, and then inserts at the lateral femoral condyle. The popliteus tendon is commonly injured in runners. Initial treatment includes rest, ice, and NSAIDs. Massage and muscle energy techniques may relieve tension in the tendon. A gradual return to sport is necessary for prolonged relief. Irritation of the popliteus bursa, which underlies the tendon, may be confused with popliteus tendinitis.

### Lateral Collateral Ligament

The LCL travels from the lateral femoral epicondyle to the fibular head. The ligament lies relatively posteriorly and is part of the posterolateral complex. The LCL controls primarily varus stress on the knee. It is strained or ruptured with excessive varus force on the knee. The LCL is relatively protected from injury compared with the MCL because varus injury is much less common than valgus injury and because the LCL is free of attachment to the knee capsule.

As with the MCL, examination may reveal mild localized edema and tenderness above and below the joint space over the ligament. Complete tears may be associated with gapping of the lateral joint space with varus stress. This test is best performed at 20° of flexion because the ligament is most lax in this position. The LCL is easily palpated with the knee flexed 90° and the hip flexed, abducted, and externally rotated.[36] Plain films may show avulsion of the fibular end and varus stress views may reveal joint gapping. MRI is excellent at imaging the LCL, and ligamentous disruption is best seen on T2-weighted coronal views of the knee.

Treatment is similar to that of the MCL. Elite athletes may require construction of nonhealing grade III tears. Protective bracing is protective in initial stages. Nonoperative treatment usually suffices. The RICE protocol is used initially, and exercise treatment consists of maintaining normal knee joint range of motion and strength while the ligament heals. Fibular bursa irritation may be confused with LCL strain.

### Lateral Meniscus

The lateral meniscus is relatively protected from injury compared with the medial meniscus. It has no attachment to the lateral joint capsule or lateral collateral ligament and is thus relatively mobile and protected from concomitant injury with these structures. The mechanism of injury may include a sharp valgus stress and knee rotation in the longitudinal axis that crush or tear the meniscus. It may occasionally be injured with the ACL, MCL, and LCL in the triad of O'Donoghue by a similar mechanism. As in medial meniscal injury, complaints of knee catching or locking predominate. In the child or adolescent with lateral meniscal pain, hereditary discoid meniscus should be considered. Cysts of the lateral meniscus may cause lateral knee pain. Older patients may present with insidious onset of lateral knee pain, possibly indicating a degenerative meniscus.

Examination reveals lateral joint line tenderness due to synovial and capsular inflammation. McMurray's test is positive, particularly with varus stress and internal tibial rotation. The Apley grinding and distraction tests also may indicate meniscal injury. Lateral meniscal tears, especially posterior horn tears, are less reliably seen on MRI than medial meniscal tears. Tears are classified as complete or partial, radial or vertical, or "bucket-handle." Meniscal cysts are easily identified by MRI and are most commonly found on the lateral meniscus. The discoid meniscus is thickened in the superior inferior dimension and appears round instead of the normal C-shape on axial MRI cuts.

Like medial meniscal tears, lateral meniscal tears are often surgically resected to relieve symptoms of locking. Physical therapy focuses on normal joint range of motion and muscle length and strength. Superficial or deep heat may be useful as an adjunct to soft tissue stretching. Residual gait abnormalities from acute injury are detected and corrected. Proprioceptive, plyometric, and task-specific exercises complete the rehabilitation program. NSAIDs may be used to decrease swelling and inflammation during rehabilitation.

### Iliotibial Band Syndrome

ITB syndrome is a common cause of lateral knee pain. The ITB originates from the fascia of the gluteus medius, gluteus maximus, and tensor fascia lata. It passes over the lateral femoral condyle on its way to attach to Gerdy's tubercle on the tibia. Pain is caused by friction of the ITB over the lateral femoral epicondyle. Runners, particularly those who run on banked surfaces, are susceptible. Repetitive hip abduction overload may predispose to ITB tightness, possibly leading to lateral knee pain. Foot supination may produce varus stress on the knee and increase tension on the ITB.

Examination typically reveals maximal tenderness over the lateral femoral epicondyle with knee range of motion, especially at about 30° of flexion.[71] Ober's test may be positive. The gluteus medius or other hip abductors may be weak on manual muscle testing. MRI is not necessary for diagnosis; however, it may show increased signal intensity in T2-weighted images indicative of edema and inflammation within the ITB or lateral femoral condyle.

Initial treatment includes rest, ice, and NSAIDs. Physical rehabilitation focuses on ITB stretching followed by hip abductor strengthening. Heat may be useful to aid ITB stretching after inflammation has subsided. Orthotics may be necessary to help control excessive foot supination. The patient must be taught a home stretching program to be followed rigorously before and after exacerbating activities.

### Nerves
The peroneal nerve may be susceptible to injury from a direct blow to the lateral knee, rotational knee injury,[88] and stretch from inversion ankle injury.[69] The peroneal nerve may be made more susceptible to compression, particularly at the fibular head, by concomitant peripheral neuropathy or L5 radiculopathy. EMG may be useful to differentiate these etiologies. Lateral leg pain and weakness of foot everters and dorsiflexors may be found on examination. Treatment is expectant, and medications such as tricyclic antidepressants may be helpful for neuropathic pain. Splinting and bracing for functionally limiting weakness also may be indicated.

## MEDIAL TIBIAL STRESS SYNDROME
"Shin splints" is the term used to describe pain in the distal third of the posteromedial aspect of the tibia. This condition is common in athletes who perform ballistic activities such as running and dancing. Recently Detmer described three types of medial tibial stress syndrome:[84,86]

Type 1    Local stress fracture
Type 2    Patients with medial tibial pain due to periostitis and periostalgia
Type 3    Pain due to deep posterior compartment syndrome

Studies by Detmer have shown increased uptake in bone scans in the area of the origin of the soleus. In most cases, however, bone scans are negative, not even showing a stress reaction; therefore, the diagnosis of medial tibial stress syndrome is made by the history of pain in the distal third of the tibia with point tenderness over the tibia.[22] The evaluation of patients includes a history of new activities, such as first-time runners in high school. It also may include the typical stress fracture history of increased activity, such as a summer sport camp or early double session for a new season.

The physical examination points to the exact area of pain. Evaluation of biochemical abnormalities is essential. Excessive pronation, pes planus, pes cavus, tarsal coalition, tight hamstrings, tight heel cords, and tight ITBs adversely affect the biomechanics, causing increased stress along the tibia, which may result in periostitis and possibly a stress fracture.[86]

Treatment includes NSAIDs, physical modalities, and flexibility and strengthening exercises of the lower limbs. In the case of an athlete during the season, work-up should be aggressive, including radiographs and bone scan. If the tests are compatible with a positive scan and stress fracture, rest for 6 weeks and slow return to activity are indicated. In the case of negative radiographs and bone scans, aggressive treatment with physical modalities is indicated. Neuromuscular massage with irritant cross-fiber techniques, followed by aggressive strengthening and stretching, can alleviate symptoms immediately with no rest needed. Correction of feet problems by orthotics may be beneficial and needs to be evaluated.[106]

## COMPARTMENT SYNDROME
Pain in the lower limbs after activities may be due to compartment syndrome. Acute compartment syndrome is a medical and surgical emergency and differs from chronic compartment syndrome. Acute compartment syndrome is secondary to trauma such as fracture, crush injury, and vascular occlusion. Pain is out of proportion to the injury. Pulses may be diminished only late in the course of an acute condition. Compartment pressures of 5–15 mmHg are normal. In acute compartment syndrome

pressures less than 30–50 mmHg are borderline. Pressures greater than 50 mmHg constitute a surgical emergency, and decompression is indicated.[67] While the patient awaits testing, the leg should not be elevated or bandaged, because either strategy decreases local arterial pressure and worsens the symptoms. If treated within 12 hours, the prognosis is good (85–90% success rate). After 12 hours, the amputation rate may be as high as 40%, and the incidence of functional abnormalities may be as high as 80%.[86]

Chronic compartment syndrome is more common and presents with pain in the involved muscle group. Symptoms are present with muscle activity and subside with cessation of activities. Resting compartmental pressure may rise from the normal pressure of 5–15 mmHg to 25–30 mmHg. The cause of this condition is thought to be injury to the microcirculation caused by microtrauma. The involved structures include the lymphatics, blood vessels, and the muscles themselves. Build-up of intestinal fluid results from increased vascular permeability and myositis.

Anterior compartment syndrome is seen in runners, walkers, cross-country skiers, and soccer players. The pain is located in the anterolateral middle one-third of the leg.

Deep posterior compartment syndrome is described as pain in the posterior medial border of the tibia. It is usually associated with increased activity and is usually bilateral. Patients may have paresthesias in the medial border of the foot and toes. If weakness is present in the posterior tibial muscles with a decreased pulse, acute compartment syndrome may be present.[22]

Superficial posterior compartment syndrome is rare. It involves the gastrocnemius and soleus muscles and is associated with soreness in the upper part of the posterior leg after exercising. It if becomes severe, patients have paresthesias in the lateral aspect of the foot with weak plantarflexion.[96]

Diagnosis of chronic compartment syndrome is difficult and is usually made after numerous other syndromes have been diagnosed and treated unsuccessfully.[18] The nonoperative treatment includes rest, NSAIDs, biomechanical intervention such as stretching and strengthening exercises, and orthotics. If conservative treatment is unsuccessful, operative fasciotomy is indicated. Success rates are up to 90% with fasciotomies. Most complications are seen with injuries to the sensory nerves that pass through the compartments.[106]

## ANKLE AND FOOT INJURIES

### Inversion Ankle Sprains

Inversion ankle sprains are the most common injury in athletes. They account for 38–45% of all injuries; 85% of all ankle injuries are sprains; and 85% of ankle sprains are inversion sprains to the lateral ligaments. Basketball has the highest incidence of inversion ankle sprains; nearly 50% of all basketball injuries are ankle sprains.[30,31,42,51]

Three major ligament complexes support the ankle: tibiofibular ligaments, deltoral ligament complex, and lateral ligament complex. The lateral ligament complex of the ankle consists of three separate ligaments: the anterior talofibular (ATFL), posterior talofibular (PTFL), and calcaneofibular (CFL). The anterior talofibular is the most commonly injured tendon. The orientation of the ATFL from the anterior-inferior border of the fibula to the neck of the talus makes it tense throughout plantarflexion.[49] The CFL crosses two joints. It originates at the tip of the fibula to the tubercle of the calcaneus in a posterior-inferior direction under the peroneal tendons. The PTFL runs from the lateral tubercle of the talus lateral to the flexor hallucis longus groove. It is the strongest ligament of the three.

The ankle is most stable in dorsiflexion; increasing plantarflexion allows more inferior talar translation and talar inversion. Injuries occur with full weight-bearing on the plantarflexed and internally rotated ankle. If there is a decrease in the talar weight-bearing surface, the ligaments absorb added stress. This scenario frequently occurs with unpredictable landings in basketball, cutting in football, and landing in gymnastics.[33,42,57]

Ankle sprains have been classified as grade I, grade II, and grade III. Grade I ankle sprains signify a stretched ATFL but no frank ligament tears. The patient presents with mild swelling, little or no ecchymosis, point tenderness on the ligament, and mild loss of motion. Grade II sprains involve a compete tear of the ATFL with a partial tear of the CFL. The patient presents with swelling, ecchymosis, and tenderness over the lateral ankle. Grade III sprains involve a complete tear of both the ATFL and CFL and are associated with capsular disruption. If the PTFL is also torn, ankle dislocation results. The patient presents with diffuse swelling, ecchymosis in the lateral ankle and heel, and tenderness over the anterolateral capsule. Moderate-to-severe laxity with anterior drawer or inversion may be present.[33]

Imaging for ankle sprains includes stress radiology, arthrography, and MRI. There is great controversy over what type of stress views to take and even how to interpret what is abnormal. The current consensus is that anesthetized stress radiographs are helpful in acute injuries.

A side-to-side difference in anterior drawer greater than 5 mm or a talar tilt greater than 10° correlates with a grade III ankle sprain. These techniques cannot distinguish between an ATFL tear and an ATFL tear with CFL tears.[75,87] An MRI gives better anatomic information, but it is not needed in most cases, especially if there is no ankle dislocation and conservative care is to be initiated.[24,48,61] Concurrent injuries, as well as the differential diagnosis of lateral ankle pain, include fracture of the distal fibula, fracture of the talar dome, fracture of the os calcus, subluxation of the peroneal tendon, and torn peroneal retinaculum.[34]

An avulsion fracture at the base of the fifth metatarsal also may be present, as well as a stretch injury to the peroneal or sural nerves and injury to the knee, including proximal fibular or tibial injury.

Treatment of ankle sprains follows the typical sports medicine model: control of inflammation, restoration of joint range of motion, improved muscle strength and endurance, sport-specific biomechanical skill patterns, and maintenance program[46,78,81,107] (Tables 5 and 6; see also Table 1).

Grade III lesions have the same results when treated with or without surgery, according to a study by Kannus and Renstrom.[53] This study summarized the results of all relevant prospective and controlled studies. Patients treated with conservative methods of taping, early motion, and rehabilitation exercise recovered from injury and returned to preinjury level of activity in a shorter time. The success rate was 80–90%.

Garrick has shown that ankle taping and high-top shoes decrease the incidence of ankle sprains without increasing other lower limb injuries.[31] Laughman showed that ankle taping decreased range of motion by 26% and placed the ankle in a more dorsiflexed position.[58] Ankle braces have been shown to be more effective than taping both before and after activity, but they are rarely used by teams in a prophylactic fashion.[80,91]

**TABLE 5.**
Ankle-specific Exercises*

| | |
|---|---|
| Dorsiflexion | Tubing strength exercises |
| Eversion | Closed kinetic chain |
| Inversion | Plyometrics |
| Plantarflexion | |

* Isometric and isokinetic strengthening, including tubing.

**TABLE 6.**
Proprioceptive Exercises*

| | |
|---|---|
| Biomechanical ankle platform system (BAPS board) | Pool running |
| Rolling slant board | Closed kinetic chain exercises |
| Slide and glide | Plyometrics |

* Required after sprains; should be performed prophylactically to prevent future sprains.

## Instability

Patients with a history of recurrent ankle sprains, ankle pain, swelling, giving way, and decreased function may have instability. Physical examination reveals an anterior drawer sign and talar tilt. Treatment consists of the above-mentioned rehabilitation program, if the patient has not already been treated with special attention to strengthening the peroneal muscles and proprioceptive training.[6,12,15]

Other causes need to be excluded, including occult osteochondritis, posttraumatic and degenerative arthritis, peroneal tendon tears or subluxation, deltoid ligament tears, synovitis, loose bodies, and tarsal coalition. Synovial impingement of the ATFL from scar tissue may cause lateral ankle joint impingement.

Surgical stabilization is recommended if the patient remains symptomatic after treatment, including excellent rehabilitation.

## Achilles' Tendon Injuries

Achilles tendinitis is a common injury in basketball and racquet sports. Achilles tendinitis is divided into the insertional and noninsertional categories. Noninsertional Achilles tendinitis is classified as pure peritendinitis, peritendinitis with tendinosis, and tendinosis. Rupture of the Achilles' tendon may occur with either of the latter two conditions.

The rupture usually occurs in the lower third of the Achilles' tendon, which has the least amount of blood supply. Pure peritendinitis is inflammation of the tenosynovium with no involvement of the tendon itself. Tendinosis involves fibrous and muscle degeneration of the tendon in vulnerable areas.[95]

All three stages are chronic, and recurring tenderness is localized to areas of the swelling. Treatment consists of the sports medicine model with ice, rest, NSAIDs, and closed kinetic chain exercises. Special considerations include a heel cup or heel wedges to decrease the force on the Achilles' tendon. If a pronated foot is present, orthotics are needed. Corticosteroid injection is contraindicated because it may lead to rupture.

Insertional Achilles tendinitis is treated similarly, but it may be more difficult to treat and may require surgical intervention. Retrocalcaneal apophysitis (Sever's disease) minimizes insertional Achilles tendinitis in adolescents. Pain is at the heel where the Achilles' tendon inserts. Radiographs show fragmentation sclerosis of the calcaneal apophysis. Symptomatic treatment includes heel pads, lower limb stretches, and ice. This condition is self-limiting.

Ruptures of the Achilles' tendon are uncommon. Patients report a sudden impact of pain in the posterior aspect of the lower leg that feels like a shot in the back of the leg. They have difficulty with ambulating, if they are able to ambulate at all. The Thompson test is positive. This test is performed by having the patient kneel on the table with the feet relaxed over the edge. The examiner compresses the calf while observing for plantarflexion of the foot. If there is no plantarflexion, the test is positive. Other findings include inability to perform toe raises and a defect in the tendon. Treatment may be conservative or surgical. Recent studies have shown excellent surgical results, with a decrease in rehabilitation time.

## Posterior Tibialis Tendinitis

There are two types of posterior tibialis tendinitis. Holmes and Mann reported that in the older population posterior tibialis tendinitis is associated with hypertension, diabetes, obesity, corticosteroid exposure, or major surgery around the ankle. Pain is reported on the medial aspect of the mid foot. Patients present with weakness of inversion of the foot and inability or difficulty in performing toe raises.

The second type of posterior tibialis tendinitis occurs in younger patients, who have pain not only between the medial malleolus and navicular bone but also along the posttibial muscle and distal leg. McDermott reports that this condition is associated with genu varum. Patients can perform heel raises, but only with pain.[67]

Nonoperative treatment includes neuromuscular massage, orthotic devices to limit heel valgus (UCB heel cup), and a soft longitudinal arch support. MRI helps to distinguish between tendinitis and rupture. Strengthening exercises of the foot are also needed.

## Flexor Hallucis Longus Tendinitis

Flexor hallucis longus tendinitis occurs with overuse in repetitive, forceful push-off of the forefoot. Chronic inflammation may cause stenosis as the tendon passes through the medial and lateral tubercles of the posterior talus. Active plantarflexion or passive forced dorsiflexion of the first toe may reproduce pain at the posterior medial area of the ankle. MRI, which offers excellent resolution of this tendon, is helpful in diagnosis. Nonoperative treatment includes NSAIDs, rest, ice, neuromuscular massage, and flexibility and strengthening exercises.

## Peroneal Longus Tendinitis

The function of the peroneal longus tendon is primarily plantarflexion of the first metatarsal and secondarily eversion of the foot. Lateral push-off requires an intact tendon. Tendinitis is diagnosed by placing the foot in dorsiflexion and inversion and asking the patient to invert the foot. Weakness or pain in the area of the cuboid indicates inflammation or a tear of the peroneus longus tendon. A tear usually occurs at the point where the tendon turns from the lateral aspect of the foot medially at the sesamoid adjacent to the cuboid tunnel.[67] Treatment of the tear is surgical, whereas tendinitis is treated with physical modalities and a strengthening program.

## CONCLUSION

Soft tissue injuries to the lower limbs are common in both amateur athletes and weekend warriors. A thorough history of the mechansim of injury and a complete examination consisting of palpation and assessment of motor strength and instability lead to an accurate diagnosis in most cases. Treatment addressing the limitations of flexibility, strength, and instability corrects most problems and gives excellent results.

## REFERENCES

1. American Medical Association, Committee on the Medical Aspects of Sports: Standard Nomenclature of Athletic Injuries. Chicago, American Medical Association, 1966.
2. de Andrade JR, Grant C, Dixon AS: Joint distention and reflex muscle inhibition in the knee. J Bone Joint Surg 47A:313–322, 1965.
3. Apley AG: The diagnosis of meniscus injuries—Some new clinical methods. J Bone Joint Surg 29B:78, 1947.
4. Arnoczsky SP, Warren RF: Microvasculature of the human meniscus. Am J Sports Med 10:90–95, 1982.
5. Arnoczky SP: Anatomy of the anterior cruciate ligament. Clin Orthop 172:19–25, 1983.
6. Balduini FC, Tetzlaff J: Historical perspectives on injuries of the ligaments of the ankle. Clin Sports Med 1:3–12, 1982.

7. Bealle S, Garner T, Oxley D: Anterolateral compartment syndrome related to drug induced bleeding: A case report. Am J Sports Med 25:597, 1987.
8. Berqust TH: Imaging of Orthopedic Trauma, 2nd ed. New York, Raven Press, 1991.
9. Bianchi M: Acute tears of the posterior cruciate ligament: Clinical study and results of operative treatment in 27 cases. Am J Sports Med 11:308–314, 1983.
10. Bose K, Kanagasuntherman R, Osman MBH: Vastus medialis oblique: An anatomic and physiological study. Orthopaedics 3:880–883, 1980.
11. Braddom R: Prevention and treatment of bicycle injuries. In Buschbacher RM, Braddom RL (eds): Sports Medicine and Rehabilitation: A Sport-Specific Approach. Philadelphia, Hanley & Belfus, 1994.
12. Brostrom L: Sprained ankles. VI: Surgical treatment of "chronic" ligament ruptures. Acta Chir Scand 132:551–565, 1966.
13. Butler DL, Noyes FR, Good ES: Ligamentous restraints to anterior-posterior drawer in the human knee. J Bone Joint Surg 62A:259–270, 1980.
14. Calliet R: Hip joint pain. In Calliet R (ed): Soft Tissue Pain and Disability, 2nd ed. Philadelphia, F.A. Davis, 1988.
15. Chapman MW: Sprains of the ankle. AAOS Instr Course Lect 24:294–308, 1975.
16. Chu DA: Rehabilitation of the lower extremity. Clin Sports Med 14:205–222, 1995.
17. Clancy WG, Shelbourne KD, Zoellner GB, et al: Treatment of knee joint instability secondary to rupture of the posterior cruciate ligament. Report of a new procedure. J Bone Joint Surg 65A:310–322, 1983.
18. Clanton TO, Solcher BW: Chronic leg pain in athletes. Clin Sports Med 13:743–760, 1994.
19. Clark JM, Sidles JA: The interrelation of fiber bundles in the anterior cruciate ligament. J Orthop Res 8:180–188, 1988.
20. Clendenin MB, DeLee JC, Heckman JD: Interstitial tears of the posterior cruciate ligament of the knee. Orthopaedics 3:764–772, 1980.
21. Danylchuk KD, Finlay JB, Krcek JP: Microstructural organization of human and bovine cruciate ligament. Clin Orthop 131:294–298, 1978.
22. Detmer DE: Chronic shin splints: Classification and management of medial tibial stress syndrome. Sports Med 3:436, 1986.
23. Ekberg O, Persson NH, Abrahamsson PA, et al: Longstanding groin pain in athletes: Multidisciplinary approach. Sports Med 6:56–61, 1988.
24. Ferkel R, Flannigan B, Elkins B, et al: Magnetic resonance imaging of the foot and ankle: Correlation of normal anatomy with pathological conditions. Foot Ankle 11:289–305, 1991.
25. Fulkerson J: Awareness of the retinaculum in evaluating patellofemoral pain. Am J Sports Med 10:147, 1982.
26. Fulkerson J, Tennant R, Javin J, et al: Histologic evidence of the retinacular nerve injury associated with patellofemoral malalignment. Clin Orthop 197:196, 1985.
27. Galway RD, Beaupre A, MacIntosh DL: Pivot shift: A clinical sign of symptomatic anterior cruciate ligament insufficiency [abstract]. J Bone Joint Surg 54B:763–764, 1972.
28. Gardner E: The innervation of the hip joint. Anat Rec 101:353–371, 1948.
29. Garrick JG, Requa RK: Role of external support in the prevention of ankle sprains. Med Sci Sports 5:200–203, 1973.
30. Garrick JG: Epidemiologic perspective. Clin Sports Med 1:13–18, 1982.
31. Garrick JG: The frequency of injury, mechanism of injury, and epidemiology of ankle sprains. Am J Sports Med 5:241–242, 1977.
32. Goldman AB, Pavlov H, Rubenstein D: The Segond fracture of the proximal tibia: A small avulsion fracture that reflects ligamentous damage. AJR 151:1163–1167, 1988.
33. Gronmark T, Johnsen O, Kogstad O: Rupture of the lateral ligaments of the ankle: A controlled clinical trial. Injury 11:215–218, 1980.
34. Gross ML, Nasser S, Finerman GAM: The hip and pelvis. In DeLee JC, Drez D Jr (eds): Sports Medicine: Principles and Practice, vol 2. Philadelphia, W.B. Saunders, 1994.
35. Hallisey MJ, Doherty N, Bennett WF, et al: Anatomy of the junction of the vastus lateralis tendon and the patella. J Bone Joint Surg 69A:545–549, 1987.
36. Hoppenfeld S: Physical Examination of the Spine and Extremities. Norwalk, CT, Appleton-Century-Crofts, 1976, p 182.
37. Hughston JC: Subluxation of the patella. J Bone Joint Surg 50A:1003–1026, 1968.
38. Hughston JC, Walsh WM, Puddu G: Patellar subluxation and dislocation. Philadelphia, W.B. Saunders, 1984.
39. Hungerford DS, Barry M: Biomechanics of the patellofemoral joint. Clin Orthop 114:9–15, 1979.
40. Inman VT, Ralston HJ, Todd F: Human Walking. Baltimore, Williams & Wilkins, 1981.
41. Insall JN: Anatomy of the knee. In Install JN (ed): Surgery of the Knee. New York, Churchill Livingstone, 1984, pp 1–20.
42. Jackson DW, Ashley RL, Powell JW: Ankle sprains in young athletes. Clin Orthop Rel Res 101:201–215, 1974.

43. Jacobson KE, Flandry FC: Diagnosis of anterior knee pain. Clin Sports Med 8:179–195, 1989.
44. Jacobson T, Allen WC: Surgical correction of the snapping iliopsoas tendon. Am J Sports Med 18:470–474, 1990.
45. Jakob RP, Hassler H, Staeubli HU: Observations on rotary instability of the lateral compartment of the knee. Acta Orthop Scand 191(Suppl):1–32, 1981.
46. Jaskulla R, Fischer G, Schedl R: Injuries of the lateral ligaments of the ankle joint: Operative treatment and long-term results. Arch Orthop Trauma Surg 107:217–221, 1988.
47. Jenkins DB (ed): Hollinshead's Functional Anatomy of the Limbs and Back. Philadelphia, W.B. Saunders, 1991.
48. Johannsen A: Radiological diagnosis of lateral ligament lesion of the ankle. Acta Orthop Scand 49:295–301, 1978.
49. Johnson EE, Markold KL: The contribution of the anterior talofibular ligament to ankle laxity. J Bone Joint Surg 665A:81, 1983.
50. Johnson JC, Bach B R: Use of knee braces in athletic injuries. In Scott WN (ed): Ligament and Extensor Mechanism Injuries of the Knee: Diagnosis and Treatment. St. Louis, Mosby, 1991, p 169.
51. Johnson KA, Teasdall RD: Sprained ankles as they relate to basketball. Clin Sports Med 12:363–372, 1993.
52. Kannus P, Jarvinen M: Conservatively treated tears of the anterior cruciate ligament: Long term results. J Bone Joint Surg 69A:1007–1012, 1987.
53. Kannus P, Renstrom P: Current concepts review: Treatment for acute tears of the lateral ligaments of the ankle. J Bone Joint Surg 73A:305–312, 1991.
54. Kapenkji FIA: The Physiology of the Joints. New York, Churchill Livingstone, 1970, pp 114–123.
55. Kerlan RK, Glousman RE: Tibial collateral ligament bursitis. Am J Sports Med 16:334, 1988.
56. Kisner C, Colby LA (eds): Therapeutic Exercise: Foundations and Techniques. Philadelphia, F.A. Davis, 1987.
57. Lassiter TE, Malone TR, Garett WE: Injury to the lateral ligaments of the ankle. Orthop Clin North Am 20:629–640, 1989.
58. Laughman RK, Carr TA, Chao EY, et al: Three-dimensional kinematics of the taped ankle before and after exercise. Am J Sports Med 8:425–431, 1980.
59. Lawson S: Compartment Pressures in Nordic Skiers. Masters thesis, University of Alberta, Edmonton, Alberta, 1989.
60. Lieb FJ, Perry J: Quadriceps function: An anatomical and mechanical study using amputated limbs. J Bone Joint Surg 50A:1535–1548, 1968.
61. Link S, Erickson S, Timins M: MR imaging of the ankle and foot: Normal structures and anatomic variants that may stimulate disease. AJR 161:607–612, 1993.
62. Liu SH, Jason WJ: Lateral ankle sprains and instability problems. Clin Sports Med 13:793–810, 1994.
63. Logan JG, Rorabeck CH, Castle GSP: The measurement of dynamic compartment pressures during exercise. Am J Sports Med 11:220, 1983.
64. Magee D: Orthopedic Physical Assessment. Philadelphia, W.B. Saunders, 1992.
65. Maigne R: Manipulations and mobilizations of the limbs. In Basmajian JV (ed): Traction and Massage. Baltimore, Williams & Wilkins, 1992.
66. Maquet PGJ: Biomechanics of the Knee. New York, Springer-Verlag, 1976.
67. McDermott EP: Basketball injuries of the foot and ankle. Clin Sports Med 12:373–394, 1993.
68. McMurray TP: The semilunar cartilages. Br J Surg 29:407, 1942.
69. Meals RA: Peroneal nerve palsy complicating ankle sprain. J Bone Joint Surg 59A:966, 1977.
70. Muller W: The Knee: Form, Function and Ligament Reconstruction. New York, Springer-Verlag, 1983.
71. Noble HB, Hajek MR, Porter M: Diagnosis and treatment of iliotibial band tightness in runners. Phys Sportsmed 10:67, 1984.
72. Nordin M, Frankel VH: Biomechanics of the knee. In Frankel VH, Nordin M (eds): Basic Biomechanics of the Musculoskeletal System. Philadelphia, Lea & Febiger, 1980, p 152.
73. Noyes FR, Bassett RW, Grood ES, et al: Arthroscopy in acute traumatic hemarthrosis of the knee: Incidence of ACL tears and other injuries. J Bone Joint Surg 62A:687–695, 1980.
74. Noyes FR, Modar PA, Matthews DS, et al: The symptomatic anterior cruciate deficient knee. I: The long term functional instability in athletically active individuals. J Bone Joint Surg 65A:163–174, 1983.
75. Nyska M, Amir H, Porath A, Dekel S: Radiological assessment of a modified anterior drawer test of the ankle. Foot Ankle 13:400–403, 1992.
76. Ober FB: The role of the iliotibial and fascia lata as a factor in the causation of low-back disabilities and sciatica. J Bone Joint Surg 18A:105, 1936.
77. O'Donoghue DH: Surgical treatment of fresh injuries to the major ligaments of the knee. J Bone Joint Surg 32A:721–738, 1950.
78. Orava S, Kujala UM: Rupture of the ischial origin of the hamstring muscles. Am J Sports Med 23:702–714, 1995.

79. Palmitier R, An K, Scott S, et al: Kinetic chain exercise in knee rehabilitation. Clin Sports Med 11:6, 1991.
80. Palutsis RS, Duncan J, Jacobson KE, Liu SH: Comparison of ankle supports for control of talar tilt. Presented at the 60th Annual Meeting of the American Academy of Orthopaedic Surgeons, San Francisco, February 18–23, 1993.
81. Panariello R: The closed kinetic chain in strength training. Nat Strength Condition J 13:1, 1991.
82. Parolie JM, Bergfield JA: Long term result of non-operative treatment of isolated posterior cruciate ligament injuries in athletes. Am J Sports Med 14:35–38, 1986.
83. Pecina MM, Krmpotic-Nemanic JK, Markiewitz AD (eds): Tunnel Syndromes. Boca Raton, FL, CRC Press, 1991.
84. Puranen J: The medial tibial syndrome: Exercise ischaemia in the medial fascial compartment of the leg. J Bone Joint Surg 56B:712, 1974.
85. Ray JM, Clancy WG, Lemon RA: Semimembranosus tendonitis: An overlooked cause of medial knee pain. Am J Sports Med 16:347, 1988.
86. Reid DC: Exercise induced leg pain. In Sports Injury Assessment and Rehabilitation. New York, Churchill Livingstone, 1992, p 269.
87. Rijke AM, Jones B, Vierhout PA: Stress examination of traumatized lateral ligaments of the ankle. Clin Orthop Rel Res 210:143–151, 1986.
88. Saal JA: The pseudoradicular syndrome. Spine 13:926–930, 1988.
89. Sammarco GJ: The dancer's hip. In Ryan AJ, Stephens RE (eds): Dance Medicine: A Comprehensive Guide. Chicago, Pluribus Press, 1987.
90. Sandberg R, Balkfors B: Partial rupture of the anterior cruciate ligament: Natural course. Clin Orthop 220:176–178, 1987.
91. Shapiro MS, Kabo JM, Mitchell PW, et al: Ankle sprain prophylaxis: An analysis of the stabilizing effects of braces and tape. Am J Sports Med 22:1–5, 1994.
92. Shin DY, Lennard TA: Proximal lower extremity blocks. In Lennard TA (eds): Physiatric Procedures in Clinical Practice. Philadelphia, Hanley & Belfus, 1995, pp 150–162.
93. Slocum DB, Larson RL: Rotary instability of the knee: Its pathogenesis and clinical test to demonstrate its presence. J Bone Joint Surg 50A:211–225, 1968.
94. Solomonov M, Baratta R, Zhoud BH, et al: The synergistic action of the anterior cruciate ligament and thigh muscles in maintaining joint stability. Am J Sports Med 15:207–213, 1987.
95. Sona CA, Mandelbaum BR: Achilles tendon disorder. Clin Sports Med 13:811–824, 1994.
96. Stack C: Superficial posterior compartment syndrome of the leg with deep venous compromise. Clin Orthop 220:223, 1987.
97. Stanish WD, Curwin S, Rubinowich M: Tendinitis analysis and treatment. Clin Sports Med 4:593–608, 1986.
98. Strobel M, Stedtfeld HW: Diagnostic Evaluation of the Knee. Berlin, Springer-Verlag, 1990.
99. Teitz CC, Kronmal RA, et al: Evaluation of the prophylactic braces to prevent injury to the knee in collegiate football players. J Bone Joint Surg 69A:2–9, 1987.
100. Torg JS, Conrad W, Kalen V: Diagnosis of anterior cruciate ligament instability in the athlete. Am J Sports Med 4:8484–8493, 1976.
101. Travell JG, Simons DG (eds): Myofascial Pain and Dysfunction: The Trigger Point Manual. The Lower Extremities. Baltimore, Williams & Wilkins, 1992.
102. Voloshin AS, Wosk J: Shock absorption of meniscectomized and painful knees: A comparative in-vivo study. J Biomech Eng 5:7–93, 1976.
103. Waters PM, Millis MB: Hip and pelvic injuries in the young athlete. Clin Sports Med 7:513, 1988.
104. Wiberg G: Roentgenographic and anatomic studies of the femorapatellar joint, with special references to chondromalacia pain. Acta Orthop Scand 12:319–410, 1941.
105. Wiley JP, Clement DB, Doyle DL, et al: A primary care perspective of chronic compartment syndrome of the leg. Physician Sporstmed 15:111, 1987.
106. Windsor RE, Dreyer SJ, Lester JP: Overuse injuries of the leg, ankle and foot. Phys Med Rehabil Clin North Am 5:195–214, 1994.
107. Yack H, Collins C, Whieldon T: Comparison of closed and open kinetic chain exercise in the anterior cruciate ligament-deficient knee. Am J Sports Med 21:1, 1993.

# 9

# Soft Tissue Injuries of the Upper Extremities

MICHAEL WEINIK, DO
LORI WASSERBURGER, MD
STEVEN WIESNER, MD
RONALD VANDERNOORD, MD

The soft tissues of the upper extremities, including tendons, ligaments, bursae, and muscles, are subject to tremendous stresses as a result of single or repetitive loading and torsional, angular, or tractional forces. Making this system even more susceptible to injury are the limitations in ligamentous support necessary to allow full, functional range of motion for carrying out activities of daily living, including occupational and sport-specific demands. Accurate diagnosis and appropriate care and rehabilitation must be based on a detailed history of the mechanism of injury, understanding of relevant anatomy and functional biomechanics, precise physical examination, and selection of appropriate diagnostic tests to confirm the clinical impressions. Only then can one implement a comprehensive care plan (conservative or surgical), including rehabilitative measures that allow timely healing and safe return to leisure and work-related activities.

## WRIST

The wrist is arguably the most complex and intricate joint of the human body. Proper function in all three degrees of freedom (flexion and extension, supination and pronation, radial and ulnar deviation) requires precise alignment and constrained movement of the carpal bones through intrinsic and extrinsic ligamentous integrity and smooth, coordinated action of the dorsal and volar forearm musculature. Alterations in any one of these relationships place the other structures of the wrist and the tendons and nerves that either cross over or through the wrist at increased risk for injury. Although knowledge of the mechanism of injury and clinical evaluation are invaluable, such diagnostic tools as plain radiographs, stress views, magnetic resonance imaging (MRI), bone scan, arthrogram, arthroscopy, arthrocentesis, and anesthetic injections may prove necessary to make a clear and accurate diagnosis. Rehabilitation of wrist injuries also must be specific and detailed to allow adequate healing, protection, and restoration of function.

### Anatomy

The wrist or carpus is composed of a total of eight bones arranged in a proximal and distal row. The unique shape of these bones and the bowstring effect of the flexor

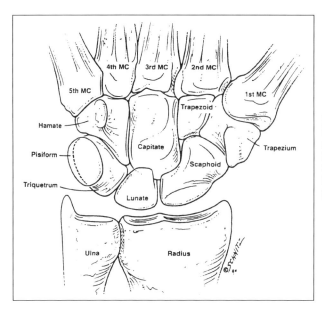

**FIGURE 1.**
Bony anatomy of the wrist.
(From Sternberg BD, Plancher KD: Clinical anatomy of the wrist and elbow. Clin Sports Med 14:301, 1995, with permission.)

retinaculum create a bony transverse arch that defines the carpal tunnel. The more mobile and proximal row of carpal bones consists of the scaphoid, lunate, triquetrum, and pisiform. The less mobile distal row consists of the trapezium, trapezoid, capitate, and hamate. The proximal row articulates with the radius and triangular fibrocartilage complex (TFCC) proximally and the distal carpal row distally (Fig. 1). The ulna does not directly articulate with the proximal carpal bones, from which it is separated by the TFCC. The distal row articulates with the metacarpal bones. Stability of the carpus is achieved through the intricate fit of the eight individual bones and an extensive system of intrinsic interosseous (intercarpal) and extrinsic (extracapsular) ligaments. This system is further defined by either dorsal or palmar location (Table 1). The palmar

**TABLE 1.**
Wrist Ligaments

| | |
|---|---|
| **Extrinsic ligaments** | |
| Palmar ligaments | Dorsal ligaments |
|     Radial collateral ligament |     Radiotriquetral ligament |
|     Palmar radiocarpal ligament |     Radiolunate ligament |
|         Radioscaphoidcapitate |     Radioscaphoid ligament |
|         Radioscaphoidlunate | |
|         Radiolunate | |
|     Ulnocarpal ligament complex | |
|         Ulnar collateral ligament | |
|         Ulnolunate | |
|         Radioulnar | |
|         Triangular fibrocartilage | |
| **Intrinsic ligaments** | |
| Palmar ligaments | Dorsal ligaments |
|     Lunatotriquetral ligament |     Capitohamate ligament |
|     Scapholunate ligament |     Trapeziocapitate ligament |
|     Arcuate or V ligament |     Trapeziotrapezoid ligament |
|         Triquetrohamate |     Dorsal intercarpal ligament |
|         Triquetrocapitate | |
|         Scaphocapitate | |

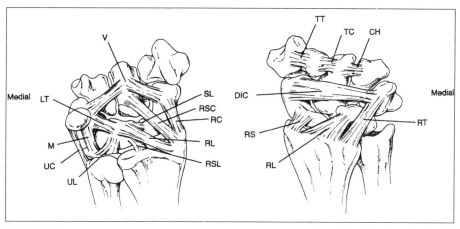

**FIGURE 2.**
Wrist ligaments (right hand). *Left,* Palmar ligaments. Extrinsic: M = meniscus homolog; RC = radial collateral; RL = radiolunate; RSC = radioscaphocapitate; RSL = radioscapholunate; UC = ulnar collateral; UL = ulnolunate. Intrinsic: LT = lunatotriquetral; SL = scapholunate; V = deltoid. *Right,* Dorsal ligaments. Extrinsic: RL = radiolunate; RS = radioscaphoid; RT = radiotriquetral. Intrinsic: CH = capitohamate; DIC = dorsal intercarpal; TC = trapeziocapitate; TT = trapeziotrapezoid. (From Bednar JM, Osterman AL: Carpal instability. J Am Acad Orthop Surg 1:14, 1993, with permission.)

extrinsic ligaments are far thicker and stronger than the dorsal ligaments and are considered the main ligamentous stabilizers of the carpal bones. Further support is gained through the overlying flexor and extensor retinaculum[53] (Figs. 2 and 3).

To understand the patterns of wrist injuries, a basic knowledge of normal wrist kinematics is necessary. Wrist joint motion in the planes of flexion and extension as well as radial and ulnar deviation is centered at the head of the capitate in the distal row.[90] Normal wrist motion from full flexion to extension averages 150°, with approximately 50% at the radiocarpal joint and 50% at the midcarpal joint.[32,71] Normal wrist motion from full radial deviation to ulnar deviation averages 50°, with 60% at the midcarpal joint and 40% at the radiocarpal joint.[67] At a position of full radial deviation, the proximal row of carpal bones is in a flexed posture. In moving to an ulnar deviated position, the proximal row of carpal bones rotates into an extended posture[47] (Fig. 4). The

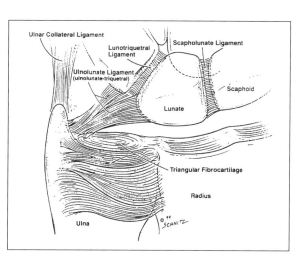

**FIGURE 3.**
Triangular fibrocartilage complex. (From Sternberg BD, Plancher KD: Clinical anatomy of the wrist and elbow. Clin Sports Med 14:300, 1995, with permission.)

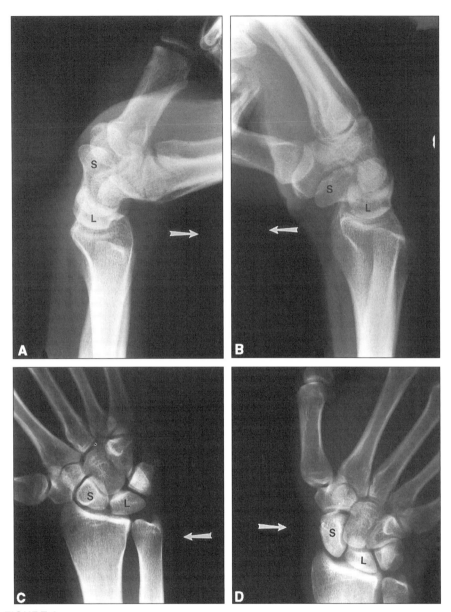

**FIGURE 4.**
Motion studies of the right wrist with the wrist extended *(A)* and flexed *(B)* in the lateral projection and the radial *(C)* and ulnar *(D)* deviation on the posteroanterior views. Note the changes in the shape of the scaphoid (S) and its relationship to the lunate (L) on these normal studies. (From Berquist TH: Wrist disorders: What should we be looking for with imaging techniques? J Hand Ther 9:110, 1996, with permission.)

primary movers of the wrist (flexor carpi ulnaris, flexor carpi radialis, extensor carpi radialis longus and brevis, extensor carpi ulnaris, and abductor pollicis longus) are positioned peripherally to the center of wrist motion (the head of the capitate) and thereby create a strong lever arm for wrist motion.[47,59,81] The function of the proximal row of carpal bones has been described as an intercalcated, geometrically variable link between the distal row of carpal bones and the more proximal radius and TFCC.[6,41,67] None of the primary movers of the wrist attach to the proximal carpal row, which functions as a slider arm to translate and control motion of the carpus. The function and efficacy of this system depend on the integrity of the carpal ligamentous structures and unique geometry of each carpal bone.

### Triangular Fibrocartilage Injury

The triangular fibrocartilage and its meniscoid homolog lie between the distal ulnar and proximal row of carpal bones and thus are subject to axial loading and sheering forces that, depending on the magnitude, may result in acute traumatic avulsions and perforation or chronic, age-related degenerative changes.[55,59] Triangular fibrocartilage tears should be suspected in patients who complain of pain along the ulnar aspect of the wrist with supination or pronation. Grip strength also may be reduced.[83]

Physical examination reveals point tenderness between the proximal carpal row, ulna, and triquetrum.[46,48] Combined ulnar deviation, axial loading, and rotation increase shear through the TFCC and produce pain and crepitance (Fig. 5). A neutral rotation posteroanterior radiograph may reveal positive ulnar variance; this relative lengthening of the ulna may increase loadbearing through the TFCC. Wrist arthrography has been reported to be 95% accurate[65] and may reveal contrast within the substance of the TFCC (incomplete tear) or a communicating defect between the distal radioulnar joint and radiocarpal joint (complete tear).[19] Magnetic resonance images (MRIs) of higher tesla strength with dedicated wrist surface coils and interpretation by an experienced radiologist increase diagnostic yields and avoid false-positive and false-negative findings.[18,39,56,75] Arthroscopy further increases diagnostic yield because of its ability to specify the size and location of TFCC tears and to assess for ligamenous tears, chondromalacia, and carpal instability.[15,83] As with the meniscus of the knee, the location of the tears influences the potential for healing. Tears located more on the periphery of the triangular fibrocartilage have the highest potential for healing with conservative measures because of the relatively better vascular supply along the edges of the fibrocartilage. Conservative care includes immobilization in a long-arm plaster cast in neutral forearm rotation for 4–6 weeks. Tears that remain symptomatic should be referred for surgical consultation. Tears located on the periphery may be repaired, whereas tears that are more centrally located are usually debrided because of poor healing potential.

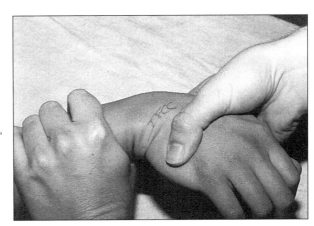

**FIGURE 5.**
TFCC grind or load test. (From Skiven T: Clinical examination of the wrist. J Hand Ther 9:102, 1996, with permission.)

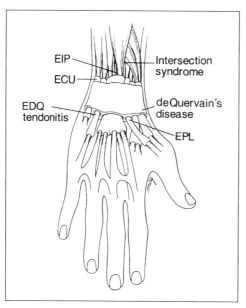

**FIGURE 6.**
Tendinopathies of the wrist. (From Kiefhaber TR, Stern PJ: Upper extremity tendinitis and overuse syndromes in the athlete. Clin Sports Med 11:43, 1992, with permission.)

## Tendinopathies

The mechanisms of injury and healing of both acute and overuse injuries to tendinous structures are discussed at length elsewhere in this book. However, in general it is believed that tendons are most susceptible to injury when loads are placed quickly and in a torsional direction.[62] Because the wrist has multiple planes of combined motion and is exposed to repetitive and frequently heavy loads, the tendons that cross it are uniquely susceptible to injury (Fig. 6).

### De Quervain's Tenosynovitis

One of the most common tendinopathies of the wrist, de Quervain's tenosynovitis involves stenosis of the extensor pollicis brevis and abductor pollicis longus tendons as they pass through the first dorsal compartment of the wrist. It is frequently seen in athletes or laborers who perform repetitive wrist radial and ulnar deviation (Fig. 7). Golf (particularly in regard to the proximal hand), fly fishing, javelin, discus, and tennis and other racquet sports are commonly offending activities.[69,86]

The patient presents with complaints of pain and, less frequently, swelling along the radial aspect of the wrist. Point tenderness and crepitus may be noted just proximal to the radial styloid.[22,50] Finkelstein's maneuver, in which the thumb is flexed and held

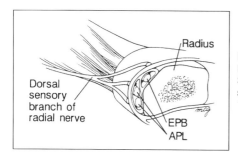

**FIGURE 7.**
First dorsal compartment. (From Kiefhaber TR, Stern PJ: Upper extremity tendinitis and overuse syndromes in the athlete. Clin Sports Med 11:44, 1992, with permission.)

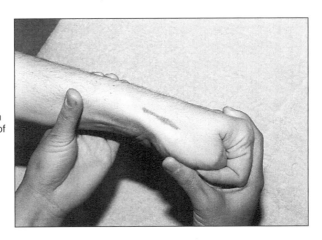

**FIGURE 8.**
Finkelstein's test to detect de Quervain's tenosynovitis. (From Skiven T: Clinical examination of the wrist. J Hand Ther 9:98, 1996, with permission.)

in palmar adduction while the wrist is ulnarly deviated, places the extensor pollicis brevis and abductor pollicis longus tendons in maximal excursion and typically reproduces or exacerbates the patient's discomfort (Fig. 8).

First-line conservative treatment includes activity modification, selected physical modalities (e.g., iontophoresis with 4% dexamethasone, ultrasound, cryotherapy), and oral antiinflammatory agents. If these measures prove ineffective, a peritendinous corticosteroid injection of the first extensor compartment should be performed. Success rates vary between 62% and 100%.[42,85] A low-temperature thermoplastic thumb spica is applied for 10–14 days. If well-formed, the thumb spica need not immobilize the interphalangeal joint. Suboptimal results may warrant a repeat injection, given the fact that the extensor pollicis brevis and abductor pollicis longus tendons are separated by a longitudinal septum within the first extensor compartment in as many as 30% of patients.[26] Surgical decompression of the first extensor compartment is reserved for recalcitrant cases.

### Intersection Syndrome

Another cause of dorsal wrist pain is intersection syndrome, which is so named because the abductor pollicis longus and extensor pollicis brevis cross over the extensor carpi radialis longus and brevis tendons. This condition has been noted in weightlifters, players of various racquet sports, and canoeists.[86] Rowers also are frequently affected, particularly in the wrist that "feathers" or rotates the blade during each stroke. Of interest, intersection syndrome is not often associated with rowing on a stationary ergometer because no repetitive wrist dorsiflexion or "feathering" motion is required.[10]

The pathophysiology of intersection syndrome remains controversial. Theories include formation of an adventitial bursa between the extensor carpi radialis brevis and abductor pollicis longus;[87] hypertrophy of the abductor pollicis longus and extensor pollicis brevis muscles, which results in compression of the underlying extensor carpi radialis brevis and longus tendons;[84] and tenosynovitis of the wrist extensors as they pass through the second dorsal compartment[28] (Fig. 9).

Symptoms at presentation often include pain and swelling along the radial dorsal forearm at a point approximately 4–6 cm proximal to the distal radius. Pain is usually worse with thumb and/or wrist extension.[28] Palpable and occasionally audible crepitus is appreciated with wrist motion.[38,77]

Conservative treatment is essentially identical to that for de Quervain's tenosynovitis except that the low-temperature thermoplastic wrist orthosis should have slightly

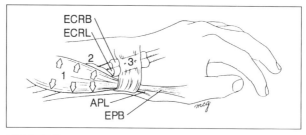

**FIGURE 9.**
Intersection syndrome may be caused by any of the following:
(1) An exertional compartment syndrome of the abductor pollicis longus (APL) and extensor pollicis brevis (EPB) or degenerative changes within these muscles. (2) Inflammation or adventitial bursa formation at the intersection of the APL and EPB and the extensor carpi radialis longus (ECRL) and extensor carpi radialis brevis (ECRB). (3) Stenosing tenosynovitis of the ECRL and ECRB. (From Kiefhaber TR, Stern PJ: Upper extremity tendinitis and overuse syndromes in the athlete. Clin Sports Med 11:43, 1992, with permission.)

deeper gutters to ensure limitation of both wrist and thumb motion. Such measures are successful in as many as 95% of cases.[62] Some authors recommend up to 6 weeks of conservative management before surgical intervention is considered. Surgical options include abductor pollicis longus and extensor pollicis brevis fasciotomies, debridement of adventitial bursae and inflammatory tissue, and second extensor compartment release and tenosynovectomy.[38,77,89]

### Extensor Carpi Ulnaris Tendinitis and Subluxation

The second most common tenosynovitis of the wrist[86] involves the extensor carpi ulnaris tendon, which lies within the sixth extensor compartment beneath its own subsheath and the common extensor retinaculum. Extensor carpi ulnaris tendinitis has been reported in sports that require repetitive motion, such as racquet sports, rowing, and baseball.[69] Rupture of the tendon has been noted in the trailing (proximal) hand of baseball batters as it assumes forced supination, flexion, and ulnar deviation.[20,59,60]

Extensor carpi ulnaris tendinitis has been associated with repetitive motion through the fibroosseus tunnel of the sixth extensor compartment, fibrosis of the subsheath[38,77] as a result of subluxation of the extensor carpi ulnaris tendon,[62] an anatomic variant of an accessory slip to the extensor mechanism of the fifth digit,[2] and triangular fibrocartilage complex injury[58] (Fig. 10).

Presenting symptoms include pain and swelling along the dorsal ulnar aspect of the wrist. Numbness in the distribution of the dorsal ulnar sensory nerve has been noted as well, presumably secondary to local inflammation.[38] Extensor carpi ulnaris tendinitis is exacerbated by resisted wrist dorsiflexion and tendon subluxation produced by combined supination and ulnar deviation[77] (Fig. 11). Tendon subluxation is extremely important to note on clinical examination because conservative treatment of tendinitis may be highly efficacious,[58] whereas conservative treatment of tendon subluxation is rarely successful.[20]

Conservative treatment of extensor carpi ulnaris tendinitis includes oral antiinflammatory agents and splinting in a well-molded ulnar gutter splint with extended dorsal flare and the wrist in neutral to slight palmar flexion. Corticosteroid injection of the tendon sheath may be warranted for patients who are symptomatic during activities of daily living.[36] Conservative treatment of extensor carpi ulnar tendon subluxation

**FIGURE 10.**
The extensor carpi ulnaris is bound to the ulna by a substantial subsheath that is separate and distinct from the overlying extensor retinaculum. Sixth dorsal compartment tendinitis, tenosynovitis, or stenosing tenosynovitis may develop from overuse or as secondary manifestation of a tear in the triangular fibrocartilage complex (TFCC). (From Kiefhaber TR, Stern PJ: Upper extremity tendinitis and overuse syndromes in the athlete. Clin Sports Med 11:43, 1992, with permission.)

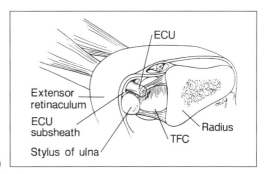

with a long arm cast and the wrist in slight dorsiflexion and full pronation has been described.[86] Surgical intervention includes radial release of the subsheath and repair of the extensor retinaculum.[31]

### Flexor Carpi Radialis Tendinitis

As a prime mover of the wrist, the flexor carpi radialis tendon is subject to repetitive trauma due to the motion of the carpal bones beneath it as well as the rigid and narrow confines of the fibroosseous tunnel through which it must pass to its insertion on the base of the second and third metacarpals. This narrow tunnel is bordered inferiorly by the scaphoid and trapezius, radially by the trapezial tuberosity, and superiorly by the transverse carpal ligament. The flexor carpi radialis tendon occupies 90% of the tunnel.[8,27] Repetitive trauma within the tunnel may cause primary tenosynovitis.[23] The flexor carpi radialis tendon must pass over or closely along the radiocarpal joint, scaphoid-trapezium-trapezoid joint, and carpometacarpal joints. Thus, any degenerative or inflammatory process of the underlying joints may result in secondary tendinitis.[8,27,36] Severe, invasive synovitis may even cause tendon rupture.[82]

Presenting symptoms are pain and swelling along the radial volar aspect of the wrist, just proximal to the volar crease. Pain may be elicited by resisted wrist flexion and radial deviation or by abrupt, passive wrist extension.[45]

Conservative treatment includes immobilization in a modified thumb spica (with or without restriction of the first metacarpal phalangeal joint; restriction is necessary with tendinitis of the first carpal metacarpal joint), oral antiinflammatory medications, and, in recalcitrant cases, corticosteroid injection of the fibroosseous tunnel. Patients who fail such methods require surgical release of the fibroosseus tunnel.[23,27]

**FIGURE 11.**
Test position for extensor carpi ulnaris subluxation involves forearm supination and ulnar deviation. (From Skiven T: Clinical examination of the wrist. J Hand Ther 9:104, 1996, with permission.)

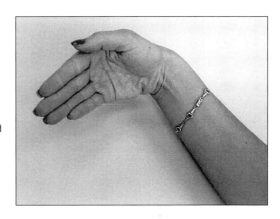

Flexor tendon rupture need not be repaired; debridement is sufficient for effective pain relief.[38]

### Flexor Carpi Ulnaris Tendinitis

Flexor carpi ulnaris tendinitis has been reported in golf, badminton, and squash, presumably because of the repetitive stresses in such sports.[33] Presenting symptoms include pain and swelling just distal to the pisiform,[62] but pain may radiate to the hypothenar eminence and or through the ulnar forearm to the medial and posterior lateral aspect of the elbow. Paresthesias in the ulnar nerve distribution of the hand also may be noted.[36]

Symptoms may be exacerbated by passive wrist extension and resisted flexion and ulnar deviation. Calcific tendinitis has been described and occasionally may be seen on a slightly supplanted, oblique lateral radiograph.[14] Pisotriquetral joint laxity and associated arthritis, which may produce similar symptoms,[33] can be differentiated by eliciting pain and crepitance with medial lateral displacement of the pisiform on the triquetrum. Pisotriquetral joint degeneration may be seen on a lateral radiograph with the wrist in slight supination and extension.[38]

Conservative treatment includes antiinflammatory medications, peritendinous corticosteroid injection, and splinting the wrist in 25° of flexion. Such measures may prove successful in 35% of patients with flexor carpi ulnaris tendinitis; in recalcitrant cases, excision of the pisiform and 5-mm Z-plasty lengthening of the flexor carpi ulnaris tendon are recommended.[61]

## Wrist Ganglions

Ganglions are the most common benign soft tissue tumor of the wrist and occur more commonly on the dorsal surface.[30] A history of trauma is found in only 15% of patients with dorsal ganglions and is particularly uncommon in patients with occult ganglions.[29] Dorsal ganglions arise from the scapholunate interosseus ligament, whereas volar ganglions arise from the flexor carpi radialis tendon sheath[51] and radiocarpal and scaphotrapezial joints.[1] Most extraosseous tumors about the wrist are benign, including synovial chondromatosis and cavernous and capillary hemangiomas, but malignant tumors such as peripheral nerve tumors and liposarcomas occur in rare cases.[9,74]

Presenting symptoms may include a palpable, soft-to-firm, cystlike mass that may vary in size and tension at the extremes of wrist motion. Occult wrist ganglions may not be palpable on physical examination but should be suspected in patients under the age of 35 years. Pain may include localized tenderness, and discomfort may be either constant or associated with activity only.[70] Deficits in wrist range of motion and grip strength have been described.[30]

Diagnosis is often based on clinical findings; however, occult wrist ganglions may go undetected until they are visualized either directly or, at times, microscopically.[30] Diagnosis by ultrasound and MRI with dedicated wrist coils has been described. MRI is particularly helpful for detecting occult ganglions and assessing the previously operated wrist.[25,35,80]

Conservative treatment includes aspiration, preferably with an 18-gauge needle, to facilitate return of the often viscous fluid; injection with lidocaine and corticosteroid; activity modification; and immobilization for 7–10 days. If conservative measures fail, incision and curetting[29] or excision of the cyst, including a small V-shaped portion of the scapholunate ligament, has been recommended.[70] Both procedures may be followed by immobilization in a wrist orthosis for 7–14 days; thereafter, controlled but frequent mobilization exercises (10 minutes every other hour while awake) may be started.[69]

## Ligamentous Injuries

Normal wrist motion necessitates the coordinated and controlled motion of the carpal bones within each row, between each row, and between the carpal metacarpal and carpal radial–TFC complex articulations. Acute traumatic ligamentous tears, chronic ligamentous attenuation, bone fracture, inflammatory arthritis, synovitis, or tendinitis may alter this delicate balance of motion. Attempts to classify such instabilities remain controversial and in a state of continual evolution. The foundational work of Linscheid and associates[48] has recently been expanded by Hodge,[34] who classifies carpal instabilities as follows:

- Carpal instability dissociative (CID): disruption of motion between carpal bones within the same row. CID may result from injury to the intrinsic ligaments or their bony attachments (i.e., avulsion fracture).
- Carpal instability nondissociative (CIND): disruption of motion of the carpal rows, with preservation of normal motion within each row. CIND is usually due to injury to the extrinsic ligaments, joint capsule, or their bony attachments.
- Carpal instability combined (CIC): disruption of motion between the individual carpal bones within a row and concurrent disruption of motion of either one or both carpal rows.
- Carpal instability adaptive (CIA): adaptive positioning of the carpal bones as allowed by uninjured ligaments.

Hodge[34] subclassifies these injuries by chronicity, constancy, etiology, location, direction, and pattern. A detailed discussion of these categories is beyond the scope of this chapter.

The usual mechanism of wrist injury is a fall on outstretched arm with forced wrist dorsiflexion, ulnar deviation, and supination. Mayfield[52] reproduced similar forces in the cadaver model and found a progressive pattern of perilunar instability. He staged the pattern as follows: (1) scapholunate diastasis, (2) dorsal dislocation of the capitate, (3) lunotriquetral dissociation, and (4) lunate dislocation.

Although Hodge's work allows classification of a large number of different wrist ligamentous injuries, only the major types seen clinically are discussed below.

### Scapholunate Ligament Injury

Scapholunate ligament injury is the most common pattern of carpal instability. Patients often present with a history of a fall on an extended arm with forced wrist dorsiflexion, ulnar deviation, and supination. Acute symptoms include pain, swelling, and tenderness over the dorsal radial aspect of the wrist as well as point tenderness over the scapholunate joint (just distal to Lister's tubercle). In chronic injury, patients may complain of dull achy wrist and forearm pain that worsens with repetitive or forceful activities. Watson's test may reveal dynamic scapholunate instability. In this maneuver, volar pressure is placed on the scaphoid tuberosity, and the wrist is passively drawn from full ulnar deviation to radial deviation, thereby blocking normal flexion of the scaphoid. Pain and a click or clunk, as the scaphoid is subluxated, are indicative of a positive test (Fig. 12). Comparison with the uninvolved wrist may prove helpful; however, the incidence of contralateral scapholunate ligament disruption has been reported in cadaver studies to be as high as 66%.[79]

A supinated anteroposterior radiograph of the wrist may reveal a scapholunate joint space greater than 2 mm, indicating diastasis of the joint. In addition, a cortical ring sign may be seen when the distal pole of the volarly flexed scaphoid is viewed on end[4] (Fig. 13). Lateral view of the wrist reveals an increased scapholunate angle of 70+° as the lunate extends and the scaphoid flexes, producing the pattern of dorsal intercalated segmental instability (DISI)[49] (Fig. 14). Midcarpal joint arthrogram reveals contrast dye filling the scapholunate joint. Minor degrees of subluxation may require

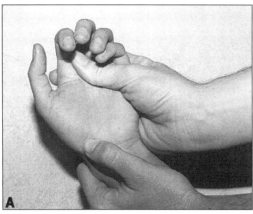
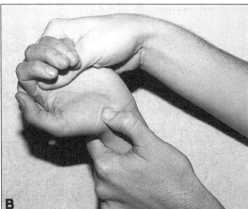

**FIGURE 12.**
Watson's scaphoid shift test to assess scaphoid stability. *Top,* Starting position is with the wrist in ulnar deviation. *Bottom,* Wrist is moved into radial deviation with constant thumb pressure over the volar scaphoid. (From Skiven T: Clinical examination of the wrist. J Hand Ther 9:104, 1996, with permission.)

cine fluoroscopic or arthroscopic evaluation for detection of instability. MRI with dedicated coils has been reported to be approximately 80% accurate in the diagnosis of scapholunate ligament tears.[83]

### Lunotriquetral Ligament Injury

Injury of the lunotriquetral ligament has been described with dorsiflexion and rotational stresses to the wrist.[12,66] Patients often present with pain on the dorsal ulnar aspect of the wrist and note clicking with ulnar circumduction. Grip weakness also may be present.[30] Physical examination reveals point tenderness over the lunotriquetral joint (just distal to the ulnar head). The lunotriquetral ballottement test is helpful in differentiating this injury from triangular fibrocartilage complex injury. The lunate is immobilized between the thumb and index finger of one hand while the index finger and thumb of the other hand mobilize the triquetrum and pisiform in a dorsal-to-volar direction. A positive test reproduces the patient's pain and clicking sensation[63] (Fig. 15). As with most ligamentous injuries, comparison with the uninvolved side may prove helpful; however, cadaver studies have revealed a 53% prevalence of lunotriquetral ligament tears in the contralateral wrist.[79]

A posteroanterior radiograph of the wrist may reveal a triangular-shaped and palmar-flexed lunate, which may overlap the triquetrum. Diastasis of the lunotriquetral joint may not be seen; however, rotation and extension of the triquetrum produce a step deformity of the normally smooth arc of the proximal row (Fig. 16). On lateral radiograph

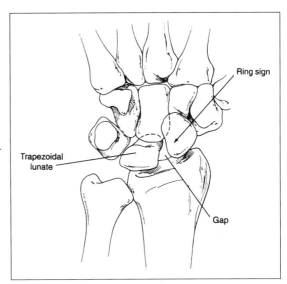

**FIGURE 13.**
Scapholunate dissociation. The scaphoid is palmar flexed, producing a cortical ring sign. A gap is present between the scaphoid and the lunate. The lunate appears trapezoidal. (From Bednar JM, Osterman AL: Carpal instability. J Am Acad Orthop Surg 1:14, 1993, with permission.)

the lunate and scaphoid assume a flexed posture as the capitate and triquetrum are extended; this produces a scapholunate angle of less than 30° and the characteristic volar intercalated segment instability pattern (VISI)[63] (Fig. 14). Midcarpal arthrography may reveal contrast dye in the lunotriquetral joint, communicating with the radiocarpal joint. MRI is reported to be only 50% accurate in the diagnosis of lunotriquetral ligament injury.[83] The lunotriquetral joint may be injected with lidocaine to assess its contribution

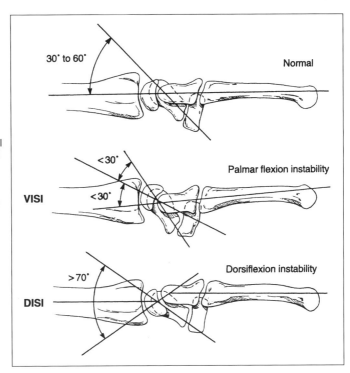

**FIGURE 14.**
Scapholunate angle measurement in normal wrist, volar intercalated segment instability (VISI), and dorsal intercalated segment instability (DISI). (From Bednar JM, Osterman AL: Carpal instability. J Am Acad Orthop Surg 1:14, 1993, with permission.)

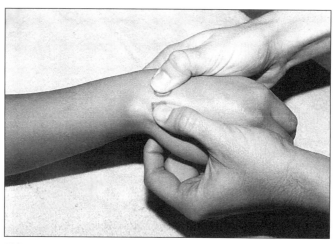

**FIGURE 15.**
Ballottement test for lunotriquetral instability. (From Skiven T: Clinical
examination of the wrist. J Hand Ther 9:103, 1996, with permission.)

to ulnar wrist pain complaints.[30] As with other wrist ligamentous injuries, arthroscopy
may help to delineate the extent of injury, dynamic stability, and other concurrent injuries, such as chondromalacia and triangular fibrocartilage complex damage, all of
which influence treatment decisions and prognosis.[79]

### Triquetrohamate Ligament Injury

Triquetrohamate ligament injuries often occur in wrist dorsiflexion from either an
acute traumatic insult[48] or chronic repetitive attenuation.[73] Clinical presentation varies
with the chronicity of injury. A new injury may present with acute ulnar pain, swelling,
and point tenderness over the triquetrohamate interspace. In chronic injury an often
painful, audible click or clunk may be appreciated with ulnar wrist deviation.[12]

A helpful diagnostic maneuver is the midcarpal instability test, in which pressure
is directed on the dorsal wrist at the distal end of the capitate by the examiner's thumb.

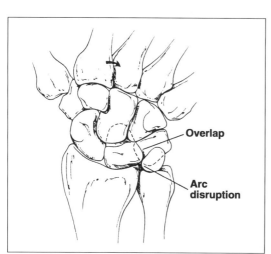

**FIGURE 16.**
Lunotriquetral instability. Shortened
scaphoid and cortical ring sign are
present without scapholunate widening.
Lunate appears triangular. Lunotriquetral widening is not present. (From
Bednar JM, Osterman AL: Carpal
instability. J Am Acad Orthop Surg 1:15,
1993, with permission.)

Axial loading and ulnar deviation are then introduced. A painful click is indicative of midcarpal instability.[73]

Tears of the triquetrohamate ligament (ulnar arm of the arcuate ligament) result in midcarpal instability and usually in a nondissociative VISI pattern on plain radiograph.[12]

### Extrinsic Ligament Injury

True dislocations of the carpus or wrist occur through disruption of the extrinsic ligaments, often associated with high-energy hyperextension injuries that also cause intrinsic damage.[52] As many as 40% of intraarticular distal radius fractures may be associated with wrist extensor ligamentous injuries.[83] This acute injury presents as a painful, swollen wrist with marked limitations of motion. Nerve compression symptoms, particularly the median nerve, are often reported.[76] Chronic cases often present with vague, diffuse pain but no significant swelling. A sudden painful clunk is often reported with radial to ulnar deviation. Examination of the contralateral wrist may help to differentiate an old isolated ligamentous injury from a generalized hyperlaxity state. Gross malalignments may or may not be readily apparent. In cases of ulnar extrinsic ligament injury, a carpal supination deformity may be noted (Fig. 17).

**FIGURE 17.**
Relocation test for ulnocarpal instability. *Top,* Instability is characterized by volar sag and supination of the wrist. *Bottom,* Relocation of the carpus is accomplished by volar-to-dorsal glide and pronation of the carpus. (From Skiven T: Clinical examination of the wrist. J Hand Ther 9:103, 1996, with permission.)

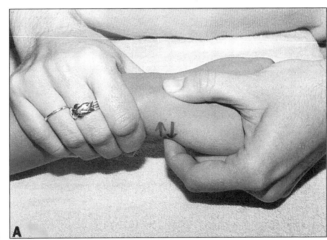

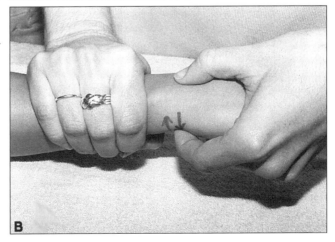

Plain radiographs may be unrevealing if spontaneous reduction has occurred. A posteroanterior view with either radial or ulnar deviation may reveal disruption of the radiocarpal articulation. Lateral radiographs usually demonstrate a VISI pattern, but a DISI pattern may be seen in rare cases. MRI with dedicated coils may prove helpful in acute injuries,[88] and arthrography may demonstrate a tear of the volar capsule. This tear may scar over in time and render later arthrograms normal.[83] Arthroscopy allows direct visualization of the injured extrinsic ligaments.

### Treatment and Rehabilitation

Treatment of carpal instabilities remains controversial. Decisions about nonoperative vs. surgical treatment are influenced by chronicity of the injury, location of the injured ligament, degree of ligamentous disruption, presence or absence of associated bony injury or arthritic changes, position and stability of displaced segments, and anticipated functional demands on the wrist after repair (e.g., laborer, typist).[17] Many believe that scapholunate tears are best addressed through surgical means such as direct ligamentous reconstruction, intercarpal bony fusion, plating, compression screws, Kirschner wires and plaster, or capsulodesis.[4,16,37,88] Lunotriquetral and triquetrohamate ligament injuries are often amenable to nonoperative treatment such as custom-molded thermoplastic splinting or plaster casting in a long-arm cast for at least 6–8 weeks.[12,88] If conservative measures fail, ligamentous injuries can be addressed through the surgical interventions noted above.[4]

Before initiation of rehabilitative therapies, the surgical procedure and its expected outcome must be clearly understood. After surgical intervention and subsequent immobilization, limitations in wrist motion are to be expected (in fact, desired in the case of a fusion procedure) by the patient and therapist. Therapy should not be initiated until the surgeon judges the tensile strength of ligamentous repairs to be adequate; likewise, bony fusions should be assessed by tomograms to ensure solid consolidation and to judge alignment of the carpus. Cooney recommends immobilization in a thumb spica cast for an average of 8 weeks for either ligamentous repair or bony fusion, followed by a thumb spica splint for an additional 4–6 weeks.[17]

Even before removal of the cast, the patient should become an active participant in the rehabilitative program. Elevation of the involved wrist, minimal use of a sling, and range-of-motion exercises for the shoulder and elbow (if not casted) should be taught and encouraged. Low-weight, high-repetition resistive exercises for the shoulder girdle musculature are recommended to avoid inadvertent deconditioning during wrist immobilization.

Early therapeutic interventions after postoperative casting should be aimed at the control and mobilization of edema and release of soft tissue that may have become adherent and adaptively shortened during postoperative immobilization.[69] Therapeutic massage and compressive wraps, sleeves, or gloves may facilitate removal and control of edema. Myofascial release and other deep tissue mobilization techniques help to restore gliding between tissue planes before joint mobilization is attempted.[78]

In most patients, restoration of motion equal to the uninvolved wrist is not the goal; rather, painfree motion in a functional range (approximately 40° of flexion, 40° of extension, and 40° of combined radial to ulnar deviation) may be a more realistic early goal.[68] Cannon and others[13,44] advocate active range-of-motion (AROM) exercises for 1 month after cast removal and then progression to passive range-of-motion exercises (PROM). Overly aggressive or too frequent stretching (high-load brief or high-load prolonged stress) may cause microtrauma and inflammation that impede healing.[11,72] Low-load prolonged stress is the preferred form of passive joint mobilization. It is believed to allow permanent remodeling and lengthening of scar tissue, whereas high-load prolonged stress and high-load brief stress may lead to tissue failure.[21] Thus, rigid casting or splinting at the end of the elastic limits of the contracted tissue may provide benefit over some forms of dynamic splinting, which may engage this endpoint only intermittently.[5]

Laseter[43] reports that a key important principle in wrist rehabilitation is reestablishment of independent wrist extension without the assistance of the digit extensors. This substitution pattern, which follows prolonged immobilization of the wrist, must be abolished early if overall hand function is to improve. Isolated wrist extension should be taught with the fingers in flexion and the patient monitoring the metacarpal joints to ensure no assistance from the digit extensors. Occasionally, functional neuromuscular electrical stimulation of the extensor is necessary to facilitate this retraining.[57] Likewise, wrist flexion should be performed with the digits in an extended postion and relaxed. Wrist radial and ulnar deviation should be performed with the forearm pronated and the hand flat on the table to avoid substitutive patterns in these planes of motion.

The addition of progressive resistive strengthening exercises should be delayed until 4–6 months after surgical repair of the wrist, because grip-strengthening exercises load the carpus and produce significant stress across the site of fusion or ligament repair.[13,40] Resistive training should begin with isometric strengthening of the forearm musculature, followed by isotonic concentric and then isotonic eccentric strengthening. Combined and functional specific resistive training should be withheld until strength and endurance are comparable to the uninvolved side.

Bony fusions should be protected by either a cast or orthosis until solid consolidation of the fusion is confirmed by tomograms. Likewise, ligamentous repairs should be protected for a minimum of 3 months before return to work or sporting activities.[17] On return to athletic play, a fiberglass short-arm thumb spica cast covered with at least $\frac{1}{4}$-inch, closed-cell, high-density foam may afford adequate protection in contact sports.[24] When slight motion is allowable and necessary or when rigid casting is not allowed by sport governing bodies, a silicone rubber short-arm thumb spica cast may be substituted. These casts are typically covered in $\frac{1}{2}$-inch, closed-cell, high-density foam.[3,7]

## ELBOW

The elbow joint and its associated neurovascular and soft tissue structures may be injured as a result of repetitive upper extremity forces or an acute, single traumatic event. Relevant anatomy and functional biomechanical principles are presented to aid in formulating a working diagnosis and implementing a rehabilitation plan. Treatment initially involves controlling the inflammatory process, followed by a therapeutic exercise program. To provide timely healing, safe return to preinjury status, and diminished risk for reinjury, the treatment program must also address functioning of the upper extremity kinetic chain, sport technique, training regimens, and proper equipment use.

### Anatomy and Biomechanics

The elbow joint does not act in isolation but rather as an integral component of the upper extremity kinetic chain. The joint serves as the anatomic link between the shoulder and hand, thereby allowing hand placement as well as upper extremity force transmission and absorption.[83]

The distal humerus consists of two condyles that form the articular surface of the trochlea and capitellum (Figs. 18 and 19). The laterally situated capitellum serves as a buttress for lateral compression and rotational forces, as commonly encountered in throwing motions.[94] The lateral epicondyle is located proximal to the capitellum and serves as an attachment site for the supinator-extensor muscle groups as well as the lateral collateral ligament. Situated above the capitellum is the radial fossa, which accommodates the radial head during flexion. The medial epicondyle is situated proximal to the trochlea and

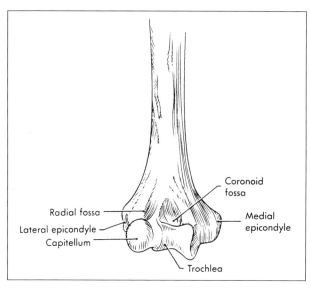

**FIGURE 18.**
Anterior view of the distal humerus. (From Anderson TL: Anatomy and physiology of the elbow. In Nicholas JA, et al (eds): The Upper Extremity in Sports Medicine. St. Louis, Mosby, 1995, p 265, with permission.)

serves as the attachment site for the medial collateral ligament as well as the flexor-pronator muscles. Superior and anterior to the trochlea lies the coronoid fossa, with the olecranon fossa situated posteriorly. The trochlea of the humerus articulates with the olecranon of the ulna, thereby defining the plane of flexion and extension.[67]

The ulnohumeral joint is formed by the articulation of the greater sigmoid notch of the ulna and the trochlea (Fig. 20). The opening of the sigmoid notch is angled 30° posteriorly, allowing maximal range of motion while maintaining articular conformity.[16,44] The coronoid process forms the distal and anterior aspect of the notch, with

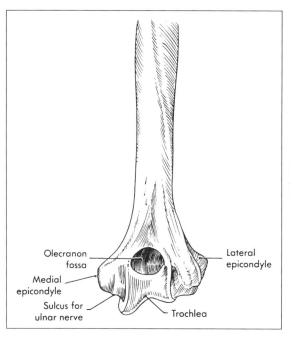

**FIGURE 19.**
Posterior view of the distal humerus. (From Anderson TL: Anatomy and physiology of the elbow. In Nicholas JA, et al (eds): The Upper Extremity in Sports Medicine. St. Louis, Mosby, 1995, p 266, with permission.)

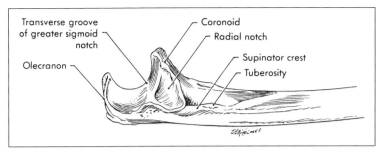

**FIGURE 20.**
Lateral view of the proximal ulna. (From Anderson TL: Anatomy and physiology of the elbow. In Nicholas JA, et al (eds): The Upper Extremity in Sports Medicine. St. Louis, Mosby, 1995, p 267, with permission.)

the olecranon forming the proximal and posterior aspect. The radial notch, also known as the lateral or lesser sigmoid notch, is located along the lateral aspect of the coronoid process. The radial head articulates with the radial notch and is stabilized by the annular ligament, which attaches to the anterior and posterior margins of the notch. The medial aspect of the coronoid process provides the attachment site for the anterior portion of the medial collateral ligament and the ulnar portion of the pronator teres.[16,56] The cylindrical radial head articulates with the capitellum as well as the proximal ulna. The radial neck is distal to the head, with the radial tuberosity forming the most distal aspect of the neck.

The elbow joint is commonly described as a hinge joint, but complex motions are allowed through the combined movements of both flexion-extension and pronation-supination. Specifically, the ulnohumeral (trochlear) articulation is considered a uniaxial hinge joint, allowing 1° of freedom, namely flexion and extension. The radiohumeral and proximal radioulnar articulations allow axial rotation and may be considered pivot-type joints. The axis of elbow flexion-extension is through the center of the trochlea and capitellum, with the axis of supination-pronation situated within the center of the radial head and the capitellum and along a line through the base of the ulnar styloid.[49,55]

## Ligamentous and Capsular Stability

The collateral ligaments are specialized thickenings of the medial and lateral capsule. The medial collateral ligament (MCL) is composed of three bands: a major anterior oblique band, a thin posterior portion, and a nonfunctional transverse ligament (Fig. 21). The proximal attachment of the MCL is at the inferior surface of the medial epicondyle in a somewhat medial position, with the anterior band positioned posterior to the axis of rotation. The ligamentous fibers of the anterior portion insert along the medial aspect of the coronoid process, and the posterior band inserts on the medial aspect of the posterior olecranon. The anterior oblique band is the prime stabilizer of the joint medially; a portion of the anterior band, due to its continuum of fiber insertions, remains taut throughout the range of elbow motion.[74,78] Sectioning of the posterior band, which is lax until approximately 60° of flexion, causes minimal change in elbow stability.[55] Because the transverse ligament arises and inserts onto the ulna, it does not contribute to elbow stability.[59]

The lateral ligamentous complex is not as clearly defined and has a more variable pattern than the medial structures (Fig. 22). According to Morrey, the complex is comprised of the radial collateral ligament, lateral ulnar collateral ligament, accessory lateral collateral ligament, and annular ligament.[56]

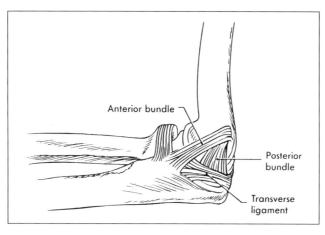

**FIGURE 21.**
Medial collateral ligaments of the elbow. (From Anderson TL: Anatomy and physiology of the elbow. In Nicholas JA, et al (eds): The Upper Extremity in Sports Medicine. St. Louis, Mosby, 1995, p 269, with permission.)

The lateral collateral ligament complex provides stability to varus stress. While the radial collateral ligament is taut throughout flexion and extension, the accessory collateral ligament is taut only with varus stress and is unrelated to flexion and extension positions. The lateral ulnar collateral ligament provides the primary restraint to posterolateral rotatory instability.[16,69]

The annular ligament originates and inserts onto the anterior and posterior margins of the radial notch and maintains contact of the radius with the ulna, thereby limiting distal migration of the radius. Because of the tapered nature of the ligament distally, it assumes the shape of a funnel and constitutes about four-fifths of the fibroosseous ring, with the remainder of the ring formed by the radial notch. The ligamentous complex in concert with the radial notch functions at the limits of biomechanical tolerance; thus, disruption of the anatomic structures may lead to loss of articular congruity with subsequent deficits in forearm rotation.[3,56]

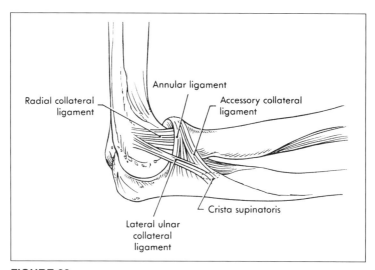

**FIGURE 22.**
Lateral collateral ligaments of the elbow. (From Anderson TL: Anatomy and physiology of the elbow. In Nicholas JA, et al (eds): The Upper Extremity in Sports Medicine. St. Louis, Mosby, 1995, p 268, with permission.)

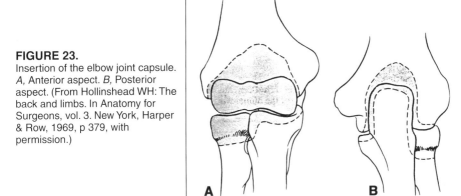

**FIGURE 23.**
Insertion of the elbow joint capsule.
*A,* Anterior aspect. *B,* Posterior
aspect. (From Hollinshead WH: The
back and limbs. In Anatomy for
Surgeons, vol. 3. New York, Harper
& Row, 1969, p 379, with
permission.)

The anterior joint capsule inserts proximally above the level of the coronoid and radial fossae, distally and medially to the anterior aspect of the coronoid, and laterally to the annular ligament (Fig. 23). The anterior capsule is taut in extension and lax in flexion. Posteriorly, the capsule attaches just superior to the olecranon fossa and the medial and lateral margins of the trochlea. The posterior capsule is redundant, allowing full range of motion at the elbow and accumulation of fluid secondary to inflammatory conditions. [5,56]

## Muscles

The extensors of the wrist and fingers originate from a common tendinous origin at the lateral distal humerus and epicondyle and consist of the extensor carpi radialis brevis (ECRB), extensor carpi radialis longus (ECRL), extensor carpi ulnaris (ECU), and extensor digitorum communis musculature (EDC). The brachioradialis is discussed on the basis of its functional role rather than its anatomic position. [68]

The flexor-pronator muscle group includes the pronator teres, flexor carpi radialis, flexor carpi ulnaris, and palmaris longus. The muscles arise from the medial epicondyle via a common flexor tendon. The pronator teres is the most proximal and superficial of this group. The two heads arise from the medial epicondyle and coronoid process of the ulna. Their insertion is at the junction of the proximal and middle portions of the lateral aspect of the radius through a common musculotendinous unit. An arch is formed by the two heads through which the median nerve courses on its way to the forearm, thereby creating a potential site for entrapment. The muscle serves as a primary pronator of the forearm as well as a weak elbow flexor. The flexor carpi radialis and palmaris longus, when present, function as wrist flexors and also may assist with forearm pronation. [72] The flexor carpi ulnaris is the most posterior of these muscles and functions as a wrist flexor and ulnar deviator because of its insertion into the pisiform. The ulnar nerve passes between its two heads, creating a potential site for compressive neuropathy. [34,56]

The primary elbow flexor muscles include the brachioradialis, biceps brachii, and brachialis, with secondary contributions by the pronator teres and flexor carpi ulnaris. [24] The brachioradialis originates from the lateral border of the humerus and the lateral intermuscular septum and inserts at the lateral aspect of the distal radius. It provides the greatest mechanical advantage of the elbow flexors, adding speed and power. The biceps brachii is a major flexor of the elbow with the two heads joining into a common tendon that passes in front of the elbow to insert on the radial tuberosity. Because the tuberosity is situated on the ulnar surface of the radius, the biceps in producing flexion also rotates the radius to provide supination. Thus, in the pronated position the biceps functions more as a supinator than as an elbow flexor. The brachialis, although having the largest cross-sectional area of the flexors, suffers from a poor mechanical advantage as it crosses close to the axis of rotation. Unlike the biceps, however, the brachialis attaches to the ulnar tuberosity and does not contribute to pronation or supination; thus, it is equally effective in flexing the forearm, regardless of the position of rotation.[34,56]

The primary elbow extensor is the triceps brachii, which is composed of three heads, two of which originate along the posterior aspect of the humerus. The long head originates from the infraglenoid tuberosity of the scapula. The three heads combine to insert onto the olecranon, with the attachment separated by the olecranon bursa. Although various bursae have been described about the elbow, the most commonly involved bursal structure is the superficial olecranon bursa, which may be injured by direct trauma and repetitive pressure or inflammatory conditions.

The anconeus originates from the lateral epicondyle with insertion along the lateral side of the olecranon and ulna. It assists in stabilization of the elbow joint during flexion and forearm rotation motions and also serves as a secondary elbow extensor.[34]

The supinator originates from the lateral aspect of the lateral epicondyle, lateral collateral ligament, and posterolateral surface of the ulna just below the radial notch (crista supinatoris). It courses in a downward and lateral manner to insert diffusely onto the radius. As the name implies, the muscle serves as a supinator of the forearm. Unlike the supination action of the biceps, its effectiveness is not altered by the position of the elbow. It is believed, however, to be a weaker supinator than the biceps. The radial nerve divides the fibers into superfical and deep layers, with the arcade of Frohse referring to the thickened edge of the superficial component.[34,56]

## Elbow Injuries and Rehabilitation Management

### Lateral Elbow Injuries

Although the most common injury to the lateral elbow complex is lateral epicondylitis, the differential diagnosis also includes entrapment neuropathies, namely posterior interosseous involvement, which may mimic lateral epicondylitis or coexist with it; lateral compression injuries, which primarily involve the bony structures and result from abnormal compression forces at the radiocapitellar region; and referred pain processes[30] (Table 2).

**Lateral Epicondylitis.**   The athlete with lateral epicondylitis (Table 3) is most commonly involved in racquet sports. Various factors that increase the likelihood of developing lateral epicondylitis in tennis players include older age, lower skill level, frequency of play, force and flexibility deficiencies of the forearm extensor muscles, and lack of coordinated functioning of the upper extremity kinetic chain.

**TABLE 2.**
Differential Diagnosis of Lateral Elbow Pain

| |
|---|
| Lateral epicondylitis |
| Radial tunnel syndrome/posterior interosseous nerve entrapment |
| Musculocutaneous nerve entrapment |
| Posterolateral rotatory instability/lateral collateral ligament disruption |
| Osteochondritis dissecans |
| Radiocapitellar degenerative changes/loose body formation |
| Fractures (radial head, capitellum/distal humerus, lateral epicondyle) |
| Cervical radiculopathy/referred pain process |

**TABLE 3.**
Components of Tissue Injury in Lateral Epicondylitis

| |
|---|
| **Method of presentation**<br>Insidious onset with gradually increasing symptoms and/or acute exacerbation of a chronic injury. |
| **Tissue injury complex**<br>Microtears in the extensor carpi radialis brevis tendon with angiofibromatous changes. |
| **Clinical symptoms complex**<br>Tenderness over the lateral epicondylar region with associated swelling, pain with resisted wrist extension that may extend distally into the forearm, and weakness of grip strength. |
| **Functional biomechanical deficit**<br>Wrist extensor muscle inflexibility and weakness, weak shoulder external rotation, tight shoulder internal rotators. |
| **Functional adaptation complex**<br>Poor backhand technique, change in racquet (grip size, composition, string tension) or playing surface. |
| **Tissue overload complex**<br>Wrist extensor group, shoulder rotators, and scapular stabilizers |

Adapted from Kibler WB, Chandler TJ, Stracener ES: Musculoskeletal adaptations and injuries due to overtraining. Sport Sci Rev 20:99–126, 1992.

Most tennis players with lateral epicondylitis have developed altered backhand mechanics, whereby the elbow leads into the backhand swing. Excessive spin and repetitive peripheral rather than central ball-racquet contact may lead to excessive rotational torque to the racquet, thereby increasing the demand on the wrist extensor musculature to control the abnormal forces.[12,33,68,76] When altered sport mechanics develop, the biomechanically inefficient position transfers forces to the extensor muscles of the forearm rather than to the larger shoulder and trunk muscles. Dysfunction within the entire kinetic chain may ultimately include not only strength and flexibility deficits of the wrist and finger extensors but also weakness in the posterior shoulder musculature.[42]

The patient may present with pain and tenderness localized approximately 1 cm medial and distal to the lateral epicondyle over the origin of the extensor carpi radialis brevis.[67,70] The pain commonly increases with resisted wrist or digit extension, especially with the elbow extended, and with gripping activities and end-range passive wrist flexion (Fig. 24). Anteroposterior and lateral elbow radiographs may be considered to assess degenerative changes at the radiocapitellar joint and to better delineate bony articulation.[22]

The pathophysiology of lateral epicondylitis involves the forearm extensors, most commonly the extensor carpi radialis brevis and less commonly the extensor carpi radialis longus and anterior portion of the extensor communis tendon. Nirschl described the pathologic process involving the tendon origin as angiofibroblastic tendinosis, which results from tensile overuse, fatigue, weakness, and possibly avascular changes secondary to anoxia and vascular thrombosis. Such changes appear consistent with a degenerative process rather than primary inflammation.[63,65] If progressive insult occurs, partial and, more rarely, complete tears in the extensor radialis brevis may develop.

**Controlling the Inflammatory Process.**    A period of relative rest in which the athlete avoids activities that increase symptoms is implemented. Total immobilization should be avoided because of the potential for further loss of motion and the increased risk for additional atrophy and strength loss in an already weakened muscle-tendon complex.[68] In the highly acute phase, however, the use of a wrist orthosis, with the wrist positioned in approximately 15° of extension, may be helpful to rest the extensor musculature.[13] Icing techniques and nonsteroidal antiinflammatory medication may be effective during the initial healing period. Additional modalities, including high-voltage galvanic stimulation, iontophoresis, and whirlpool, may help to control pain and inflammation.[23,43]

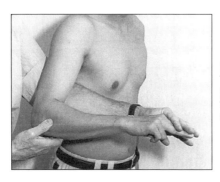

**FIGURE 24.**
Test for lateral epicondylitis. The test is positive when pain is elicited approximately 1 cm medial and distal to the lateral epicondyle with resisted wrist or third digit extension.

**Restoration of Normal Tissue Functioning.**   As the acute symptoms diminish, a therapeutic exercise program is initiated. For lateral epicondylitis, specific attention is directed to the wrist and finger extensors. A comprehensive muscle reconditioning program is provided, and multiplane and multijoint exercises are incorporated to simulate functional activities (Table 4).

To improve wrist flexion mobility, which is often limited by the tight extensor musculature, the wrist extensors are placed on a passive stretch with the elbow extended[6,85,91] (Fig. 25). Heating modalities, including ultrasound and phonophoresis; myofascial release techniques; and joint mobilizations and distractions can be used to improve soft tissue mobility and joint range of motion.[17,46]

As pain-free range of motion is obtained, strength training is initiated. For the patient with lateral epicondylitis, multiple angle isometric exercises within the pain-free range and manual resistance exercises, focusing initially on the wrist extensors are provided. A progressive resistance program is then incorporated[91] (Figs. 26 and 27). The muscles of pronation-supination and radial-ulnar motions can be strengthened through the use of a weighted rod[32,91] (Fig. 28). As functional range of wrist and elbow motion is obtained, isokinetic devices may be useful in delineating strength imbalances and upgrading high-velocity endurance patterns.[21,68,82]

Proprioceptive neuromuscular facilitation techniques incorporating diagonal patterns with dynamic stabilization and slow reversal holds are used to improve elbow control and to upgrade functional patterns.[88,92] The use of wall pulleys may be considered to simulate the forehand, backhand, and overhead motions. Complex concentric-eccentric strengthening and endurance routines can be implemented through the use of resistive tubing.[45,91]

**Kinetic Chain Performance.**   Anatomic and functional deficits of the upper extremity kinetic chain need to be evaluated since the force and power provided by the trunk and lower extremities must be efficiently transferred through the shoulder complex to the elbow, forearm, wrist, and hand. As the cervical spine serves as the fulcrum for the shoulders as the body rotates in relation to the ball, cervical dysfunction may inhibit efficient kinetic chain motion. When the cervical spine and shoulder fail to provide proximal stabilization for upper extremity functioning, deficits develop distally. For example, the effects of agonist-antagonist imbalances of tight internal shoulder rotators and weak external rotators transfer into abnormal overload patterns at the elbow and must therefore

**TABLE 4.**
Flexibility and Strengthening of the Relevant Muscle Groups in Elbow Dysfunction

| | | |
|---|---|---|
| Elbow flexion-extension | Wrist flexion-extension | Hand intrinsics |
| Forearm pronation-supination | Wrist radial-ulnar deviation | |

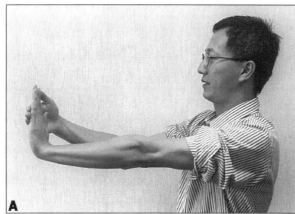

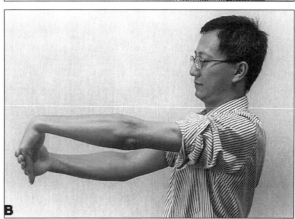

**FIGURE 25.**
Wrist stretching exercises.

be addressed.[20,72,90] Epidemiologic studies in tennis players identify a high prevalence of shoulder and elbow injuries, highlighting the necessity of a comprehensive rehabilitation approach. Priest and Nagel reported that among tennis players, 74% of men and 60% of women had a history of shoulder or elbow injuries of the dominant arm, with both the shoulder and elbow of the dominant arm involved in 21% of men and 23% of women.[73]

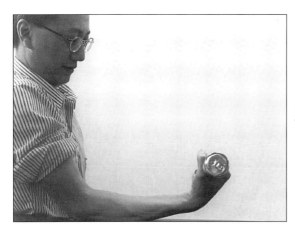

**FIGURE 26.**
Wrist flexion strengthening.

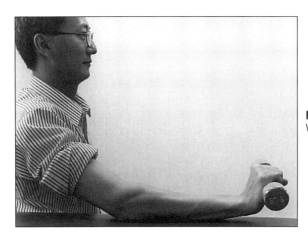

**FIGURE 27.**
Wrist extension strengthening.

**Safe Return to Sport Activity.** Attention is directed to proper technique, equipment modification, and sport-specific skill reacquisition. Interval training guidelines have been described by various authors for throwing athletes, tennis players, and golfers.[4,21,32,45,79] Progression in frequency, intensity, and duration of the particular activity should be guided by symptoms. Gradual progression of the athlete through sport-specific activities allows safe return to play with diminished risk for reinjury.[32]

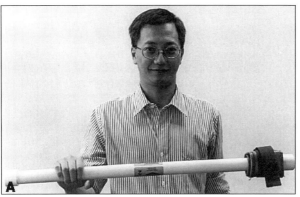

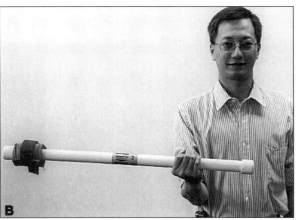

**FIGURE 28.**
A and B, Forearm pronation and supination strengthening.

**TABLE 5.**
Methods to Decrease Abnormal Force Transmission
to the Elbow Complex in Tennis Players

| |
| --- |
| Proper backhand mechanics, including a two-handed stroke |
| Racquet characteristics: |
|     Low-range string tension: 50–55 lb of tension |
|     Midsize racquet heads |
|     Proper grip size/grip padding |
|     Lightweight graphite composite construction |
| Playing surface |
|     Slower clay surface |
| Newer ball |
| Counterforce bracing |

For tennis players, controlling abnormal force transmission to the elbow is necessary for both proper tissue healing and prevention of reinjury. Various interventions have been described to diminish abnormal energy absorption secondary to the ball-racquet interface[38,45,63,68] (Table 5). Correction of improper backhand stroke and use of the two-handed backhand may decrease lateral epicondylar stress. Lowering string tension by 3–5 pounds, using racquets with midsized heads constructed of lightweight graphite, and playing with fresh balls may further decrease stress at the elbow.[22,33,47,68] Proper grip size allows the largest handle that the athlete's hand can comfortably control.[1] As described by Nirschl, grip size is determined by measuring from the tip of the ring finger along the radial border to a point on the proximal palmar crease[64] (Fig. 29).

Counterforce bracing has been advocated for decreasing the load at the epicondylar muscles.[31,66,68] Snyder-Mackler documented reduction in ECRB and EDC muscle activity with the use of an air-filled bladder counterforce orthosis.[81] The orthosis also may be used during the acute phase to diminish force production on the injured muscle-tendon unit, thereby decreasing pain and inflammation and assisting with healing.

Throughout the rehabilitation program, the physician and therapist must also identify activities in the patient's daily setting that may limit anticipated recovery. Finally, flexibility, strength, and muscular endurance of the uninvolved extremity as well as maintenance of overall body conditioning must not be overlooked at any stage in the rehabilitation process.

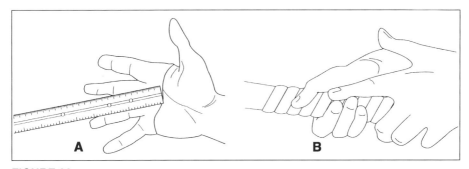

**FIGURE 29.**
A, Proper grip size may be determined by measuring along the radial side of the ring finger from the distal palmar crease to the fingertip. B, Alternatively, hold the racquet and see if a finger fits into the gap between the thumb and fingers. (From Liu YK: Mechanical analysis of racquet and ball during impact. Med Sci Sports Exerc 15:388, 1983, with permission.)

**Additional Treatment Considerations.** Local steroid injections may be considered for athletes who fail to respond to the above treatment program after 8–12 weeks or patients with marked inflammation. Injections, like passive modalities and nonsteroidal antiinflammatory medication, should be considered as a tool to control pain and the inflammatory response so that the patient can participate more actively in the full rehabilitation program. Because steroids depress fibroblastic and chondroblastic protein synthesis, with increased risk for further connective tissue weakening and poor tendon healing, judicious use is recommended.[14,67] Injections should be spaced at least 1 month apart, with no more than three injections to the same region within 1 year.[15,28,40] Finally, for the most recalcitrant cases, in which symptoms last for more than 6–12 months despite an appropriate rehabilitation approach, surgical release and debridement may be necessary.[15,19,40,63,68]

### Medial Elbow Injuries (Table 6)

**Flexor-Pronator Strain, Medial Epicondylitis, and Medial Collateral Ligament Sprain.** Patients with flexor-pronator muscle strains present with pain, tenderness, and swelling radial to the medial epicondyle, whereas in patients with medial epicondylitis pain is more localized to the medial epicondyle. Symptoms increase with resisted wrist flexion and forearm pronation.[15,45] In golfers, stress to the flexor-pronator complex occurs with forceful and repetitive wrist flexion as the right-handed player forces the club head down at the ball with the right arm rather than pulling the club through with the left arm and trunk.[6] Medial epicondylar and flexor-pronator regional pain may occur during the tennis forehand, serve, and overhead shot as a result of combined valgus elbow stress, wrist flexion, and forearm pronation.[61] Players who commonly apply a top spin to their stroke also increase their risk for medial epicondylitis due to repetitive forced pronation motion.[22]

Repetitive valgus stress may lead to capsular and medial collateral ligamentous disruption (microtearing or complete rupture), osteophytic spur formation, and ulnar neuropathy. In addition to ulnar nerve compromise, the differential diagnosis of medial elbow pain includes more proximal neuropathic involvement, namely cervical radiculopathy, especially C8 lesions; lower trunk brachial plexus injuries; and thoracic outlet syndrome.[72] In throwing athletes, injury to the medial collateral ligament most commonly leads to pain complaints during the acceleration phase, with electromyographic (EMG) analysis showing the greatest activity in the pronator teres during this phase.[58] Medial elbow complex symptoms may also be noted at ball release and point of ball impact.[16,18]

**TABLE 6.**
Differential Diagnosis of Medial Elbow Pain

| |
|---|
| Medial epicondylitis |
| Flexor-pronator group strain/tear, Bennett's fascial compression syndrome |
| Medial collateral ligament disruption (sprain/tear) |
| Medial epicondylar avulsion fracture |
| Valgus extension overload complex |
| Ulnar neuropathy/cubital tunnel syndrome |
| Osteophytic spurring |
| Loose bodies |
| Cervical radiculopathy (C8/T1) |
| Brachial trunk/plexus injury/thoracic outlet syndrome |
| Referred pain process |

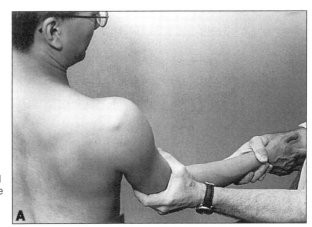

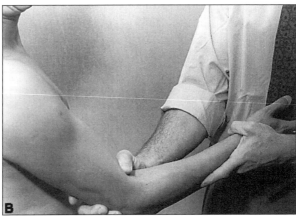

**FIGURE 30.**
Stability testing of the collateral ligaments of the elbow. With the elbow held in 20–30° flexion and the humerus firmly stabilized, a valgus stress is applied to test the medial collateral ligaments *(A)* or a varus stress test is applied to test the lateral collateral ligaments *(B).*

When the MCL has been injured, tenderness is noted approximately 2 cm distal to the medial epicondyle.[16] To assess ligamentous integrity, valgus stress testing is performed. Once the humerus is stabilized, a valgus force is applied to the elbow, which is flexed 20–30° to eliminate the articular stability provided by the olecranon (Fig. 30). With a positive result, medial opening with a less distinct endpoint in comparison with the uninvolved extremity is noted.[18,39,41] The examiner also may palpate the medial joint line beneath the medial collateral ligament while performing the stress test to precipitate pain.

To assist in differentiating ligamentous involvement from medial epicondylitis and pronator-flexor sprains, resistance against wrist flexion and forearm pronation does not commonly lead to pain with pure collateral compromise. Laxity is not noted on stress testing when only the flexor-pronator muscle group is involved.[94] Radiographs may show medial spurring off the proximal ulna, and heterotopic calcification may be seen after frank avulsion fractures.[94] To define more accurately the integrity of the medial collateral ligament, additional diagnostic evaluation may include MRI and computed tomographic (CT) arthrography.[54,86]

Treatment concepts for medial epicondylitis and flexor-pronator group strains are similar to those described for lateral epicondylitis. When the symptoms are highly acute, the wrist may be immobilized in 10° of palmar flexion to decrease tension on the flexor mass. In more severe cases, a splint blocking forearm rotation can also be considered.[77] As the pain diminishes, a therapeutic flexibility and strengthening program is begun with specific attention to the flexor-pronator group, upgrading to involve the entire kinetic chain.[91] Underlying biomechanical abnormalities, such as the pitcher who "opens up" prematurely with the dominant arm trailing behind the rotation of the trunk during the pitching motion, must also be addressed.[40] As with lateral epicondylitis, surgical intervention is indicated in recalcitrant cases in which conservative treatment has not provided adequate pain relief or functional improvement.[87] When significant disruption of the medial collateral ligament develops, reconstruction of the medial collateral ligament with the palmaris longus or short toe extensor tendon is pursued.[79]

### Posterior Elbow Injuries

**Extensor Musculotendinous and Bursal Compromise** (Table 7).    Triceps tendinitis most commonly results from repetitive overload of the extensor muscles due to hyperextension forces, as seen in pitchers, shot-putters, weightlifters, and gymnasts. In gymnasts, the elbow is exposed to additional stress as it is placed into hyperextension during upper extremity weightbearing activities (e.g., vaulting, balance beam, floor events). The athlete commonly presents with elbow pain that may be associated with loss of elbow motion. Conservative management includes controlling the inflammatory process and elbow strengthening, with attention to the biceps group so that the elbow need not assume a hyperextended position.[2,51,52]

Olecranon bursitis most commonly develops from repetitive pressure applied to the posterior elbow region but also may result from acute impact. The athlete presents with swelling in the posterior aspect of the elbow, which may be painless. Pain is more commonly associated with an acute event or infection. The patient may report discomfort with flexion past 90°, but range of motion is usually within functional limits. Radiographs may identify soft-tissue calcification, and with acute trauma, an olecranon or trochlear fracture may be seen. Aspiration with analysis of fluid from the swollen bursa is indicated when septic arthritis is suspected; however, in the noninfectious setting aspiration alone may not prevent fluid reaccumulation. Treatment includes rest through splinting, compression, cryotherapy alternating with warm soaks, and nonsteroidal antiinflammatory medication. A pad over the bursae may decrease recurrences. Surgical excision may be necessary in chronic cases.[16,50,75]

Triceps rupture with associated avulsion fractures may result from forceful and uncoordinated triceps contracture, as seen during a fall or direct impact to the elbow. Triceps disruption also has been seen in weightlifters and may be associated with anabolic steroid use or local steroid injections. Most tears occur at the tendon insertion; fewer cases are noted at the musculotendinous junction. Clinical presentation includes pain and ecchymosis over the triceps insertion, which may be associated with a palpable defect. Elbow extension is limited with increased pain response. Radiographs may identify a small fleck of bone avulsed from the olecranon. Surgical intervention is the treatment of choice.[9,16,80,84]

**Valgus Extension Overload Syndrome.**    In throwing athletes, most injuries to the posterior compartment result from repetitive valgus forces generated at the posterior

**TABLE 7.**
Differential Diagnosis of Posterior Elbow Pain

| | |
|---|---|
| Triceps tendinitis/rupture | Valgus extension overload syndrome |
| Olecranon bursitis | Osteophytes |
| | Loose body formation |
| Olecranon fractures | |
| | Dislocation |
| Olecranon apophysitis | |

medial aspect of the elbow during the acceleration phase. Additional extension sheer stess is created during the follow-through/deceleration phase as the triceps acts on the olecranon, leading to olecranon compression and impingement against the posteromedial portion of the fossa.[5,93] The syndrome may lead to loss of proper articulate congruity due to the hypertrophy of the distal humerus as well as osteophyte formation at the posteromedial aspect of the olecranon tip.[5,8,40] Abnormal compression at the radiocapitellar joint may develop, especially when the medial collateral ligament has been injured.[22,60]

Pain and tenderness are localized to the posteromedial aspect of the elbow, often with swelling. The symptoms increase with extension and valgus stress testing. Patients also may report crepitus, catching, and frank locking when a loose fragment is free within the joint.[5,93] Pitchers often describe pain that increases early in the game, leading to loss of control, early ball release, and highly thrown pitches. Tennis players report similar symptoms with overhead serves as they reach full extension.[41]

The valgus extension overload test is helpful in determining whether pain is the result of posteromedial osteophytes abutting against the medial margin of the olecranon fossa. The test is performed by forcing the elbow into extension while exerting a valgus stress, thereby simulating the position of the arm during the acceleration phase. At the same time, the examiner palpates over the posteromedial olecranon tip to elicit tenderness as well as crepitation (Fig. 31). In a positive test, pain is reproduced at the posteromedial olecranon process.[7,93] To assess for degenerative changes at the radiohumeral joint, the elbow is supinated and pronated in varying degrees of flexion. While performing this motion, the examiner palpates the head of the radius, feeling for crepitus, popping, or reproduction of pain.[2,7]

Radiographic evaluation includes standard anteroposterior and lateral views. An axial projection is helpful in identifying posteromedial osteophytes. Although radiographs can detect osteophytes and loose bodies, CT scans help to determine the three-dimensional anatomy.[71]

Management includes control of the inflammatory process, therapeutic exercise, and proper throwing mechanics. Attention is directed to balanced triceps and biceps

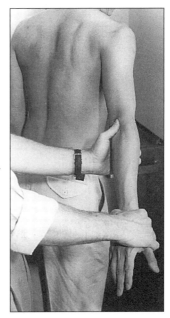

**FIGURE 31.**
Valgus extension overload test.

functioning and strengthening of the wrist flexors and forearm pronators.[6] Early loss of elbow extension must be treated aggressively. As normal tissue function is restored, higher-level eccentric-concentric training, using resistive tubing and weighted balls, can be initiated to simulate functional activities and train the athlete to transfer energy more efficiently and to stabilize the joints of the upper extremity kinetic chain.[92] An interval throwing program is ultimately provided. The athlete is advanced only when progress occurs without an increase in symptoms, as discussed under anterior elbow injuries. When chronic bony sequelae develop, surgical intervention is usually required.[15,63,89]

**Elbow Instability and Dislocations.**    Elbow subluxations and dislocations commonly result from falls onto an outstretched hand. The elbow undergoes an axial compressive force during flexion as the body approaches the ground as well as a supination and valgus moment as the body rotates internally on the elbow. Most elbow dislocations occur posteriorly, based on the final resting position of the olecranon relative to the distal humerus. Anterior dislocations occur in only 1–2% of patients with dislocations.[6]

The patient with a complete posterior dislocation presents with the limb in 45° of flexion and the olecranon situated posteriorly. Differentiation between posterior dislocation and supracondylar fracture may be difficult initially because of associated swelling and olecranon positioning. With a supracondylar fracture the normal alignment of the olecranon relative to the epicondyles is maintained. In the posterior dislocation, this relationship is altered; the olecranon is displaced from the plane of the epicondyles.[48]

Reduction, management of associated fractures, ongoing assessment of neurovascular status (with particular attention to the brachial artery and median and ulnar nerves), and early protected range of motion to minimize the risk of flexion ankylosis form the basis of treatment.[36,37] When arterial injury is present, emergent management directed at repairing the vascular insult is mandatory to minimize the risk for compartment syndrome.

Harrelson describes a rehabilitation program following reduction of a posterior elbow dislocation.[32] Posterior splint immobilization at 90° of flexion is provided. The splint may be removed for active elbow flexion-extension and supination-pronation exercises after 3–4 days; valgus stress is avoided. By 10 days to 2 weeks the splint should be discontinued and a full elbow flexibility and strengthening program pursued. A hinged brace also may be used postoperatively, allowing 15–90° of motion, for up to 4 weeks if stability is a concern.[6] On return to play the elbow may be braced or taped to limit elbow hyperextension and to provide protection from valgus forces. In unstable dislocations, the medial collateral ligament is repaired, and a longer period of joint protection is provided.[6]

### Anterior Elbow Injuries (Table 8)

Elbow hyperextension injuries may lead to anterior capsular disruption with damage to the elbow flexor muscles, median nerve, and brachial artery. Patients present with swelling anteriorly and inability to extend the elbow fully because of pain. Distal biceps tendinitis develops as a result of repetitive flexion and supination motions that lead to tenderness at the distal bicipital tendon insertion site with pain and weakness on resisted supination and flexion. Conservative management of capsular strains and bicipital tendinitis includes a brief period of immobilization, usually less than 5 days. A comprehensive therapeutic exercise program is then provided, ensuring full elbow range of motion and flexion and supination strength.[35,92]

Although rare, distal biceps ruptures may occur, usually due to a single traumatic event, with underlying degenerative tendinous changes associated with previous corticosteriod injections.[25] The tendon is generally avulsed from its insertion onto the radial tuberosity by eccentric contraction against an extension force that overloads the tendon.

**TABLE 8.**
Differential Diagnosis of Anterior Elbow Pain

| | |
|---|---|
| Anterior capsular strain/tear | Annular ligament disruption |
| Brachialis tendinitis | Loose body formation |
| Biceps tendinitis, distal biceps rupture | Adhesions/synovitis |
| Ectopic bone formation | Distal physeal humeral fracture |

Clinical signs include sudden onset of pain and asymmetry of the anterior arm muscu-lature. Supination and forearm weakness with associated antecubital ecchymosis are noted on examination. Treatment is surgical, as nonoperative management may lead to significant strength deficits.[10,50]

**Flexion Contractures.**    Morrey classifies the causes of elbow stiffness into three categories: (1) extrinsic causes, which include contractures of the joint capsule, sur-rounding musculature, and collateral lateral ligaments as well as ectopic bone forma-tion; (2) intrinsic causes, which include intraarticular adhesions, disruption of articular congruity, and loss of articular cartilage; and (3) combined causes, as seen with immo-bilization (extrinsic component) after an intraarticular fracture (intrinsic compo-nent).[57,58] The development of a complex regional pain syndrome also should be considered in the differential diagnosis of mobility loss and contracture development.

When relatively minimal mobility loss develops, management may include my-ofascial and soft tissue work, joint mobilization and proprioceptive neuromuscular tech-niques, flexiblity and joint range-of-motion exercises, and deep heating modalities to improve collagen extensibility. A passive stretch may be created by having the patient hold a 2–4-pound weight or a resistive band while resting the arm on a point proximal to the elbow joint. Stretching must be performed in a manner that ensures that the healing tissues are not overstretched and that the pain response is not increased. The proper degree of sustained stretch facilitates collagen fiber elongation, because pain and protec-tive muscle guarding are minimized. Aggressive high-force stretching is avoided to de-crease the risk of myositis ossificans with further pain and loss of motion.[4,32,62]

In the chronic setting and in patients with more significant loss of motion, dy-namic orthotics, static adjustable splints, and serial casting may be used. These tech-niques allow for gradual increase in range of elbow motion through the use of low-intensity, prolonged controlled force generation and are most effective in the ab-sence of intraarticular pathology[29,53,77] (see Fig. 30). In the most marked cases of elbow arthrofibrosis, surgical intervention is required.

## SHOULDER

Anatomically, the shoulder is designed for increased mobility and has a greater range of motion than any joint in the body. Because the shoulder girdle is not con-structed to control or prevent excessive motion, it is a leading target for injury. Soft tis-sues of the shoulder girdle (muscle, tendon, ligament, bursa), bone, and nerve tissue have specific functions, mechanisms of injury, and healing responses.[15]

Shoulder injuries are not uncommon in the workforce, through either repetitive mi-crotrauma or acute trauma. Soft tissue injuries of the shoulder commonly occur in con-tact sports such as football and hockey and are more likely to result in dislocations and fractures.[52] Noncontact sports such as swimming, racquet sports, volleyball, baseball, and weightlifting are also frequently associated with shoulder injuries but are more likely to result in repetitive microtrauma.[27,29,31,32,60] Downhill skiing, waterskiing, and board sports (snow board, wakeboard, surfboard, and skateboard ) also result in various impact injuries to the shoulder.[39,56]

Common soft tissue shoulder injuries include (1) various forms of glenohumeral instability; (2) rotator cuff, capsular, and bursal impingement injuries; (3) biceps tendinitis and tears; (4) glenoid labral injuries; (5) acromioclavicular joint injuries and arthritis; (6) sternoclavicular subluxations and dislocations; (7) isolated fractures or fractures associated with soft tissue injuries; (8) peripheral nerve and plexus injuries; (9) thoracic outlet syndrome; and (10) muscle tears. Most often the clinical history (mechanism of injury or pathomechanics) yields a preliminary diagnosis, which may be confirmed by further testing.

## Anatomy

Understanding the intricate anatomy and biomechanics of the shoulder girdle is imperative to mastering the complexities of a specific diagnosis and the rehabilitation process. Articulations of the shoulder girdle complex include the glenohumeral, acromioclavicular, and sternoclavicular joints and scapulothoracic, sternocostal, and costotransverse articulations (Fig. 32). The scapulohumeral group of muscles spans from the scapula to the humerus and includes the rotator cuff muscles (supraspinatus, infraspinatus, teres minor, and subscapularis) as the prime movers. The scapulohumeral group of muscles includes the deltoid, teres major, and coracobrachialis. The humeral group of muscles attaches from the trunk to the humerus and includes the pectoralis major, coracobrachialis, and latissimus dorsi. Lastly, the scapulothoracic stabilizer group of muscles runs from the trunk to the scapula itself and includes the trapezius, levator scapula, rhomboids, serratus anterior, and pectoralis minor. Recognition of how these groups interact, with selective strengthening and stretching of affected muscles, is part of the total rehabilitation package.

The glenohumeral joint is the synovial joint of the humerus and glenoid fossa of the scapula. No more than one-third of the head of the humerus is in contact with the glenoid fossa of the scapula at any point of motion.[32,58] The glenoid labrum, a fibrocartilaginous material that provides depth to the glenoid fossa, attaches to the rim of the

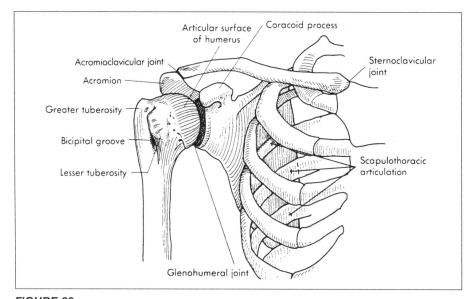

**FIGURE 32.**
Osseous anatomy of the shoulder. (From Hurley JA: Anatomy of the shoulder. In Michaels JA, et al (eds): The Upper Extremity in Sports Medicine, 2nd ed. St. Louis, Mosby, 1995, p 24, with permission.)

glenoid fossa of the scapula to assist in stabilizing the glenohumeral joint. The synovial-lined joint capsule originates from the glenoid labrum and attaches to the anatomic neck of the humerus. Capsular volume is approximately twice the size of the humeral head.[47] The redundant distal medial recess allows unrestrained movements in overhead arcs. The capsule is thickened anteriorly and inferiorly by the glenohumeral ligaments. Four ligament complexes help to support the glenohumeral joint:

1. The coracohumeral ligament (CHL) arises from the coracoid to insert on the greater and lesser tuberosities.

2. The superior glenohumeral ligament (SGHL) originates below the CHL, investing in the capsule to insert on the lesser tuberosity.

3. The middle glenohumeral ligament (MGHL) arises from the anterior glenoid and crosses inferior to the SGHL, inserting at the lower lesser tuberosity.

4. The inferior glenohumeral ligament (IGHL) originates from the anterior glenoid, inserting below the MGHL. The IGHL complex is the main stabilizer that limits anterior translation in the abducted shoulder[8] (Fig. 33).

Static translation of the glenohumeral joint is primarily restrained by the glenoid labrum and glenohumeral ligaments.[55] The rotator cuff also contributes to the stability of the capsule. The supraspinatus reinforces the capsule superiorly, the subscapularis anteriorly, and the infraspinatus and teres minor posteriorly. The long head of the biceps brachii also reinforces the capsule superiorly; it arises from the supraglenoid tubercle and labrum and passes through the intertubercular sulcus. The glenoid attachment is supported inferiorly by the long head of the triceps brachii. Dynamic compression forces provided by these surrounding muscles and tendons are the most important mechanism for stability in the midrange of glenohumeral motion, because the capsule and ligaments are lax at this range.[42]

There are two areas of relative avascularity in the suprahumeral region: the supraspinatus tendon near its insertion on the greater tuberosity and the long head of the biceps near its origin from the supraglenoid tubercle.[59] These avascular zones must be

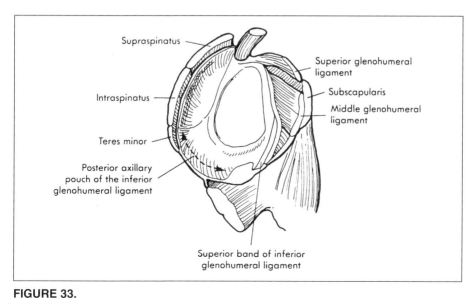

**FIGURE 33.**
Anatomy of the glenoid labrum and supporting structures. (From Hurley JA: Anatomy of the shoulder. In Michaels JA, et al (eds): The Upper Extremity in Sports Medicine, 2nd ed. St. Louis, Mosby, 1995, p 30, with permission.)

taken into consideration in rehabilitating patients with impingement or instability with concurrent impingement problems.

Eight bursae are found in the shoulder region. Most, except the subscapular bursa, do not communicate with the shoulder joint. The subacromial, subdeltoid, and subcoracoid bursae are often contiguous with one another. They separate the rotator cuff from the coracoacromial arch and do not communicate with the capsule if the rotator cuff is intact. These bursae normally allow smooth movement between the rotator cuff and overlying coracoacromial arch and deltoid; however, they also may participate in the inflammatory process. Superior rotator cuff inflammation may cause friction in the subacromial bursa, resulting in pain and inflammation. Bursae may develop adhesions to themselves or other soft tissue structures.

The acromioclavicular (AC) joint is a synovial joint formed by the medial aspect of the acromion and the distal clavicle. Appropriate scapulothoracic motion can be accomplished only with adequate gliding and rotatory motion at the AC joint. The joint is supported by the superior and inferior acromioclavicular ligament and the trapezoid and coracoid ligaments of the coracoclavicular ligament. The coracoacromial ligament spans between the coracoid process and acromion of the scapula, whereas the coracohumeral ligament extends from the coracoid process of the scapula to the top of the bicipital groove (Fig. 34). The sternoclavicular (SC) joint, also a synovial joint, is formed by the medial clavicle and the manubrim and cartilagenous portion of the first rib. The joint is supported by the anterior and posterior sternoclavicular ligaments, the costoclavicular ligament inferiorly, and the interclavicular ligament superiorly. It is divided into a medial and lateral joint by an articular disc (Fig. 35).

## Biomechanics

Glenohumeral motion accounts for 120° of the 180° of abduction range of motion. Scapulothoracic motion is responsible for the remaining 60°. After 30° of abduction, the ratio of glenohumeral-to-scapulothoracic motion is 2:1.[58] In addition, if the humerus is not capable of full external rotation, abduction is restricted by impingement of the greater tuberosity on the acromion. Abduction is accomplished by the deltoid, supraspinatus, trapezius, and serratus anterior muscles.[3] An important force couple across the glenohumeral joint is the rotator cuff and deltoid. The supraspinatus depresses the humeral head and holds it against the glenoid fossa, thereby forming a fulcrum to allow abduction and forward flexion of the arm. Ninety-seven percent of the supraspinatus contractual force is aimed at stabilizing the humeral head in the glenoid.[55,76] The remaining muscles of the rotator cuff depress the humeral head in an inferior direction within the force couple throughout the range of motion of flexion and abduction. The opposing force of the force couple is the deltoid muscle. Based on its line of pull with initiation of arm elevation, the deltoid tends to displace the humerus upward and create shear forces.[57] If the deltoid is unopposed by simultaneous, synchronous rotator cuff actions of joint compression and caudal glide, shear forces are created in the first 90° of humeral elevation. Therefore, coordinated contraction of the muscles in this force couple is necessary to allow humeral elevation without reduction in the interval between the humeral head and coracoacromial arch (impingement interval). If coordinated contraction does not occur, impingement of the suprahumeral soft tissues frequently develops.[55]

The infraspinatus and teres minor provide external rotation power, whereas internal rotation is often overpowered by the pectoralis major, latissimus dorsi, teres major, and subscapularis. The shoulder flexors are the pectoralis major, anterior deltoid, and biceps brachii.[3] The posterior deltoid, teres major, and latissimus dorsi perform extension. Adduction is accomplished by the subscapularis, infraspinatus, teres minor, pectoralis major, latissimus dorsi, and teres major.

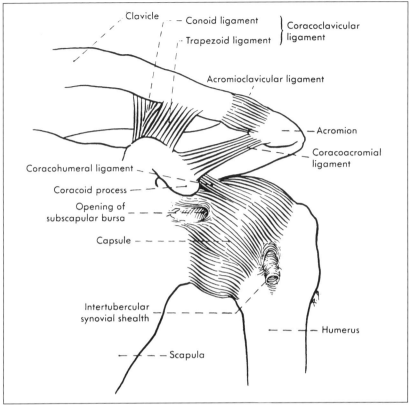

**FIGURE 34.**
Ligamentous anatomy of the shoulder. (From Bergfield JA, Parker RD: Acromioclavicular complex. In Michaels JA, et al (eds): The Upper Extremity in Sports Medicine, 2nd ed. St. Louis, Mosby, 1995, p 160, with permission.)

## Glenohumeral Instability

Instability of the shoulder is defined as loss of comfort and function of the joint because of unwanted glenohumeral translation. The different forms of shoulder instability include dislocation, or complete separation of the articular surface without immediate and spontaneous relocation; subluxation, or symptomatic translation of the humeral head on the glenoid fossa without total separation of the articular surfaces; and multidirectional instability, which requires inferior instability of the glenohumeral joint in addition to either anterior or posterior instability.[48]

Shoulder instability is not synonymous with joint laxity. Many people who have apparently excessive translation of the humerus in the glenoid fossa are asymptomatic, and many with ligamentous laxity do not have instability. Shoulder instability is classified by determining four separate factors: degree, frequency, cause, and direction. The degree of instability is classified as either subluxation or dislocation. Direction of instability may be anterior, posterior, inferior, or multidirectional. Frequency may be acute, recurrent, or chronic. The cause may be repeated microtrauma, major trauma, or voluntary injury.

Many causes of shoulder pain, as classified by Jobe, involve instability.[28,37] This classification system is useful for developing a treatment plan in athletes with anterior instability:

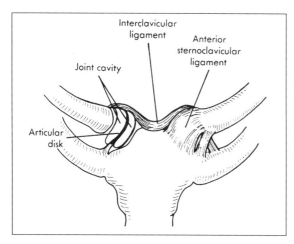

**FIGURE 35.**
Anatomy of the sternoclavicular joint and supporting structures. (From Hurley JA: Anatomy of the shoulder. In Michaels JA, et al (eds): The Upper Extremity in Sports Medicine, 2nd ed. St. Louis, Mosby, 1995, p 160, with permission.)

Group I patients have pure impingement with no instability. Impingement testing is positive, but instability tests are negative except for occasional end-range pain.

Group II patients have primary instability secondary to microtrauma to the capsule and glenoid labrum. They develop either secondary internal impingement (group IIA) of the posterior superior rim along the undersurface of the rotator cuff or secondary subacromial impingement (group IIB). Group II patients have pain with instability testing but no apprehension; pain is relieved with the relocation maneuver. Impingement signs are also positive.

Group III patients have primary instability due to generalized ligamentous hyperelasticity and secondary impingement. They demonstrate similar findings to group II patients. Examination of other joints may demonstrate generalized ligamentous laxity or bilateral signs. Even athletes may develop this entity through selective stretching out of shoulder restraints.[78] Examination under anesthesia usually demonstrates multidirectional instability.

Group IV patients have pure instability without impingement. They usually have had a single traumatic event that led to anterior subluxation or dislocation. They may exhibit pain or a sense of instability with the apprehension maneuver and relief of symptoms with the relocation test. Under anesthesia unidirectional instability is generally excessive. Group IV patients are more likely to demonstrate humeral head depression defects or labral injury, although both also may occur in group III patients.[66]

The continuum of shoulder instability was also classified by Thomas and Matson.[73] **TUBS** is the acronym for **t**raumatic instability, **u**nidirectional in nature, **B**ankhart lesion, and likely to respond to **s**urgery. **AMBRI** indicates patients with an **a**traumatic cause, **m**ultidirectional instability, **b**ilateral findings, responsiveness to **r**ehabilitation, and the need for **i**nferior capsular shift in surgical repair.

Various anterior shoulder subluxations in athletes have been described by Rowe and Zarins as the "dead arm syndrome."[66] Affected athletes may feel sudden pain with extremes of external rotation and abduction or after direct trauma to the shoulder. They typically do not complain of classic instability symptoms but may experience persistent soreness or weakness that limits athletic performance. They may display loss of muscular control over the involved arm, especially while throwing or performing racquet sports. This loss of control may result in decreased precision or intensity of a throw or stroke.

Glenohumeral (GH) dislocations constitute 50% of all dislocations and are the most common in the entire skeletal system.[50] More than 90% of GH dislocations are anterior.

The vast majority are due to trauma from a direct blow to the posterior glenohumeral joint; landing on an outstretched, externally rotated, abducted arm; or distal stress in a posterior direction on an arm in the same position. Anterior dislocations are most commonly subcoracoid but also may be subglenoid, subclavicular, or intrathoracic.

Because the humeral head is levered out of the glenoid fossa anteriorly and inferiorly, the dislocation stretches the anterior shoulder restraints, which include the capsule, glenohumeral ligaments, and subscapularis muscle. The posterolateral aspect of the humerus comes in contact with the glenoid rim. This contact may result in an impaction fracture of the humerus (Hill-Sachs lesion) or glenoid (Bankhart lesion).[23] The former occurs in 67–76% of dislocations and the latter in about 50%.[6] Patients with either lesion are more prone to recurrent dislocation or development of posttraumatic arthritis.[36,50] With anterior dislocation, fractures of the greater tuberosity occur in less than 15% of dislocations; coracoid fractures are even less common. When a primary shoulder dislocation results from high-energy impact forces, the probability of associated soft tissue injuries is greater. Either acute or recurrent dislocations may cause tears of the rotator cuff or ruptures of the capsule.

Glenohumeral dislocations may be associated with neurovascular injury. Nerves may be injured by compression or stretch. The axillary nerve is injured in 5–35% of initial anterior glenohumeral dislocations.[43] Occasionally, the radial, musculocutaneous, and median nerves and, in rare settings, the entire plexus may be involved. The axillary artery also may be injured by glenohumeral dislocation or relocation. The artery may develop intimal lacerations, thrombosis, or false aneurysms. Axillary artery injury often may be missed because peripheral pulses may remain intact as a result of collateral circulation. A high index of suspicion must be maintained; amputation rates approach 50% after axillary artery occlusion.[6]

Posterior dislocations account for approximately 2–4% of glenohumeral dislocations.[65] They may result from direct trauma to the anterior shoulder, a fall onto an adducted, externally rotated arm, electrocution, or grand mal seizure.[6] Over 50% of posterior dislocations may be missed acutely, because alignment on anteroposterior radiographs may be maintained.[63] For this reason recommended radiographic views in a trauma series include a true anteroposterior, a true scapulolateral, and an axillary view. Posterior dislocations may be associated with posterior capsular tears and fractures of the lesser tuberosity and glenoid. They are not associated with the same level of reccurence as anterior dislocations.[46] The complication of delayed arthrosis is more common after posterior dislocations.

## Rotator Cuff and Bursal Injuries

The arch of the shoulder joint is formed by the anterior acromion, coracoacromial ligament, clavicle, and acromioclavicular joint. Normally the subacromial bursa permits uniform motion between the humeral head and arch. When the arm is in the abducted, externally rotated position, the rotator cuff and subacromial bursa may be impinged between the acromial arch and greater tuberosity of the humerus. The term *impingement syndrome* was first used by Neer and Welsh.[51] Rotator cuff pathology ranges from tendinitis to partial or complete tears. Rotator cuff impingement occurs more readily with structural abnormalities or abnormal biomechanics. The shape of the acromion may predispose to impingement problems.[7] The type III (anterior hooked) and type II (gently curved) rather than the type I (flat) acromion are associated with more significant rotator cuff attrition.[7,11] Soft tissue impingement injuries are particularly common in swimming, tennis, and throwing sports such as baseball, but they are also seen in volleyball, lacrosse, rowing, and weightlifting. Such injuries are due to the repetitive positions in which the arm is placed as part of the sport. Many of these sports require the shoulder to move from abduction and external rotation into forward flexion and internal rotation.

Shoulder pain is the most common musculoskeletal complaint reported in competitive swimmers.[60] Shoulder symptoms develop in 40–80% of competitive swimmers.[29,38] Rotator cuff injuries may be seen in up to 65% of baseball players.[44]

Three stages of impingement have been described by Neer.[47] Stage I changes include edema and hemorrhage, which develop most commonly in the critical zone medial to the supraspinatus insertion.[11] These changes are usually reversible and occur at younger ages (12–25 years old). Stage II changes typically occur between ages 25–40 and are due to repetitive microtrauma. Anatomic changes include fibrosis of the subacromial bursa and rotator cuff, thickening of the coracoacromial ligament, hypertrophic subacromial bony changes or erosions, and sclerosis of the greater tuberosity. Stage III changes are most common after age 40. Partial or complete rotator cuff tears may occur, along with further degeneration of other glenohumeral structures.[54]

The long head of the biceps also may be affected by the impingement process.[26] Injuries to the biceps tendon parallel injuries to other rotator cuff tendons, ranging from tendinitis to complete ruptures. The subacromial and subdeltoid bursa are often involved in the impingement process. When abnormal biomechanics develops at the scapulothoracic articulation due to the impingement process, the scapulothoracic bursa may become inflamed. Inflammation may result in pain at the inferiomedial angle of the scapula, a snapping sensation with arm motion, and occasionally a palpable subscapular mass.

## Acromioclavicular Joint Injuries

Dislocations of the acromioclavicular (AC) joint occur less commonly than glenohumeral dislocations and account for approximately 10% of dislocations of the skeletal system.[6] A fall on the point of the shoulder, high-speed collisions with the boards in hockey, or a force directed superiorly through the humeral head are common mechanisms of injury. Acromioclavicular joint injuries in adults have been classified by Allman and Rockwood.[1,62] Type I injuries are defined as a sprain without complete disruption of the acromioclavicular ligaments. Radiographs appear normal. Type II injuries are associated with disruption of the AC ligaments and intact coracoacromial (CC) ligaments. Type I injuries demonstrate no-to-minimal displacement on anteroposterior stress radiographs. In type II injuries the clavicle is displaced superiorly by 50% of the normal AC joint height. Both type I and II injuries are successfully treated with closed reduction and application of a figure-of-eight harness during the symptomatic period, followed by rehabilitation.

Type III injuries occur when the AC and CC ligaments are torn, as demonstrated radiographically when the distance between the superior aspect of the coracoid and inferior surface of the clavicle is greater than 50% or increased by more than 5 mm compared with the normal shoulder during weighted AC joint views.[50] Type IV injuries are associated with posterior displacement of the clavicle; type V, with superior elevation of the distal clavicle and disruption of the deltoid and trapezius attachments of the clavicle; and type VI, with anterior entrapment of the distal clavicle under the acromion or coracoid process or in the biceps mechanism.[50] Type III separations with persistent pain and instability or types IV–VI may be managed with reconstruction[45,76] (Fig. 36).

## Sternoclavicular Dislocations

Sternoclavicular (SC) dislocations are not common and are usually caused by indirect trauma to the shoulder. Anterior SC dislocations are generally caused by medially directed posterolateral forces. They occur more frequently than posterior dislocations.[50] Posterior SC dislocations are typically caused by direct anterior trauma. They may be quite serious because of potential injury to the trachea and great vessels. Type I and II dislocations differ only in the degree of injury to the sternoclavicular joint, whereas type III injuries include injury to the SC and costoclavicular ligaments. They are best diagnosed

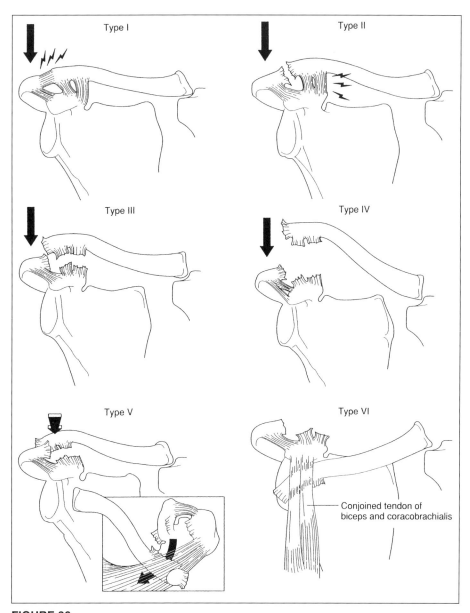

**FIGURE 36.**
Classification of acromioclavicular joint injuries. (From Reid DC: Sports Injury Assessment and Rehabilitation. New York, Churchill Livingstone, 1992, p 929, with permission.)

by computed tomography (CT), which can differentiate the direction of dislocation as well as assess injury to the trachea, great vessels, and adjacent soft tissues.[6]

## Nerve Injury

Various nerve injuries that may be a source of pain about the shoulder girdle are covered in greater depth in other chapters. Nerve injuries may result from the same trauma that causes other soft tissue injuries about the shoulder girdle. At times they mimic other soft tissue injuries, creating diagnostic dilemmas. Whether caused by radiculopathy, brachial plexus, or peripheral nerve, weakness in the C5 and C6 distribution may predipose to abnormal mechanics at the glenohumeral joint and possible impingement or instability problems. It also may prolong recovery and rehabilitation in patients with existing shoulder problems.

Radiculopathy from a disc herniation or lateral recess and foraminal stenosis also may cause shoulder pain. Not all patients with disc herniations present with axial pain. Imaging studies help to confirm a potential neurocompressive lesion. Unfortunately, most degenerative changes occur at C5–C6 and C6–C7, making it difficult to determine whether the anatomic changes seen on imaging studies are clinically relevant. The C5–C6 and C6–C7 levels potentially affect the C6 and C7 nerve roots, which contribute significantly to innervation of the glenohumeral joint and shoulder girdle. Electrodiagnostic testing may be of benefit in determining associated axonal loss. Selective injections may assist in testing out whether a given nerve root is a source of pain.

Brachial plexus injuries are frequently encountered in contact or collision sports such as football, hockey, and wrestling. It has been estimated that 50–70% of collegiate football players have at least one stinger or burner in their athletic career, and 57% suffer more than one.[10,12,61,69] Typical symptoms of a burner are sudden upper extremity burning, aching pain, or weakness for 2–15 minutes, typically in the C5 and C6 distribution. Lower-intensity aching, weakness, and paresthesias may persist from hours to months. Weakness is usually seen in shoulder abduction, external rotation in the adducted position, wrist extension, and thumb extension; there may be sensory loss in the C5 and C6 dermatome. Injury to nerves that come directly off the plexus or nerve roots (suprascapular, long thoracic, and dorsal scapular nerves) also may occur. Permanent weakness may develop with a single episode of a brachial plexus lesion; however, it tends to develop more commonly after repeated episodes.

Many of the same mechanisms of injury that create shoulder and shoulder girdle injuries also create brachial plexus traction injury. Examples include simultaneous lateral flexion forces that drive the head and neck to the side opposite the symptomatic side and forceful shoulder depression ipsilateral to the symptomatic arm.[19,33,41] The mechanism of brachial plexus upper-trunk traction is more common in high school players who sustain stingers, whereas cervical nerve root injury secondary to the extension rotation compression mechanism is more common in professional players.[22] Injury mechanisms of stingers may cause secondary problems with soft tissues about the shoulder girdle and cervical and thoracic spine. These areas of soft tissue overload and biomechanical dysfunction may make the athlete more prone to a second injury to the brachial plexus, shoulder girdle, or cervical spine.

Peripheral nerve injuries are an occasional source of pain about the shoulder girdle and proximal arm. Peripheral nerve injuries caused by sporting activities account for approximately 2.7–5.7% of all peripheral nerve injuries.[70] Lesions of the suprascapular, axillary, spinal accessory, dorsal scapular, and long thoracic nerve may be associated with pain, paresthesia, or weakness about the shoulder girdle. They may predispose the shoulder girdle to recurrent injury or prolonged rehabilitation. The suprascapular nerve may be injured by a direct blow to the base of the neck, at the suprascapular notch, or at the point where the nerve wraps around the scapular spine at the supraglenoid notch. This nerve is also vulnerable to traction injury at the plexus level.[16] It is often difficult to differentiate an isolated suprascapular nerve injury from a stinger that is diagnosed somewhat late because of the variable rate of recovery in different terminal nerves. Weakness secondary to rotator cuff lesion is often difficult to distinguish from suprascapular nerve palsy; both may be caused by similar mechanisms.

The axillary nerve is not usually injured without an associated injury such as shoulder dislocation.[62] The axillary nerve may be damaged by direct trauma at the quadrilateral space, but such injury is uncommon. When an isolated axillary nerve injury occurs, it is usually incomplete.[6,50] Injuries of the spinal accessory, dorsal scapular, and long thoracic nerves result in various types of scapular winging, which causes biomechanical dysfunction at the shoulder girdle and cervicothoracic articulations. The spinal accessory nerve may be damaged by a direct blow from sporting implements or shoulder pads, surgical trauma, or radiation.[16] Patients with lesions of the spinal accessory nerve may experience weakness in shrugging the shoulders or lateral winging of the scapula because of overpull by the serratus anterior. Because the dorsal scapular nerve comes directly off the C5 (C4) nerve roots, it is susceptible to injury in isolation or in conjunction with upper brachial plexus injuries. An isolated lesion causes weakness of the levator scapula, resulting in abduction and depression of the scapula, inferomedial rotation of its inferior angle, and hypesthesia on the dorsal aspect of the scapula. The long thoracic nerve innervates the serratus anterior, which is the primary muscle that stabilizes the scapulothoracic articulation. An injury to this nerve results in medial winging of the medial scapular border, especially the inferior angle. Scapular winging due to a nerve lesion must be distinguished from functional instability that results from altered mechanics of the scapulothoracic articulation. When this distinction remains a diagnostic dilemma, electrodiagnostic testing may be of benefit.

### Muscle Tears

Tears of the tendinous portions of the rotator cuff muscles and long head of the biceps as a result of chronic impingement are discussed above. Intrasubstance muscle tears may occur with acute trauma or chronic overload. They are not as common as lower extremity muscle tears. As in the lower extremity, acute tears often occur after an explosive contraction against an eccentric load. Pectoralis muscle tears are most common. They have been reported in weightlifters.[31] Chronic muscle overloads are common in the shoulder girdle. The muscle overloads may be part of the subclinical adaptation and biomechanical deficit seen with impingement and instability syndromes. Although they may become a secondary source of pain, they do not typically result in macrotears.

### Management of Shoulder Injuries

The most important factor in the management of shoulder injuries is to make as complete and specific a diagnosis as possible. This goal requires complete physical examination of the entire shoulder girdle as well as a brief examination of the elbow and neck for associated problems. The physical examination should focus on postural alignment, presence of deformity, and soft tissue spasm in the cervical spine, scapulothoracic articulation, and remainder of the shoulder girdle. These areas also should be assessed for range of motion, dyssynchronous motion, and hyper- or hypomobility. A screen for generalized ligamentous laxity should be included. Palpation evaluates for soft tissue and joint pain, pain over the plexus, and potential nerve entrapment sites. Impingement and instability tests should be performed (Figs. 37–39).

Manual muscle testing should evaluate strength of isolated muscle groups, focusing on the rotator cuff, scapulohumeral, and scapulothoracic muscles and C5–C6 innervated muscles distal to the shoulder. It is often difficult to distinguish true neuromuscular weakness from weakness due to pain in patients with shoulder injuries. A practical method of manual muscle testing is to start with the arm adducted at the side and the elbow at 90° in the neutral position of supination and pronation. The examiner may support and hold the elbow and humerus at the side with the arm opposite the arm tested on the athlete. (For example, if the athlete's right arm is tested, it is supported with the examiner's left arm.) Caution the athlete not to use substitution maneuvers such as shoulder shrugging or abducting the arm, unless they are being tested. From that position:

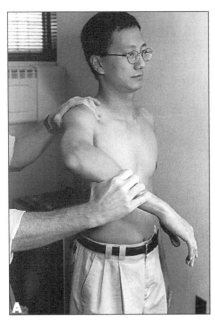 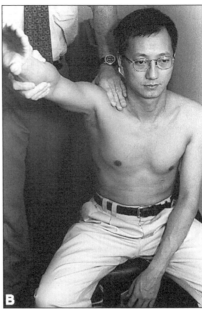

**FIGURE 37.**
Shoulder impingement tests. Positive shoulder impingement tests are noted when pain is elicited at end ranges of combined shoulder abduction and internal rotation *(A)* or with abduction within the plane of the scapula between 70° and 120° while the acromion is depressed by the tester *(B)*.

1. Internal rotation tests the pectoralis muscle (medial and lateral pectoral nerves—C5, C6, C7, C8, T1).

2. External rotation tests the infraspinatus muscle (suprascapular nerve—C5, C6).

3. Elbow flexion tests the brachioradialis and brachialis muscles (musculocutaneous and radial nerves—C5, C6).

4. Elbow extension tests the triceps muscle (radial nerve—C6, C7, C8).

5. Elbow flexion with supination tests the biceps (musculocutaneous nerve—C5, C6).

6. Isometric abduction tests the deltoid muscle (axillary nerve—C5, C6).

Testing by this method is a quick screen and is tolerated by athletes with almost any shoulder or cervical injury. If these maneuvers are tolerated, one then may test the supraspinatus (suprascapular nerve), serratus anterior (long thoracic nerve), and trapezius (spinal accessory nerve) muscles. The supraspinatus is tested in the "empty can" position and the serratus anterior and trapezius by scapular protraction and retraction. A brief sensory examination evaluates for deficits in light touch, pinprick, and proprioception. The neurologic examination includes side-to-side symmetry of reflexes, comparison of upper extremities with lower extremities, and assessment for pathologic reflexes.

Patients with pure impingement typically complain of pain during certain arcs of movement. They usually demonstrate disruption of the normal glenohumeral-to-scapulothoracic rhythm or evidence of scapular slide in the affected shoulder girdle. Impingement signs are positive, and supraspinatous muscle testing may produce pain. The drop-arm test may be positive in patients with complete rotator cuff tears. Patients with combined instability may demonstrate problems with various instability tests. Most patients without rotator cuff tears respond to conservative rehabilitation.

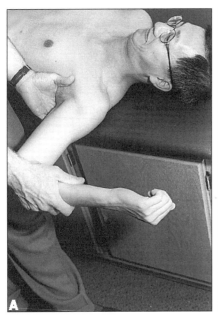 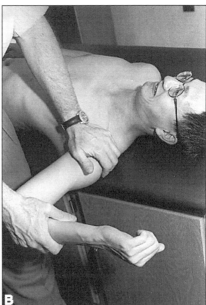

**FIGURE 38.**
Apprehension and relocation tests for anterior glenohumeral joint laxity. Apprehension of anterior dislocation of the humeral head is appreciated by the patient at end range of external rotation and 90° abduction while the tester anteriorly translates the humeral head *(A)*. This apprehension is relieved in the relocation test when posteriorly directed pressure by the tester's hand reseats the humeral head within the glenoid fossa *(B)*.

Patients with acute subluxation generally complain of acute shoulder pain or loss of control over the arm; they may report that the shoulder "slipped out of place." They have full range of motion, although certain ranges may be restricted by pain or a sense of instability. No reduction is necessary. Tests for shoulder instability should be carried out. Tests that are positive for instability may include increased anterior-posterior translation on the load-and-shift test, pain or "instability" on apprehension tests, relief on relocation tests, and a positive sulcus sign. The clunk test also may be performed to rule out functional GH instability secondary to a glenoid labrum tear and impingement. Impingement testing and strength testing should be performed to rule out simultaneous rotator cuff pathology. Depending on the severity of the subluxation, a brief period of sling immobilization vs. relative rest is adequate before initiating rehabilitation. Subsequent management after shoulder dislocation or subluxation involves relief of acute pain and inflammation, regaining of normal range of motion in a manner that protects the injured part, and strengthening of the dynamic stabilizing muscles.

The patient with an acutely dislocated shoulder typically complains of severe shoulder pain and supports the affected forearm with the opposite hand. The athlete often complains that the shoulder is "out." The initial assessment determines whether to attempt to reduce the shoulder in the direction of, or opposite to, the dislocation. If the mechanism of injury was not observed, it should be obtained from other witnesses if possible.

First-time dislocations generally require significant trauma. Therefore, any patient with a first-time dislocation should be closely questioned about the presence of sensory changes, weakness, or paresthesias, not only in the injured arm, but also on the contralateral side and lower extremities. Contralateral or lower extremity symptoms have

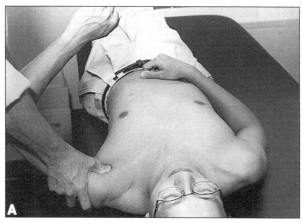

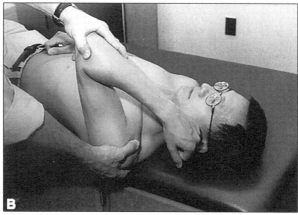

**FIGURE 39.**
Clunk tests for posterior glenohumeral joint laxity. A positive clunk test is noted when the humeral head can be displaced off the posterior rim of the glenoid fossa either by posteriorly directed pressure directly over the humeral head *(A)* or through the humerus when forward flexed to 90° *(B)*.

implications for the presence of transient quadriplegia or potential injury to the spinal cord or brain. In addition, the patient should be questioned about prior cervical spine, brachial plexus, and shoulder injuries (rotator cuff or dislocations/subluxations). If the patient has shoulder pain and persistent cervical pain, increased pain, stiffness, or neurologic symptoms with gentle active or passive cervical range of motion, the spine should remain immobilized until definitive evaluation has been completed.

Before removal of clothing or athletic equipment after an acute dislocation, documentation of the vascular integrity of the radial and ulnar arteries and a sensorimotor examination are necessary. Loss of sensation over the lateral aspect of the shoulder alone is an unreliable indicator of axillary nerve dysfunction. With protection of the glenohumeral joint and support of the shoulder and elbow, deltoid and biceps strength should be tested isometrically. Patients should be checked for deformities, abrasions, swelling, and ecchymoses. Gentle palpation should assess for soft tissue or joint crepitance and tenderness. The patient may attempt active range of motion. If it is not tolerated, the shoulder and arm should be immobilized, and a more thorough examination should be performed, starting proximally and proceeding distally through the shoulder girdle, to look for more severe injuries. Any evidence of a posterior sternoclavicular dislocation dictates transport to emergency facilities because of potential associated injury to the mediastinum.

Immediate reduction of a glenohumeral dislocation on the field rather than in a more controlled setting depends on various factors. Athletes who have suffered first-time dislocations may have an associated humeral neck or head fracture, Hill-Sach's lesion, or nerve injury. In patients with generalized joint hypermobility, it does not take as much trauma to sustain an initial dislocation; therefore, the probability of associated injuries is lower. By the second (or greater) recurrent dislocation, significantly less trauma is necessary to cause dislocation. In first-time dislocations with hyperlaxity or recurrent dislocations, it is reasonable to attempt reduction on the field. Only gentle traction and manipulation should be used to avoid potential fracture or neurovascular injury. Reduction is generally performed with the patient in the supine position. Slight traction is placed on the affected arm, which is in slight abduction/forward flexion. Then a gentle internal rotation force is applied. The restraining shoulder girdle muscles should relocate the joint. If more effort is required, the patient should be splinted for comfort and sent to a more controlled setting for reduction.

It is prudent to send patients with a primary dislocation and possible associated trauma for definitive management in a hospital setting, where radiographic procedures can be performed as necessary. The patient may require intravenous sedation. An intraarticular lidocaine injection helps to anesthetize the joint and relaxes muscles to expedite attempts at reduction. Methods described by Stenson or Kocher may be used. Stenson recommended placing the patient prone on the edge of an examination table or bed, with the affected arm hanging freely over the edge. A weight of 5–10 pounds is attached to the wrist, and the patient is allowed to relax for 15–20 minutes, with the hope that the dislocation will reduce on its own. The method described by Kocher requires one assistant to loop a sheet around the patient's thorax in the supine position and provide countertraction. The second sheet is tied loosely around the waist of the physician and looped over the patient's forearm, which is at 90° of elbow flexion. The physician then gently leans backward, applying traction force with slight abduction and forward flexion while simultaneously oscillating the humerus gently between external and internal rotation and applying outward pressure on the proximal humerus. This method is rarely used in older patients with osteoporosis because of the higher risk of bony injury to the humerus or scapula.

After appropriate reduction, neurovascular examination should be repeated. Repeat radiographs in the anteroposterior, scapulolateral plane, or axillary lateral views should verify reduction and determine the presence of additional fractures of the glenoid or proximal humerus. CT, arthrography, or MRI may be necessary to define associated injuries more completely. Displaced fractures of the greater tuberosity, large glenoid rim fractures (> 5 mm), soft tissue interposition, or rotator cuff tendon avulsion necessitates open reduction and internal fixation. If associated peripheral nerve lesions or a brachial plexus injury is suspected, the patient should undergo electrodiagnostic testing within appropriate time frames after injury.

Conservative treatment is associated with a higher percentage of good-to-excellent results in patients with atraumatic instability than in patients with traumatic shoulder instability, especially if recurrent.[66] The success rate of any conservative treatment program is contingent on the ability to correct or control the factors of glenohumeral stability. Glenohumeral stability depends on the static restraints of the capsulolabral ligamentous complex and dynamic stabilization of the rotator cuff and deltoid muscles.[42] The most significant factor determining recurrence is the athlete's age at primary dislocation.[65] In patients younger than 20 years at first dislocation, the recurrence rate is 20–55%; it is much lower in patients over 30 years of age.[24,65] Athletes younger than

20 are likely to sustain not only capsular stretching but also labral avulsion, which makes the lesions less likely to heal spontaneously. The greater the severity of the initial trauma, the higher the rate of recurrent dislocation.[66] Most dislocations recur within the first two years after the initial episode. The type or length of immobilization does not appear to affect incidence of recurrence after primary dislocation.[66]

The period of immobilization after a dislocation depends on the patient's age. It is recommended that patients under the age of 20 be immobilized for 3–4 weeks because of slow soft tissue healing about the shoulder and the possibility of glenoid labral detachment. During immobilization, external rotation and distraction of the shoulder should be avoided. With each decade, the period of immobilization should decrease. Patients over 30 years of age should be immobilized for only 10–14 days, and for patients over 40 years of age immobilization may be necessary for only a few days. Patients over the age of 40 have a significant risk of glenohumeral joint contracture. In all cases, early passive motion may be allowed, avoiding pain and external rotation. Early controlled range of motion helps to prevent contractures at the glenohumeral joint and has positive effects on collagen alignment in the articular cartilage.[18] Early motion stimulates mechanoreceptors, which may reduce the patient's perception of pain, and helps to avoid loss of dynamic stability through deconditioning of the glenohumeral joint muscles. Unweighted pendulum exercises should be encouraged early in older patients to prevent contractures at the glenohumeral joint. A specific rehabilitation program for shoulder instability should be based on the extent of damage to either dynamic or static stabilizers so that the injured athlete avoids positions that may magnify the instability and cause further damage. With anterior shoulder dislocations, one should proceed cautiously in the range of external rotation, especially when it is combined with abduction. In addition, resistance exercises that force the humeral head anteriorly should be avoided. The pace of the rehabilitation program needs to take into consideration the number of recurrences and the presence of multidirectional instability to restore preinjury level of function as rapidly and safely as possible.

## Rehabilitation

The rehabilitation program for shoulder injuries must balance knowledge of the involved structures and degree of bony and soft tissue injury with the optimal time frame needed for healing of affected structures. The injured joint must be loaded in a protected fashion to promote healing and to prevent the deleterious effects of immobilization. Immobilization increases collagen fiber cross-linkages in all of the various connective tissues.[2,53] A tendency toward shortening of the intramuscular soft tissue and contracture of the joint capsule results in increased stiffness. Muscle atrophy occurs quickly after injury and immobilization.

The injury itself may cause chemical and neural mechanisms that inhibit muscular action.[67] This inhibition initially protects the extremity from further injury; however, eventually it may further destabilize the joint. Chemical mediators may cause inhibition of the agonistic muscle and spasm in the antagonistic muscle with attempts to splint the injured extremity.[67] Such protective responses may cause further problems if they are allowed to continue. Strengthening generally should proceed within a pain-free range of motion; excessive pain during rehabilitation reinitiates chemical and neural mechanisms that inhibit muscle contraction and promote muscle spasm. Isometrics are often preferable initially because they can be used to strengthen within limitations of range of motion or pain.

Pain tends to cause neuromuscular inhibition with subsequent scapular fixation in an elevated adducted position.[54] Soft tissue rehabilitation techniques and flexibility exercises should focus on decreasing pain and normalizing tone and length in shortened tissues in the upper trapezius, levator scapula, rhomboids, teres major, and rotator cuff.

A tight posterior cuff tends to load the inferior glenohumeral ligament, which is the primary restraint that prevents symptomatic translation causing shoulder instability. In addition, tight scapulothoracic and pectoralis minor muscles create abnormal scapular and therefore glenoid positioning, altering normal glenohumeral biomechanics. Overutilization of scapular stabilizers and abnormal biomechanics also may cause overload of cervical structures. Especially with recurrent subluxations or dislocations or impingement, there is a distinct interplay between shoulder girdle and cervical dysfunction and pain.

Another important part of the rehabilitation process is strengthening of the scapular stabilizers. Several investigators have demonstrated the importance of a rehabilitation program that emphasizes shoulder stability and synchronous scapular motion.[27,34,68] Coordinated scapulothoracic motion helps to provide a stable fulcrum for rotation of the humerus and allows appropriate alignment of the humeral head and glenoid fossa. Scapular stability is provided by serial contraction of the lower trapezius, rhomboids, serratus anterior, and upper trapezius. The scapulothoracic muscles contract concentrically to secure the scapula to the thorax in a position of retraction and acromial elevation. Rotator cuff impingement can occur when the acromion is not elevated. The rotator cuff muscles must work harder to depress the humeral head, resulting in fatigue, overuse, and subclinical adaptations with subsequent symptom development. In addition, if the scapula slides laterally, the glenoid is in a more anterior position, allowing increased humeral head motion. This position creates less stress on the static restraints (especially the anterior capsule) of the glenohumeral joint.

The strengthening program should involve the scapular stabilizers (rhomboids, trapezius, serratus anterior) to maintain optimal position of the scapula during functional activities, especially during the eccentric phase of movements. Fatigue of the scapulothoracic muscles generally results in abnormal scapulothoracic rhythms, which may lead to various compensatory mechanisms in other muscles. Such mechanisms eventually create secondary impingement and shoulder girdle myofascial pain. The serratus anterior is one of the first scapulothoracic stabilizers to be affected by glenohumeral pathology. Strengthening of the serratus should be emphasized early in the rehabilitation process. It is one of last scapulothoracic muscles to regain full function; therefore, strengthening should continue throughout the rehabilitation process[15] (Fig. 40).

In the early phase of rehabilitation, manual scapular stabilization exercises should be performed one-on-one with the therapist. Retraction-protraction as well as elevation-depression patterns may be performed in a sidelying position with the therapist providing manual resistance. These exercises are often difficult for patients to master. If patients move too rapidly into progressive resistive exercises with weights, they generally do not isolate particular muscle groups and subsequently create compensatory patterns. As kinesthetic awareness of the scapula is obtained, the patient may be advanced to utilizing resistance with TheraBands or resistance equipment, but the patient must be cautioned to stabilize the scapula throughout the plane of motion. If the patient begins to fatigue and precise repetitions cannot be performed, the exercise should be discontinued. An increased number of repetitions or increased resistance should not be performed at the expense of precise repetitions. Closed-chain kinetic exercises also may be performed to train the scapular stabilizer muscles.[72] Loading the glenohumeral joint in an axial plane decreases tensile stresses on the capsule while creating compressive forces in the joint, enhancing joint stability.[14] Closed-chain kinetic activities also stimulate mechanoreceptor activity at the glenohumeral joint, thus enhancing proprioception as well.[72]

The next phase of rehabilitation focuses on restoring dynamic stability to the glenohumeral joint and should await adequate scapular stability. The rotator cuff muscles work to maintain proper centering and compressive forces of the humeral head in

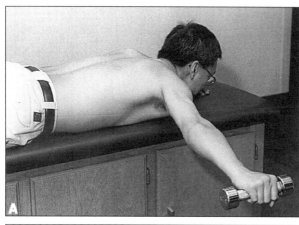
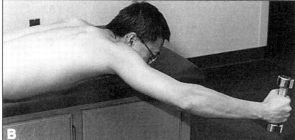
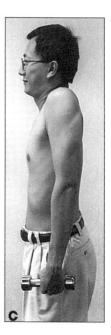
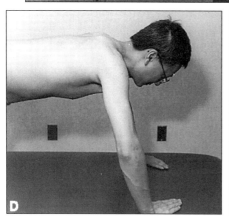
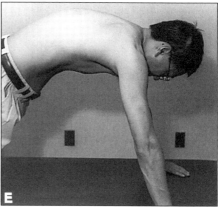

**FIGURE 40.**
Scapular stabilizing exercises. *A,* Rhomboids. *B,* Lower trapezius. *C,* Upper trapezius. *D,* Serratus anterior, push-up. *E,* Serratus anterior, push-up with a plus.

the glenoid fossa, enhancing its stability.[4,68,75] Lack of rotator cuff control leads to abnormal glenohumeral rhythm as well as potential superior head migration, which may result in secondary impingement problems. Rotator cuff strengthening initially avoids the abducted position, which may improve blood flow to the avascular zone of the rotator cuff. Therefore, strengthening of the rotator cuff and deltoid first through isometric and then through isotonic exercise in the pain-free range of motion should be initiated (Fig. 41). The preferred position is 20–45° of abduction.[59] Ideally, range of motion and strengthening exercises should be performed in the scapular plane, which

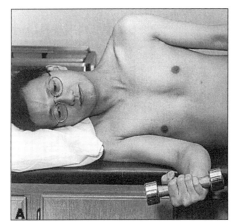
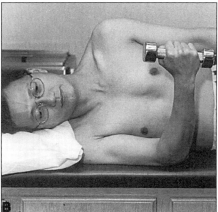

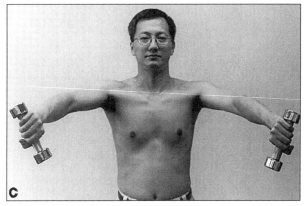

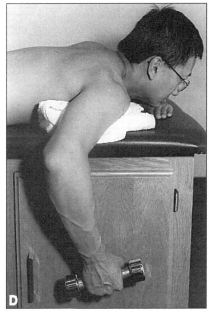
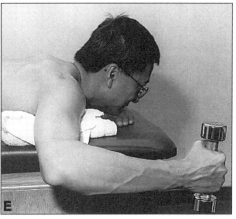

**FIGURE 41.**
Rotator cuff strengthening. *A* and *B*, Subscapularis.
*C*, Supraspinatus. *D* and *E*, Infraspinatus and teres
minor.

is 30–45° anterior to the coronal plane. Stress on the anterior and posterior capsule as well as rotator cuff is minimized,[30] and this position involves a high degree of congruence between the humeral head and glenoid.[68] The deltoid and supraspinatus muscles are provided a more direct line of action in the scapular plane, enhancing muscle force and decreasing subacromial impingement as the arm is abducted.[20,30,71] Rotator cuff weakness in patients with chronic impingement or instability may lead to changes in the subacromial bursa and rotator cuff tendon that in turn lead to further impingement symptoms and degenerative changes in the glenoid labrum. Muscular imbalance of the external and internal rotators should be identified and corrected. With the shoulder in the neutral position, the ratio of external-to-internal rotation strength is 66%; in 90° of abduction, it should be 78%.[71]

As with rehabilitation of scapular muscles, retraining the rotator cuff should include eccentric strengthening in addition to concentric activities. Athletic activities frequently require eccentric activity of the shoulder prime movers. This is nowhere more evident than in throwing. Posterior rotator cuff muscles fire significantly during the deceleration and follow-through phase of throwing to control the arm eccentrically.[13] As pain decreases, strength and conditioning improve, and apprehension disappears, the athlete may begin to work into overhead ranges of motion for strengthening.

Strength in the biceps brachii is important because it has a stabilizing function for the humerus in the abducted and externally rotated position.[26] The proximal portion of the triceps also acts as a decelerator of the arm. Strengthening of the pectoralis major and latissimus dorsi is necessary because they are prime accelerators of the humerus and upper extremity. Overstrengthening of the internal rotators, such as the latissimus dorsi and pectoralis major, tends to increase anterior glenohumeral translation. It is important to avoid muscle imbalance in the primary and secondary dynamic stabilizers.

In the rehabilitation of any joint, it is important to restore normal joint proprioception as well as complex movement patterns. Proprioceptive neuromuscular facilitation patterns may be used to restore both.[35] Combining flexion, abduction, and external rotation strengthens the deltoid supraspinatus, infraspinatus, and teres minor, the muscles that tend to be deficient in patients with instability. Strengthening in this pattern requires a negative apprehension test and adequate range-of-motion strength. Rhythmic stabilization emphasizes cocontraction of the antagonistic and agonistic dynamic stabilizers.

The final phase of rehabilitation progressively trains the patient in sport- or work-specific activities. For throwing sports, the shoulder must be trained at end-range external rotation and horizontal abduction, as seen in the cocking phase of throwing. Once strength and endurance are adequate, athletes may progress to a throwing program. Fatigue must be respected because it may lead to loss of dynamic stability, compensatory motion patterns, and tissue overload from increased humeral head translation. The rehabilitation program should increase progressively the speed of contractions with isokinetic training. Progression through each phase of rehabilitation is contingent on meeting objective parameters of strength and range of motion and addressing the athlete's subjective complaints.

## Summary

Evaluation and treatment of injuries to the shoulder require the clinician to have knowledge of normal anatomy and optimal biomechanics as well as pathoanatomy and mechanics of injury. Appropriate initial assessment is necessary, and subsequent management is based on repeat evaluations and timing and selection of diagnostic studies. The injured area is initially braced or protected, as necessary, and activity is restricted. The rehabilitation program progresses through the phases of pain and inflammation reduction, restoration of function, and maintenence. The rate of progression through each phase of rehabilitation is contingent on individual goals, subjective complaints, and meeting appropriate objective parameters of strength, range of motion, and precise technique of sporting activities, if applicable.

## REFERENCES

### Wrist
1. Angelides AC, Wallace PF: The dorsal ganglion of the wrist: Its pathogenesis, gross and microscopic anatomy, and surgical treatment. J Hand Surg 1A:228–235, 1976.
2. Barfred T, Adamson S: Duplication of the extensor carpi ulnaris tendon. J Hand Surg 11A: 423–425, 1986.
3. Bassett FH, Malone T, Gilchrist RA: A protective splint of silicone rubber. Am J Sports Med 7:358–360, 1979.
4. Bednar JM, Osterman AL: Carpal instability: Evaluation and treatment. J Am Acad Orthop Surg 1:10–17, 1993.
5. Bell-Krotoski JA, Figarola JH: Biomechanics of soft tissue growth and remodeling with plaster casting. J Hand Ther 8:131–137, 1995.
6. Berger RA, Kauer JMG, Landsmeer JML: Radioscapholunate ligament: A gross and histologic study of fetal and adult wrist. J Hand Surg 16A:350–355, 1991.
7. Bergfeld JA, Weiker GG, Andrish JT, et al: Soft playing splint for protection of significant hand and wrist injuries in sports. Am J Sports Med 10:293–296, 1982.
8. Bishop AT, Gabel G: Flexor carpi radialis tendinitis. Part I: Operative anatomy. J Bone Joint Surg 76A:1009–1014, 1994.
9. Bogumill GP, Sullivan DJ, Baker GI: Tumors of the hand. Clin Orthop 108:214–222, 1975.
10. Boland AL, Hosea TM: Rowing and sculling and the older athlete. Clin Sports Med 10:245–256, 1991.
11. Brand PW: The forces of dynamic splinting: Ten questions before applying a dynamic splint to the hand. In Hunter JM, et al (eds): Rehabilitation of the Hand. St. Louis, Mosby, 1990, pp 1095–1100.
12. Brooks AA: Ligamentous injuries and fractures of the wrist. In The Hughston Clinic Sports Medicine Book. Baltimore, Williams & Wilkins, 1995, pp 353–360.
13. Cannon NM (ed): Diagnosis and Treatment Manual for Physicians and Therapists. 3rd ed. Indianapolis, Hand Rehabilitation Center of Indiana, 1991.
14. Carroll RE: Acute calcium deposits in the hand. JAMA 157(5):422-426, 1955.
15. Cooney WP: Evaluation of chronic wrist pain by arthrography, arthroscopy and arthrotomy. J Hand Surg (Am) 18:815, 1993.
16. Cooney WP, Dobyns JH, Linschield RL: Fractures and dislocation of the wrist. In Rockwood CA, Green DP (eds): Fractures, 3rd ed. Philadelphia, J.B. Lippincott, 1991, pp 563–579.
17. Cooney WP, Linscheid RL, Dobyns JH: Carpal instability: Treatment of ligament injuries of the wrist. AAOS Instr Course Lect 45:33–44, 1996.
18. Dalinka MK, Meyers S, Kricun ME, et al: Magnetic resonance imaging of the wrist. Hand Clin 7:87–98, 1991.
19. Dell, P C: Traumatic disorders of the distal radioulnar joint. Clin Sports Med 11:141–159, 1992.
20. Eckardt WA, Palmer AK: Recurrent dislocation of the extensor carpi ulnaris tendon. J Hand Surg 6A: 629–631, 1981.
21. Fess EE, Phillips C: Hand Splinting: Principles and Methods, 2nd ed. St. Louis, Mosby, 1987.
22. Finkelstein H: Stenosing tendovaginitis at the radial styloid process. J Bone Joint Surg 12A:509–540, 1930.
23. Fitton JM, Shea FW, Goldie W: Lesions of the flexor carpi radialis tendon and sheath causing pain in the wrist. J Bone Joint Surg 50A:359–363, 1968.
24. Foreman S, Gieck J: Rehabilitative management of injuries to the hand. Clin Sports Med 1:239–252, 1992.
25. Fritz RC, Brody GA: MR imaging of the wrist and elbow. Clin Sports Med 14:315–330, 1995.
26. Froimson A: Tenosynovitis and tennis elbow. In Green DP (ed): Operative Hand Surgery, 3rd ed. New York, Churchill Livingstone, 1992, pp 1989–2006.
27. Gabel G, Bishop AT, Wood MB: Flexor carpi radialis tendinitis. Part II: Results of operative treatment. J Bone Joint Surg 76A:1015-1018, 1994.
28. Grundberg AB, Reagan DS: Pathologic anatomy of the forearm: Intersection syndrome. J Hand Surg 10A:299-302, 1985.
29. Gunther SF: Dorsal wrist pain and the occult scapholunate ganglion. J Hand Surg 10A:676, 1985.
30. Halikis MN, Taleisnik J: Soft tissue injuries of the wrist. Clin Sports Med 15:235–259, 1996.
31. Hajj AA, Wood MB: Stenosing tenosynovitis of the extensor carpi ulnaris. J Hand Surg 11:519–520, 1986.

32. Heck CV, Hendryson IE, Carter RR: Joint Motion: Method of Measuring and Recording. Chicago, American Academy of Orthopedic Surgeons, 1965.
33. Helal B: Raquet player's pisiform. Hand 10:87–90, 1978.
34. Hodge JC, Gilula LA, Larsen CF, Amadio PC: Analysis of carpal instability. II: Clinical applications. J Hand Surg 20A:765–776, 1995.
35. Hoglund M, Tordai P, Engkvist O: Ultrasonography for the diagnosis of soft tissue conditions in the hand. Scand J Plast Reconstr Surg Hand Surg 25:225, 1991.
36. Johnson RK: Soft tissue injuries of the forearm and hand. Clin Sports Med 5:701–707, 1985.
37. Kleinman WB: Management of chronic rotary subluxation of the scaphoid by scapho-trapezial-trapezoid arthrodesis: Rationale for technique, postoperative changes in biomechanical technique and results. Hand Clin 3:113–133, 1987.
38. Kiefhaber TR, Stern PJ: Upper extremity tendinitis and overuse syndromes in the athlete. Clin Sports Med 11:39–55, 1992.
39. Koman LA, Mooney JF III, Poehling GG: Fractures and ligamentous injuries of the wrist. Hand Clin 6:477–491, 1990.
40. Krakauer JD, Bishop AT, Cooney WP: Surgical treatment of scapholunate advanced collapse. J Hand Surg 19A:751–759, 1994.
41. Landsmeer JMF: Study on anatomy of articulation. I: The equilibrium of the intercalated bone. Acta Morph Neer Scand 3:287–303, 1961.
42. Lapidus PW, Guidotti FP: Stenosing tenovaginitis of the wrist and fingers. Clin Orthop 83:87–90, 1972.
43. Laseter GF, Carter PR: Management of distal radius fractures. J Hand Ther 2:114–128, 1996.
44. Levine WR: Rehabilitation techniques for ligament injuries of the wrist. Hand Clin 8:669–681, 1992.
45. Lister G: The Hand, 2nd ed. Edinburgh, Churchill Livingstone, 1984.
46. Linscheid RL, Dobyns JH: Athletic injuries of the wrist. Clin Orthop 198:141–151, 1985.
47. Linscheid RL, Dobyns JH: Carpal instability. Curr Orthop 3:106–114, 1989.
48. Linscheid RL, Dobyns JH, Beabout JW, Bryan RS: Traumatic instability of the wrist: Diagnosis, classification and pathomechanics. J Bone Joint Surg 54A:1612–1632, 1972.
49. Linscheid RL, Dobyns, Beckenbaugh RD, et al: Instability patterns of the wrist. J Hand Surg 8:682–686, 1983.
50. Loomis LK: Variations of stenosing tenosynovitis at the radial styloid process. J Bone Joint Surg 33A:340–346, 1951.
51. Mirabello SC, Loeb PE, Andrews JR: The wrist: Field evaluation and treatment. Clin Sports Med 11:1–25, 1992.
52. Mayfield JK: Patterns of injury to the carpal ligaments. A spectrum. Clin Orthop 187:36–42, 1984.
53. Mayfield JK, Johnson RP, Kilcoyne RF: The ligaments of the human wrist and their functional significance. Anat Rec 186:417–428, 1976.
54. Mayfield JK, Johnson RP, Kilcoyne RK: Carpal dislocations: Pathomechanics and progressive perilunar instability. J Hand Surg 5A:226–241, 1980.
55. Mikic ZD: Age changes in the triangular fibrocartilage of the wrist joint. J Anat 126:367–384, 1978.
56. Mooney JF III, Siegel DB, Koman LA: Ligamentous injuries of the wrist in athletes. Clin Sports Med 11:1:129–139, 1992.
57. Mullins PA: Use of therapeutic modalities in upper extremity rehabilitation. In Hunter J, et al (eds): Rehabilitation of the Hand: Surgery and Therapy, 4th ed. St. Louis, Mosby, 1995, pp 1495–1520.
58. Osterman AL, Moskow L, Low DW: Soft tissue injuries of the hand and wrist in racquet sports. Clin Sports Med 7: 329–348, 1988.
59. Palmer AK, Werner FW: The triangular fibrocartilage complex of the wrist: Anatomy and function. J Hand Surg 6:153–162, 1981.
60. Palmer AK, Werner FW: Biomechanics of the distal radioulnar joint. Clin Orthop 187:26–35, 1984.
61. Palmieri TJ: Pisiform area pain treatment by pisiform excision. J Hand Surg 7:477–480, 1982.
62. Plancher KD, Peterson RK, Steichen JB: Compressive neuropathies and tendinopathies in the athletic elbow and wrist. Clin Sports Med 15:331–371, 1996.
63. Reagan DS, Linscheid RL, Dobyns JH: Lunotriquetral sprains. J Hand Surg 9A:502–514, 1984.
64. Rettig AC: The wrist and hand. In Stover CN, McCarroll JR, Mallon WJ (eds): The Medical Aspects of Golf. Philadelphia, F.A. Davis, 1994.
65. Roth JH, Haddad RG: Radiocarpal arthroscopy and arthrography in the diagnosis of ulnar wrist pain. Arthroscopy 2:234–243, 1986.
66. Ruby LK: Carpal instability. AAOS Instr Course Lect 45:3–13, 1996.
67. Ruby LK, Cooney WP, An KN: Relative motion of selected carpal bones: A kinematic analysis of the normal wrist. J Hand Surg 13A:1–9, 1988.
68. Ryu J, Cooney WP, Askew LJ, et al: Functional ranges of motion and the wrist joint. J Hand Surg 15A:409–419, 1991.
69. Sailer SM, Lewis SB: Rehabilitation and splinting of common upper extremity injuries in athletes. Clin Sports Med 2:411–446, 1995.

70. Sanders WF: The occult dorsal carpal ganglion. J Hand Surg 10B:257, 1985.
71. Sarrafian SK, Melamed JL, Goshgarian GM: Study of wrist motion in flexion and extension. Clin Orthop 126:153–159, 1977.
72. Schultz-Johnson K: Splinting the wrist: Mobilization and protection. J Hand Ther 2:165–177, 1996.
73. Schroer W, Lacey S, Frost FS, Keith MW: Carpal instability in the weight bearing upper extremity. J Bone Joint Surg 12:A1838–1843, 1996.
74. Shaffer B, Bradley JP, Bogumill GP: Unusual problems of the athlete's elbow, forearm and wrist. Clin Sports Med 15: 425–438, 1996.
75. Skahen JR III, Palmer AK, Levinsohn EM, et al: Magnetic resonance imaging of the triangular fibrocartilage complex. J Hand Surg 15A:552–557, 1990.
76. Sotereanos DG, Levy JA, Herndon JH: Hand and wrist injuries. In Fu F, Stone D (eds): Sports Injuries: Mechanisms, Prevention and Treatment. Baltimore, Williams & Wilkins, 1994, pp 937–948.
77. Stern PJ: Tendinitis, overuse syndromes, and tendon injuries. Hand Clin 6:467–476, 1990.
78. Travel JG, Simons DG: Myofascial Pain and Dysfunction. Baltimore, Williams & Wilkins, 1983.
79. Viegas SF: Arthroscopic assessment of carpal instabilities and ligamentous injuries.AAOS Instr Course Lect 44:151–154, 1995.
80. Vo P, Wright T, Hayden F, et al: Evaluating dorsal wrist pain: MRI diagnosis of occult dorsal wrist ganglion. J Hand Surg 20A:667–670, 1995.
81. Weber ER: Concepts governing rotational shift of the intercalated segment of the carpus. Orthop Clin North Am 15:193–207, 1984.
82. Weeks PM: A cause of wrist pain: Nonspecific tenosynovitis involving the flexor carpi radialis. Plast Reconstr Surg 62:263–266, 1978.
83. Whipple TL: Chronic wrist pain. AAOS Instr Course Lect 44:129–138, 1995.
84. Williams JGP: Surgical management of traumatic noninfective tenosynovitis of the wrist extensors. J Bone Joint Surg 59B:408–419, 1977.
85. Witt J, Pess G, Gelberman RH: Treatment of de Quervain's tenosynovitis. J Bone Joint Surg 73A:219–222, 1991.
86. Wood MB, Dobyns JH: Sports-related extra-articular wrist syndromes. Clin Orthop 202:93–102, 1986.
87. Wood MB, Linscheid RL: Abductor pollicus longus bursitis. Clin Orthop 93:293–296, 1973.
88. Wright TW, Michlovitz SL: Management of carpal instabilities. J Hand Ther 2:148–156, 1996.
89. Wulle C: Zum Intersection-Syndrom. Handchirurgie. Mikrochir Plast Chir 25:48–50, 1993.
90. Youm Y, McMurtry RY, Flatt AE: Kinematics of the wrist. J Bone Joint Surg 60A:423–431, 1978.

### Elbow

1. Adelsberg S: The tennis stroke: An EMG analysis of selected muscles with  rackets of increasing grip size. Am J Sports Med 14:139, 1986.
2. American Academy of Orthopaedic Surgeons: Joint Motion: Method of Measuring and Recording. Chicago: American Academy of Orthopaedic Surgeons, 1965.
3. Anderson TE: Anatomy and physical examination of the elbow. In Nicholas  JA, Hershman EB (eds): The Upper Extremity in Sports Medicine. St. Louis, Mosby, 1990, pp 273–288.
4. Anderson TE, Ciolek J: Specific rehabilitation programs for the throwing athlete. Instruc Course Lect 38: 487–491, 1989.
5. Andrews JR, Craven WM: Lesions of the posterior compartment of the elbow. Clin Sports Med 10:637–651, 1991.
6. Andrews JR, Wilk KE, Groh D: Elbow rehabilitation. In Brotzman SB (ed): Clinical Orthopaedic Rehabilitation. St. Louis, Mosby, 1996, pp  67–89.
7. Andrews JR, Wilk KE, Satterwhite YE, Tedder JL: Physical examination of the thrower's elbow. J Orthop Sports Phys Ther 17:296–304, 1993.
8. Andrews JR, Wilson FD: Valgus extension overload in the pitching elbow. In Zarins B, Andrews JR, Carson WG (eds): Injuries in the Throwing Athlete. Philadelphia, W.B. Saunders, 1985, pp 250–257.
9. Bach BR, Earren RF, Wickiewicz TL: Triceps rupture: A case report and literature review. Am J Sports Med 15:285, 1987.
10. Baker BD, Beirwagen D: Rupture of the distal tendon of the biceps brachii.  Operative versus nonoperative treatment. J Bone Joint Surg 67A:414, 1985.
11. Belhobek GH: Roentgenographic evaluation of the elbow. In Nicholas JA,  Hershman EB (eds): The Upper Extremity in Sports Medicine. St. Louis,  Mosby, 1990, pp 289–292.
12. Blackwell JR, Calahan T: Wrist positions in skilled and unskilled tennis players at ball-racket impact: Implications for onset of lateral epicondylitis (tennis elbow). First World Congress of Biomechanics, 1990.
13. Brown M: The older athlete with tennis elbow. Rehabilitation concerns. Clin  Sports Med 14:267–275, 1995.
14. Buckwalter JA: Pharmacologic treatment of soft tissue injuries. J Bone Joint Surg 77A:1902–1914, 1995.

15. Cabrera JM, McCue FC: Nonosseous athletic injuries of the elbow, forearm, and hand. Clin Sports Med 5:681–700, 1986.
16. Caldwell GL, Safran MR: Elbow problems in the athlete. Clin Sports Med 26:465–485, 1995.
17. Chinn CJ, Priest JD, Kent BE: Upper extremity range of motion, grip strength, and girth in highly skilled tennis players. Phys Ther 54:474–482, 1974.
18. Conway JE, Jobe FW, Glousman RE, et al: Medial instability of the elbow in throwing athletes. J Bone Joint Surg 74A:67–83, 1992.
19. Coonrad RW, Hooper WR: Tennis elbow: Its course, natural history, conservative and surgical management. J Bone Joint Surg 55A:1177–1182, 1973.
20. Dilorenzo CE, Parkes JC, Chmelar RD: The importance of shoulder and cervical dysfunction in the etiology and treatment of athletic elbow injuries. J Orthop Sports Phys Ther 11:402–409, 1990.
21. Ellenbecker TS: Rehabilitation of shoulder and elbow injuries in tennis players. Clin Sports Med 14:87–107, 1995.
22. Field LD, Altchek DW: Elbow injuries. Clin Sports Med 14:59–78, 1995.
23. Fillion PL: Treatment of lateral epicondylitis. Am J Occup Ther 45:340–343, 1991.
24. Fox GM, Jebson PJL, Orwin JF: Overuse injuries of the elbow. Physician Sportsmed 23:58–66, 1995.
25. Gilcreest EL: The common syndrome of rupture dislocation and elongation at the long head of the biceps brachii: An analysis of 100 cases. Surg Gynecol Obstet 58:322–340, 1934.
26. Glousman RE: Ulnar nerve problems in the athlete's elbow. Clin Sports Med 19:365, 1990.
27. Glousman RE, Barron J, Jobe FW, et al: An electromyographic analysis of the elbow in normal and injured pitchers with medial collateral ligament insufficiency. Am J Sport Med 20:311–317, 1992.
28. Gorga PP, Brown M, Al-Obaidi S: Hydrocortisone and exercise effects on articular cartilage in rats. Arch Phys Med Rehab 74:463–467, 1993.
29. Green DP, McCoy H: Turnbuckle orthotic correction of elbow-flexion contractures after acute injuries. J Bone Joint Surg 61A:1092–1095, 1979.
30. Gunn CC, Milbrandt WE: Tennis elbow and the cervical spine. Can Med Assoc J 114:803–809, 1976.
31. Harding WG: Use and misuse of the tennis elbow strap. Physician Sportsmed 20:65–74, 1992.
32. Harrelson GL: Elbow rehabilitation. In Andrews JR, Harrelson GL (eds): Physical Rehabilitation of the Injured Athlete. Philadelphia, W.B. Saunders, 1991, pp 443–472.
33. Henning EM, Rosenbaum D, Milani TL: Transfer of tennis racket vibrations onto the human forearm. Med Sci Sports Exer 24:1134–1140, 1992.
34. Hollinshead WH, Jenkins DB: Functional Anatomy of the Limbs and Back, 5th ed. Philadelphia, W.B. Saunders, 1981.
35. Hotchkiss RN: Common disorders of the elbow in athletes and musicians. Hand Clin 6:507, 1990.
36. Hotchkiss RN, Green DP: Fractures and dislocations of the elbow. In Rockwood CA, Green DP (eds): Fractures in Adults, vol 1, 3rd ed. Philadelphia, J.B. Lippincott, 1991, pp 739–841.
37. Hotchkiss RN, Weiland AJ: Valgus stability of the elbow. J Orthop Res 5:372, 1987.
38. Ilfeld FW: Can stroke modification relieve tennis elbow? Clin Orthop 276:182, 1992.
39. Jobe FW, Elattrache NS: Diagnosis and treatment of ulnar collateral ligament injuries in athletes. In Morrey BF (ed): The Elbow and Its Disorders. Philadelphia, W.B. Saunders, 1993, pp 566–572.
40. Jobe FW, Nuber G: Throwing injuries of the elbow. Clin Sports Med 5:621–636, 1986.
41. Johnston JJ, Plancher KD, Hawkins RJ: Elbow injuries to the throwing athlete. Clin Sports Med 15:307–329, 1996.
42. Kapandji AI: The Physiology of the Joints, vol. 1, 5th ed. Edinburgh, Churchill Livingstone, 1982.
43. LaFreniere JG: Tennis elbow: Evaluation, treatment and prevention. Phys Ther 59:742–746, 1979.
44. Larson SG: Phylogeny. In Morrey BF (ed): The Elbow and Its Disorders, 2nd ed. Philadephia, W.B. Saunders, 1993.
45. Leach RE, Miller JK: Lateral and medial epicondylitis of the elbow. Clin Sports Med 6:259–272, 1987.
46. Lee DG: Tennis elbow: A manual therapist's perspective. J Orthop Sports Phys Ther 8:134–141, 1986.
47. Lehman RC: Surface and equipment variables in tennis injuries. Clin Sports Med 7:229, 1988.
48. Linsheid RL, Wheeler DK: Elbow dislocations. JAMA 194:1171, 1965.
49. London JT: Kinematics of the elbow. J Bone Joint Surg 63A:529–535, 1981.
50. Mehlhoff TL, Bennett JB: Elbow injuries. In Mellion MB, Walsh WM, Shelton GL (eds): The Team Physician's Handbook. Philadelphia, Hanley & Belfus, 1990, pp 334–345.
51. Micheli LJ: Elbow pain in a Little League pitcher. In Smith NJ (ed): Common Problems in Pediatric Sports Medicine. Chicago, Year Book, 1989, pp 233–241.
52. Micheli LJ: Overuse injuries in children's sports: The growth factor. Orthop Clin North Am 14:337–360, 1983.
53. Middleton K: Range of motion and flexibility. In Andrews JR, Harrelson GL (eds): Physical Rehabilitation of the Injured Athlete. Philadelphia, W.B. Saunders, 1991, pp 141–164.
54. Mirowitz SA, London SL: Ulnar collateral ligament injury in baseball pitchers: MR imaging evaluation. Radiology 185:573–576, 1992.

55. Morrey BF: Anatomy of the elbow joint. In Morrey BF (ed): The Elbow and Its Disorders, 2nd ed. Philadelphia, W.B. Saunders, 1993, pp 16–51.
56. Morrey BF: Applied anatomy and biomechanics of the elbow joint. Instr Course Lect 35:59–68, 1986.
57. Morrey BF: Post-traumatic contracture of the elbow. Operative treatment, including distraction arthroplasty. J Bone Joint Surg 72A:601–618, 1990.
58. Morrey BF: Post-traumatic stiffness: Distraction arthroplasty. In Morrey BF (ed): The Elbow and Its Disorders, 2nd ed. Philadelphia, W.B. Saunders, 1993, pp 476–491.
59. Morrey, BF, An KN: Articular and ligamentous contributions to the stability of the elbow joint. Am J Sports Med 11:315–319, 1983.
60. Morrey BF, Tanaka S, An KN: Valgus stability of the elbow: A definition of primary and secondary constraints. Clin Orthop 265:187, 1991.
61. Morris M, Jobe FW, Perry J, et al: Electromyographic analysis of elbow function in tennis players. Am J Sports Med 17:241–247, 1989.
62. Nicola TL: Elbow injuries in athletes. Prim Care 19:283–302, 1992.
63. Nirschl RP: Elbow tendinosis/tennis elbow. Clin Sports Med 11:851–870, 1992.
64. Nirschl RP: Muscle and tendon trauma: Tennis elbow. In Morrey BF (ed): The Elbow and Its Disorders, 2nd ed. Philadelphia, W.B. Saunders, 1993, pp 537–552.
65. Nirschl RP: Prevention and treatment of elbow and shoulder injuries in the tennis player. Clin Sports Med 4:289–308, 1988.
66. Nirschl RP: Tennis elbow. Orthop Clin North Am 4:787, 1973.
67. Nirschl RP, Kraushaar BS: Assessment and treatment guidelines for elbow injuries. Physician Sportsmed 24:43–60, 1996.
68. Nirschl RP, Sobel J: Conservative treatment of tennis elbow. Physician Sportsmed 9:43–54, 1981.
69. O'Driscoll SW, Morrey BF, Korinek SL: The pathoanatomy and kinematics of posterolateral rotatory instability (pivot-shift) of the elbow. Trans ORS 15:6, 1990.
70. Plancher KD, Halbrecht J, Lourie GM: Medial and lateral epicondylitis in the athlete. Clin Sports Med 15:283–305, 1996.
71. Plancer KD, Minnich JM: Sports-specific injuries. Clin Sports Med 15:207–218,1996.
72. Press JM, Herring SA, Kibler, WB: Rehabilitation of musculoskeletal disorders. In Dillingham T (ed): The Textbook of Military Medicine. Washington DC, Bordin Institute, Office of the Surgeon General (in press).
73. Priest JD, Nagel DA: Tennis shoulder. Am J Sports Med 4:28–42, 1976.
74. Regan, WD, Korinek SL, Morrey BF, et al: Biomechanical study ligaments around the elbow joint. Clin Orthop 271:170, 1991.
75. Reilly JP, Nicholas JA: The chronically inflamed bursa. Clin Sports Med 6:345–370, 1987.
76. Roetert EP, Dillman CJ, Groppel JL, Schultheis JM: The biomechanics of tennis elbow. An integrated approach. Clin Sports Med 14:47–57, 1995.
77. Sailer SM, Lewis SB: Rehabilitation and splinting of common upper extremity injuries in athletes. Clin Sports Med 14:411–446, 1995.
78. Schwab GH, Bennet JB, Woods GW, et al: Biomechanics of elbow instability: The role of the medial collateral ligament. Clin Orthop 146:42, 1980.
79. Seto JL, Brewster CE, Randall CC, et al: Rehabilitation following ulnar collateral ligament reconstruction of athletes. J Orthop Sports Phys Ther 14:100–105, 1991.
80. Sherman DH, Snyder SJ, Fos JM: Triceps tendon avulsion in a professional body builder: A case report. Am J Sports Med 12:328, 1976.
81. Snyder-Mackler L, Epler M: Effect of standard and aircast tennis elbow bands on integrated electromyography of forearm extensor musculature proximal to the bands. Am J Sports Med 17:278–281, 1989.
82. Sobel J, Pettrone F, Nirschl R: Prevention and rehabilitation of racquet sports injuries. In Nicholas JA, Hershman EB (eds): The Upper Extremity in Sports Medicine. St. Louis, Mosby, 1990, pp 843–860.
83. Steinberg BD, Plancher KD: Clinical anatomy of the wrist and elbow. Clin Sports Med 14:299–3131, 1995.
84. Tarsney FF: Rupture and avulsion of the triceps. Clin Orthop 83:177, 1964.
85. Thomas DR, Plancher KD, Hawkins RJ: Prevention and rehabilitation of overuse injuries of the elbow. Clin Sports Med 14:459–477, 1996.
86. Timmerman LA, Schwartz ML, Andrews JR: Preoperative evaluation of the ulnar collateral ligament by magnetic resonance imaging and computed tomography arthrography. Evaluation in 25 baseball players with surgical confirmation. Am J Sports Med 22:26–31, 1994.
87. Vangsness CT, Jobe FW: Surgical treatment of medial epicondylitis. J Bone Joint Surg 73B:409, 1991.
88. Voss DE, Lonta MK, Meyers BJ: Proprioceptive Neuromuscular Facilitation: Patterns and Techniques, 3rd ed. New York, Harper & Row, 1985.
89. Ward WG, Anderson TE: Elbow arthroscopy in a mostly athletic population. J Hand Surg 18A:220–224, 1993.

90. Wells P: Cervical dysfunction and shoulder problems. Physiotherapy 68:66–71, 1983.
91. Wiesner SL: Rehabilitation of elbow injuries in sports. Phys Med Rehabil Clin North Am 5:81–113, 1994.
92. Wilk KE, Arrigo C, Andrews JR: Rehabilitation of the elbow in the throwing athlete. JOSPT 17:305–317, 1993.
93. Wilson FD, Andrews JR, Blackburn TA, et al: Valgus extension overload in the pitching elbow. Am J Sports Med 11:83–88, 1982.
94. Yocum LA: The diagnosis and nonoperative treatment of elbow problems in the athlete. Clin Sports Med 8:439–451, 1989.

## Shoulder

1. Allman FL: Fractures and ligamentous injuries of the clavicle and its articulations. J Bone Joint Surg 49A: 774–784, 1967.
2. Akeson WH, Woo SY, Amil D, et al: The connective tissue response to immobility. Clin Orthop 93:356–362, 1973.
3. Basmajian JV: The surgical anatomy and function of the arm–trunk mechanism. Surg Clin North Am 43:1471–1482, 1963.
4. Bassett RW, Brown AO, Morrey BF, et al: Glenohumeral muscle force in movement mechanics in a position of shoulder instability. J BioMech 23:405–415, 1988.
5. Bergfield JA, Herschman EB, Wilbourne AJ: Brachial plexus injuries in athletes. Presented at American Academy of Orthopedic Surgeons Annual Meeting, New Orleans, 1986.
6. Berquist TH: Imaging of Orthopedic Trauma, 2nd ed. New York, Raven, 1991.
7. Bigliani LY, Morrison DS, April EW: The morphology of the acromion and its relationship to rotator cuff tears. Orthop Trans 10: 228, 1986.
8. Bowen M, Warren R: Ligamentous control of shoulder stability based on selective cutting and static translation experiments. Clin Sports Med 10:757–782, 1991.
9. Burhhead WZ, Rockwood CA: Treatment of instability of the shoulder with exercise program, J. Bone Joint Surg 74A:896, 1992.
10. Clancy WG, Brand RL, Bergfield JA: Upper trunk brachial plexus injuries in contact sports. J Sports Med 5:209–215, 1977.
11. Crues JV, Fareed DO: Magnetic resonance imaging of shoulder impingement. Top Magn Imaging 73:39–49, 1991.
12. DiBenedetto M, Markey K : Electrodiagnostic localization of traumatic upper trunk brachial plexopathy. Arch Phys Med Rehabil 65:15–17, 1984
13. DiGiovine NM, Jobe FW, Pink M, et al: An electromyographic analysis of the upper extremity in pitching. J Shoulder Elbow Surg 1:15–25, 1992.
14. Dines DM, Levinson M: The conservative management of the unstable shoulder including rehabilitation. Clin Sports Med 14:797–816, 1995.
15. Dixit R: Nonoperative management of shoulder injuries in sport. Phys Med Rehabil Clin North Am 13:69–80, 1994.
16. Dumitru D: Electrodiagnostic Medicine. Philadelphia, Hanley & Belfus, 1995, pp 585–642.
17. Franco V, Nordin M: Basic Biomechanics of the Skeletal System. Philadelphia, Lea & Febiger, 1980.
18. Franks C, Akeson WJ, Woo S, et al: Physiology and therapy: The value of passive joint motion. Clin Orthop 185:113, 1984.
19. Funk FJ, Wells RE: Injuries of the cervical spine in football. Clin Orthop 109:50–58, 1975.
20. Greenfield BJ, Donatelli R, Wooden MJ, et al: Isokinetic evaluation of the shoulder rotational strength between the plane of the scapula and the frontal plane. M J Sports Med 18:2, 1990.
21. Hawkins RJ, Kennedy JC: Impingement syndrome in athletes. M J Sports Med 8:151–158, 1980.
22. Herring SA, Weinstein SM: Electrodiagnosis in sports medicine. Phys Med Rehabil State Art Rev 4:809–822, 1989.
23. Hill HA, Sachs MD: The grooved defect at the humeral head: A frequently unrecognized complication of dislocation of the shoulder joint. Radiology 35:690–700, 1940.
24. Hovelius L: Anterior dislocation of the humerus in teenagers and young adults. J Bone Joint Surg 69A:393–399, 1987.
25. Hunter C: Injuries to the brachial plexus: Experience of a private sports medicine clinic. J Md Osteop Assoc 91:757–760, 1982.
26. Itoi E, Kuechle DK, Newman SR, et al: Stabilizing function in the biceps in stable and unstable shoulders. J Bone Joint Surg 75A:546–550, 1993.
27. Jobe FW, Bradley JP: Rotator cuff injuries in baseball: Prevention and rehabilitation. Sports Med 6:378, 1988.
28. Jobe FW, Kvitne RS, Giangarra CE: Shoulder pain in the overhand or throwing athlete: The relationship of instability in rotator cuff impingement. Orthop Rev 18:963–975, 1989.
29. Johnson JE, Sims FH, Scott SG: Musculoskeletal injuries in competitive swimmers. Mayo Clin Proc 62:289–304, 1987.

30. Johnston TB: The movements of the shoulder joint: A plea for the use of "plane of scapula" as the plane of reference for movements occurring at the humeri scapular joint. Br J Surg 25:252–260, 1987.
31. Jones MW, Matthews JP: Rupture of the pectoralis major in weightlifters. Injury 19:219, 1988.
32. Kent BE: Functional anatomy of the shoulder complex. Phys Ther 51:867–887, 1971.
33. Khrisman OD, Snook GA, Stanitis JM, et al: Lateral flexion neck injuries in athletic competition. JAMA 192:613–615, 1965.
34. Kibler WB: The role of the scapula in the throwing motion. Cont Orthop 22:525–532, 1991.
35. Knott M, Voss DE: Proprioceptive Neuromuscular Facilitation. New York, Harper & Row, 1968.
36. Kummel BM: Fractures of the glenoid causing chronic dislocation of the shoulder. Clin Orthop 69:189–191, 1970.
37. Kvitne RS, Jobe FW, Jobe CM: Shoulder instability in the overhand or throwing athlete. Clin Sports Med 14:917–935, 1995.
38. Lo YP, Hsu YC, Chan KM: Epidemiology of shoulder impingement in upper arm sports events. Br J Sports Med 24:173–177, 1990.
39. Lowdon BJ, Pitman AJ, Pateman NA: Surfboard riding injuries. Med J Aust 2:613–616, 1983.
40. Lucas DB: Biomechanics of the shoulder joint. Arch Surg 107:425–432, 1973.
41. Marshall TM: Nerve pinch injuries in football. J Ky Med Assoc 648–649, 1970.
42. Matsen F, Harryman D, Sidles J: Mechanics of glenohumeral instability. Clin Sports Med 10:783–788, 1991.
43. Matsen FA, Thomas SC, Rockwood CA: Anterior glenohumeral instability. In Rockwood CA, Matsen FA (eds): Shoulder. Philadelphia, W.B. Saunders, 1990.
44. McLeod WD, Andrews JR: Mechanism of shoulder injuries. Phys Ther 66:1901–1904, 1986.
45. Mumford EB: Acromioclavicular dislocation. J Bone Joint Surg 23A:799–802, 1941.
46. Neer CS: Displaced proximal humerus fractures. Part I: Classification and evaluation. J Bone Joint Surgery 52A:1077–1089, 1970.
47. Neer CS: Impingement lesions. Clin Orthop 173:70–77, 1983.
48. Neer CS, Foster CR: Inferior capsular shift for involuntary inferior and multidirectional instability of the shoulder. J Bone Joint Surg. 62A:897, 1980.
49. Neer CS, Horowitz BS: Fractures of the proximal humeral epiphyseal plate in children. Clin Orthop 41:24–31, 1968.
50. Neer CS, Rockwood CA: Fractures and dislocations of the shoulder. In Rockwood CA, Green DP (eds): Fractures in Adults, 2nd ed. Philadelphia, J. B. Lippincott, 1984, pp 675–985.
51. Neer CS II, Welsh RP: The shoulder in sports. Orthop Clin North Am 8:583–591, 1977.
52. Norfray JF, Tremaine MJ, Groves HC, et al: The clavicle in hockey. Am J Sports Med 5:275–280, 1977.
53. Noyes FR: Functional properties of knee ligaments and alterations induced by immobilization. Clin Orthop 123:210–242, 1977.
54. Ozaki J, Fujimoto S, Nakagawa Y, et al: Tears of the rotator cuff of the shoulder associated with pathologic changes at the acromion. J Bone Joint Surg 70A:1224–1230, 1988.
55. Perry J: Anatomy and biomechanics of the shoulder in throwing, swimming, gymnastics, and tennis. Clin Sports Med 2:247–269, 1983.
56. Pino EC, Colville MR: Snowboard injuries. Am J Sports Med 17:778–781, 1989.
57. Poppen NK, Walker PS: Forces at the glenohumeral joint in abduction. Clin Orthop 135:165–170, 1978.
58. Poppen NK, Walker PS: Normal and abnormal motion of the shoulder. J Bone Joint Surg 58A:195–201, 1976.
59. Rathbun JB, MacNab I: The microvascular pattern of the rotator cuff. J. Bone Joint Surg 52B:540–553, 1970.
60. Richardson AB, Jobe FW, Collins HR: The shoulder in competitive swimming. Am J Sports Med 8:159–163, 1980.
61. Robertson WC, Eichman PL, Clancy WG: Upper trunk brachial plexopathy in football players. JAMA 241:1480–1482, 1979.
62. Rockwood CS : Subluxations and dislocations about the shoulder. In Rockwood CS, Green DP (eds): Fractures in Adults, 2nd ed. Philadelphia, J.B. Lippincott, 1984, pp 922–985.
63. Rogers LF: The shoulder and humeral shaft. In Rogers LF (ed): Radiology of Skeletal Trauma. New York, Churchill-Livingstone, 1992.
64. Rowe CR: Fractures of the adult shoulder. In Rowe CR (ed) The Shoulder. New York, Churchill Livingstone, 1988.
65. Rowe CR: Prognosis in dislocations of the shoulder. J Bone Joint Surg 38A:957, 1956.
66. Rowe CR, Zarins B: Recurrent transient subluxation of the shoulder. J Bone Joint Surg 68A:863, 1981.
67. Saal JA: Rehabilitation of throwing in tennis related shoulder injuries. Phys Med Rehabil State Art Rev 1:597–612, 1987.
68. Saha AK: Mechanism of shoulder movements in a plea for recognition of the "zero position" of the glenohumeral joint. Clin Orthop 173:3–10, 1983.

69. Sallis RE, Jones K, Knopp W: Burners: Offensive strategy for an underreported injury. Physician Sportsmed 20:47–55, 1992.
70. Takazawa H, Sudo N, et al: Statistical observation of nerve injuries in athletes. Brain Nerve Inj 3:11–17, 1971.
71. Tata GE, Ng L, Kramer JF: Shoulder antagonistic strength ratios during concentric and eccentric muscle actions in the scapular plane. J Orthop Sports Phys Ther 18:654–660, 1993.
72. Tippett SR: Closed chain exercise. Orthop Phys Ther Clin North Am 1:253–268, 1992.
73. Thomas SC, Matson FA: An approach to the repair of glenohumeral ligament avulsion in the management of traumatic anterior instability. J Bone Joint Surg 71A:506, 1989.
74. Vegso JJ, Torg E, Torg JS: Rehabilitation of the cervical spine, brachial plexus, and peripheral nerve injuries. Clin Sports Med 6:135–158, 1987.
75. Warner JP, Deng X, Warren RF, et al: Superoinferior translation in the intact and vented glenohumeral joint. J Shoulder Elbow Surg 2:99–105, 1993.
76. Weaver JK, Dunn HK: Treatment of acromioclavicular injuries, especially complete acromioclavicular separation. J Bone Joint Surg 54A:1187–1194, 1972.
77. Weiner DS, MacNab I: Superior migration of the humeral head. J Bone Joint Surg 52B:524–527, 1970.
78. Yamaguchi K, Flatlow EL: Management of multidirectional instability. Clin Sports Med 14:885–902, 1995.

# 10

# Complex Regional Painful Syndrome

## DENNIS M. LOX, MD

## HISTORICAL PERSPECTIVE

In 1994, the International Association for the Study of Pain (IASP) recommended replacing the terms *causalgia, reflex sympathetic dystrophy (RSD)*, and *sympathetic maintained pain* with the terms *complex regional painful syndrome (CRPS) type I*, which is not associated with a classic nerve injury, and *CRPS type II*, which is associated with a classic nerve injury as in causalgia.[1] The past century has seen much controversy and confusion since Mitchell introduced the term causalgia,[2] and the confusion has continued since 1946 when Evans coined the term reflex sympathetic dystrophy,[3] which is a variation of de Takats' 1937 discourse on reflex dystrophy of the extremity.[4] In 1986, Roberts theorized about sympathetic maintained pain via the wide dynamic range neuron and mechanoreceptor theory.[5] The American medical community has made a simplistic historical oversight in retaining the terms causalgia, RSD, and sympathetic maintained pain. *Sudeck's atrophy*[6] is the preferred term in German-speaking countries, and *algoneurodystrophy*[7] is the preferred term in French-speaking countries.

An historical perspective is necessary to appreciate fully the rationale for redefinition of these terms and the need for more stringent criteria. An overview of the different terms that have been used to identify the symptom complex is presented below:

| | |
|---|---|
| 1867 | Mitchell—causalgia[2] |
| 1900 | Sudeck—Sudeck's atrophy[6] |
| 1929 | Zur veth—peripheral acute trophoneurosis[8] |
| 1931 | Morton—traumatic angiospasm[9] |
| 1933 | Fontaine—posttraumatic osteoporosis[10] |
| 1934 | Lehman—traumatic vasospasm[11] |
| 1937 | De Takats—reflex dystrophy of the extremity[4] |
| 1940 | Homans—minor/major causalgia[12] |
| 1946 | Evans—reflex sympathetic dystrophy[3] |
| 1947 | Steinbrocker—shoulder/hand syndrome[13] |
| 1973 | Patman—mimocausalgia[14] |
| 1973 | Glick—algoneurodystrophy[7] |
| 1986 | Ochoa—ABC syndrome[16] |
| 1986 | Roberts—sympathetic maintained pain[5] |
| 1993 | Ochoa—chronic pains of sensory motor, vasomotor disturbances[16] |
| 1994 | IASP—complex regional painful syndrome[1] |

The history of this symptom complex began with Silas Weir Mitchell, a Civil War surgeon, who was appointed by Surgeon General Hammond to run the United States Army Hospital for Diseases of the Nervous System in Philadelphia because of his special interest in soldiers with nerve injuries. Mitchell was an extremely precise and dedicated physician who recorded his findings in great detail. It is less known that Mitchell quoted an Englishman, James Paget, who reported a similar symptom complex in 1864.[17] Later in 1864 Mitchell released his treatise *Gunshot Wounds and Other Injuries of Nerves* in conjunction with G.R. Morehouse and W.W. Keen.[18] In 1872, Mitchell wrote *Injuries of Nerves and Their Consequences*, based on on his lengthy experiences.[19] Mitchell was a prolific writer and even penned a short story entitled "Kris Kringle," which influenced the American holiday spirit. Mitchell was renowned worldwide. While ill in Paris as a young man, he consulted Charcot, the author of the invaluable 1877 lectures on disease of the nervous system.[20] Charcot, not knowing the identity of his patient, made recommendations in a letter to a leading neurologist in Philadelphia. When Mitchell asked to whom he was being referred, Charcot replied, "To Dr. S. Weir Mitchell." When Mitchell identified himself, Charcot replied, "Oh. Then you will not need this letter"—and tore it up.

Webb cites Percival Pott's mention of certain painful afflictions of the nerves in conjunction with injuries of the extremities[21] but gives no specific references. Pott was a prominent physician in England in the 1700s. *The Chirurgical Works of Percival Pott*[22] is a 493-page medical text encompassing various disorders, including multiple chapters on trauma and fractures. Pott also discusses how in 1756, after being thrown from his horse, he sustained a compound fracture of the tibia. His treatment options were either amputation or attempted splinting, which fortunately was successful. But there is no mention of a descriptive term resembling the symptom complex CRPS.

In his 1953 text on the management of pain, Bonica[23] cites Pott's observation that severe persistent and diffuse pain sometimes followed nerve injuries of the extremities and was more likely after partial than complete severance of a nerve. Bonica also cites *The Surgical and Physiological Works of John Abernathy*[24] as well as the work of Ambroise Paré, who apparently encountered painful disorders of peripheral nerves during his service as a surgeon for the King of France in the wars against Italy and the Civil War with the Huguenots. Paré was asked to treat King Charles IX after Antone Bortalis performed a lancet wound to induce bleeding for small pox fever. The pain was described as persistent and diffuse and was associated with contractures of the muscles. The king could neither flex nor extend his arm for 1 month, but the symptoms finally disappeared.

In 1813, Denmark described a pain syndrome that developed after a musket injury to the radial nerve.[25] The patient was in such profound pain that he begged to have his arm amputated. After amputation the symptoms resolved, and a tiny fragment of lead was found embedded in the nerve. In retrospect, the amputation would have been unnecessary if the surgeon had known about the fragment of lead and simply removed it. Amputation has been used unsuccessfully in other patients.[26]

Of note, Mitchell believed that the syndrome was an inflammatory response, not connected to the sympathetic nervous system. It was not, however, until Mitchell had the advantage of treating large numbers of soldiers with nerve injuries in a single site that he was able to describe accurately the syndrome that he later called causalgia because of the patient's persistent complaints of burning pain. Of interest, the patients would treat the burning pain by immersing their limbs in snow or wrapping a cool, moist towel around the limb. In the symptom complex that subsequently developed into sympathetic maintained pain, some patients report relief with cold and others report exacerbation. Paradoxically, heat sometimes alleviates and cold exacerbates.[27–29]

In 1900, Sudeck described a local bony atrophy noted on radiographs and thought that it was a local inflammatory reaction. He used the term Sudeck's atrophy, which has persisted.[6] In 1916, the French surgeon René Leriche[30] performed the first periarterial sympathectomy and later performed sympathetic blockade for similar conditions.

In the 1930s, Spurling[31] began using sympathetic ganglionectomy, hoping for better results. Medical history often forgets that sympathectomies used to be performed for peptic ulcer disease and seizure disorders, whereas now pharmacologic therapy may be prescribed instead. In a large study, Veldman found only a 7% success rate with sympathectomies.[29] In 1934, Lehman[11] described four cases that he believed were due to disturbance of blood supply by the sympathetic system. He also noted psychologic features. Of interest, Lehman reported a positive response to treatment with high doses of intravenous typhoid vaccine for a febrile reaction. In 1937, de Takats wrote about reflex dystrophy of the extremities,[4] which he believed was due to imbalance between anabolic and catabolic activities of the tissues, and proposed that the syndrome was caused by an exaggerated nutritional reflex. He also noted that symptoms could be treated with physiotherapy or sympathectomy of the efferent arc.

In 1946, almost 10 years later, Evans[3] coined the term reflex sympathetic dystrophy after reviewing 57 cases. He believed that RSD was a better term because not all patients complained of the burning pain noted by Mitchell and cited as a cause Livingston's concept of the vicious circle,[32] which was adapted from Lorento de No's 1938 theory of an internuncial pool of neurons. Evans noted that trigger points were found in 65% of patients and that addressing the trigger points provided effective treatment. This approach has been used for over a century by various authors, including Mitchell, who later recalled that in 1 year he gave over 40,000 local injections of morphine.[34–38] Fischer reported that after he gave one trigger point injection to a patient with chronic RSD, symptoms resolved immediately.[39] Of note, Livingston did not think that the vicious circle was perpetuated or mediated by an abnormal sympathetic reflex arc.

Numerous other physicians continued to describe a syndrome of varying pain, each noting different diagnostic criteria and thus making classification extremely difficult. In 1986, Roberts proposed the concept of sympathetic maintained pain: if sympathetic blockade alleviates the symptoms, the diagnosis is confirmed. In 1988, Frost[28] and later Treede[40] contended that failure of sympathetic blockade to alleviate symptoms established the diagnosis of sympathetic independent pain. Any unexplainable pain fell into one of the two categories.

Clinical manifestations depend to a large degree on which author is describing the condition. The 1864 descriptions of Paget and Mitchell may not be relevant to the descriptions in 1900 by Sudeck, in 1945 by de Takats, in 1946 by Evans, in 1955 by Casten and Betcher,[41] in 1981 by Tahmoush,[42] in 1981 by Kozin,[43] or in 1986 by Roberts. Indeed, the IASP proposed entirely different criteria in 1986 and 1994.

In 1955, Casten and Betcher[41] defined RSD as an excessive or abnormal response of an extremity to injury. They found four constant characteristics and proposed that all four must be present to justify the diagnosis:

1. Prolonged pain
2. Vasomotor disturbances
3. Delayed functional recovery
4. Trophic changes

In 1970, after reviewing 140 cases, Pak et al.[44] proposed the following criteria:

1. Evidence of neurovascular disturbance
2. Evidence of dystrophic changes, including atrophy, ankylosis or loss of range of motion, and osteoporosis

In 1992, Gibbons and Wilson[45] developed nine criteria:

1. Allodynia or hyperpathia
2. Burning pain
3. Edema

4. Color or hair growth changes
5. Sweating changes
6. Radiographic changes
7. Quantitative measurement of vasomotor changes
8. Positive response to bone scan
9. Positive response to sympathetic blockade

If fewer than 3 of the 9 criteria were present, the diagnosis was unlikely; if 3–4.5 were present, the diagnosis was possible; and if more than 5 were present, the diagnosis was probable. In 1993, Veldman listed three categories of symptoms[29]:

1. Diffuse pain, skin temperature changes, edema, color changes, decreased range of motion
2. Increased symptoms after use
3. Symptoms in an area larger than the area of initial injury

In 1994 the IASP developed the following criteria for diagnosis of CRPS:

1. Initiating noxious event
2. Continued pain, allodynia, or hyperalgesia
3. Evidence of edema, vasomotor changes, temperature changes
4. Exclusion of other causes

The fourth criterion is perhaps the most important of all. Pain and swelling may be due to various medical conditions. Failure to exclude a condition that is potentially treatable with sympathetic blockade or any other condition that may account for the symptoms was the impetus behind the recent move in a more positive direction. In 1986 the IASP criteria included a positive response to sympathetic blockade, but in 1994 this criterion was dropped. Progress depends on recognition of mistakes and attempts to make positive changes.

The incidence of the syndrome under its various names is extremely variable, depending on the diagnostic criteria. In a World War I study, Carter[46] found an incidence of 4 in 3,000 patients (< 1%). In a World War II study, Kirklin found an incidence of 61 in 2,850 patients (1.8%). In 1948 Sunderland[49] reported 34 cases among 278 patients but did not specify his diagnostic criteria. A large study by Rothenberg[50] during the Vietnam war identified 108 cases among 7,138 patients (1.5%). In a trauma center in New York, Plewes[51] found an incidence of 1 in 2,000 (0.05%). Among patients with cerebrovascular accidents, the incidence ranges from 12–21%[52,53] and among patients with coronary artery disease, from 1–20%. An incidence of 0.2% was noted in a study of 2,000 workers' compensation cases in New York,[54] and a 1980 study using positive response to sympathetic blockade as its diagnostic criterion reported an incidence of 11%.[55]

## PATHOPHYSIOLOGY

Lankford[56] cites numerous references[3,5,31,57,58] to support his claim that the role of the sympathetic nervous system in the pathophysiology of CRPS has been firmly established. But closer inspection reveals that all of his references are based on theory and that some, such as Evans[3] and Roberts,[5] are contradictory. In fact, all discussions of pathophysiology are based on theory rather than proof. The various theories can be divided into two general categories: peripheral and central.

Peripheral theories include four subcategories:

1. Inflammatory reaction, to which Mitchell subscribed;
2. Artificial synapse, which was developed by Doupe;[59]
3. Spontaneous discharge, which was developed by Devor;[60] and
4. Ischemic pain, which was developed by Lewis.[61]

Of interest, Mitchell's 1864 inflammatory theory was supported by Sudeck in 1900, and further research, including that of Goris[62] in 1985 and Veldman in 1993, has revived the peripheral theory.[63–65] In 1944, Doupe supported the artificial synapse theory by suggesting that the nerve impulse jumped from one sympathetic efferent to a somatic sensory ephapse. Doupe also described, rather prophetically, three types of RSD: causalgic (associated with injury to the nerve), dystrophic, and psychogenic. He was astute enough to understand the problem of lumping all patients under one heading. Certainly a patient with a peripheral nerve lesion will have pain as a sequela, and certain reactions, such as dystrophic changes and atrophy, may be inherent. An L5 radiculopathy with foot drop and an unsuccessful outcome will result in atrophy of the tissues. This scenario suggests causalgia and should be differentiated from a scenario with overt psychologic features and no objective physical findings that can be explained solely by neural injury. Hysterical paralysis has been well documented since the time of Charcot.[26]

Prevailing central theories can be classified into four subcategories:

1. In the reverberating circuit theory, constant bombardment of pain impulses causes a vicious circle of reflexes that spread through a pool of many neurons connecting upward, downward, and even across, reaching as high as the thalamus. The vicious circle theory of Livingston, proposed in 1947, is an elaboration of de No's 1938 theory based on an intranuncial pool of neurons.[33]

2. The gate control theory was proposed in 1965 by Melzack and Wall. Of interest, the larger A-fiber mechanoreceptors used in transcutaneous electrical nerve stimulation (TENS) to close the gate and decrease the pain are the same mechanism proposed by Roberts as initiating pain in his theory of sympathetic maintained pain.

3. The turbulence theory was proposed in 1976 by Sunderland,[49] who believed that abnormalities or degeneration of postganglionic sympathetic efferents resulted in retrograde transmission across the synapse of pre- and postganglionic nerve endings. Eventually the retrograde impulses reached the spinal cord and intranuncial pool of neurons, setting up the vicious circle.

4. The wide dynamic range neuron theory evolved from Roberts' 1986 hypothesis of sympathetic maintained pain (SMP).[5] Roberts believed that pain traveled first through unmyelinated C-fibers, then through the wide dynamic range neurons to pain receptors in the dorsal horn of the central nervous system and ultimately to the brain. The pain could travel by various mechanisms through either A-mechanoreceptors or unmyelinated C-fibers, both of which became sensitized by the wide dynamic range neurons. Roberts attributed allodynia to the mechanoreceptors and thought that sympathetic blockade would stop the transmission centrally. The intravenous regional block popularized by Hannington-Kiff in 1974 is in direct contrast to this theory.[67] Obviously no theory explains all features of the syndrome.

## EXPERIMENTAL MODEL

There is no veterinary correlate for causalgia, RDS, SMP, or CRPS. Beginning with Bennett in 1988,[68] however, various scientists have noted hyperalgesia and allodynic behavior in rats when a ligature is tied around the sciatic nerve. In 1991,[69] Bennett discussed the role of the sympathetic nervous system in painful peripheral neuropathy, and in the same year Janig[70] speculated whether this approach may provide an experimental model for RSD. Later disillusioned with the concept, Janig questioned the validity of the term RSD but recommended keeping it because of lack of a better alternative.[71] He commented that the medical community probably would continue to use the term in any case.

Obviously a descriptive term that implied no specific pathophysiology was needed. In 1993 Ochoa[16] suggested chronic pain with sensory and motor phenomena (CPSMP), pointing out that the sensory and motor phenomena may include various (and variable) combinations of negative and positive manifestations as well as vasomotor and sudomotor signs and symptoms. In 1994, the IASP recommended the use of CRPS type I for classic causalgia with clear evidence of nerve injury and CRPS type II for cases with no evidence of nerve injury.

It is hoped that elimination of the terms RSD and SMP will result in more rigid guidelines, better research, and ultimately better medical care. At present, unless a ligature is tied around a rat's sciatic nerve, there is no experimental model for CRPS.

## PSYCHOLOGIC FACTORS

Distinct psychogenic features have been proposed by various authors, although sympathophiles sharply denounced the possibility. The lack of a veterinary correlate supports the presence of psychologic factors. Work animals and race horses are prone to much the same injuries as humans and should have a similar incidence of the disorder. Furthermore, an equal incidence should be reported in the sports medicine literature, but the Index Medicus lists no references to athletic injury and RSD.

Pillemer and Micheli,[22] however, describe a similar condition that develops after traumatic injury in youth sports. The children, whose injuries typically heal relatively quickly, fell into two groups: (1) a small group treated over longer periods for severe debilitating injuries and (2) patients initially evaluated with relatively minor injuries (e.g., sprained ankle, tendinitis) who failed to respond to treatment. In the first group, which consisted primarily of children with first-time but serious injuries, depression in reaction to major change or loss was common. Patients responded well to psychiatric treatment and adaptive strategies. Patients in the second group, who continued to complain of severe discomfort and inability to participate in their normal routine, often went from one physician to another in search of treatment for the physical problem alone. Of those referred for psychologic intervention, only 60–70% followed through. Eventually many of these patients were lost to follow-up.

In a high percentage of 20 children diagnosed with RSD in a 3-year period, important psychologic issues were discovered during diagnosis and management. In addition to the stress of childhood athletic participation and loss of self-esteem, compromised independence and an ambivalence toward the rigors of sports training may have contributed to the development of clinical RSD.

The authors concluded that psychologic issues may be a factor in development of RSD among children active in sports. They cited the case report of a 16-year-old girl who was admitted to Children's Hospital for severe right foot pain on four different occasions within 1 month. Previously an avid participant in school gymnastics and track, she had injured her foot approximately 1 year earlier. The initial diagnosis was a minor sprain, which healed well with Ace bandaging and reduced weight-bearing. A diagnosis of RSD was made on the basis of her continued complaints. She experienced a cramping sensation in her toes while running in gym class. Various therapeutic measures, including exercise, TENS, hydrotherapy, and biofeedback, proved ineffective for relieving pain.

Psychologic assessment was requested. During consultation in her hospital bed, the patient was pale and anxious; she gripped the covers tightly around her body so that only her face was visible. She was guarded and withholding, demonstrating a general unresponsiveness to the interview that resembled her indifference to the various therapies that she had recently undergone. Rigorous psychologic testing and further history from her family revealed that depression predated the injury. She was also stressed by the persistent behavior of two brothers who insulted her and made sexually provocative comments. She also had multiple other somatic complaints, including stomach aches and frequent sore throats before school functions such as dances and was socially immature around boys. Two months before her recent hospitalization she had confided that she was attacked by a stranger. The authors note that she became receptive to the idea of psychologic intervention and was relieved when some of her issues had surfaced. This case illustrates the psychologic features that develop in chronic pain syndrome, which becomes an easy escape from the rigors and responsibilities of physical activity. In contrast, there are no reports of RSD among elite athletes, who may experience minor bruises, sprains, fractures, dislocations, and even quadriplegia.

In 1877, Charcot discussed hysteria at great length. He was particularly interested in patients with ovarian hemianesthesia whose pain was alleviated by palpation over the ovary. The diagnosis of ovarian hemianesthesia is no longer prevalent in the medical community. In the 1990s the Social Security Administration allows disability on the basis of subjective symptoms such as generalized pain, fibromyalgia, and RSD, even when physical findings are inconsistent. Any patient with no discrete medical findings should be referred for psychologic assessment.

In 1934, Lehman reported a patient who was successfully treated with a typhoid vaccine. The patient was involved in Workers' Compensation litigation with the support of his mother and an overzealous attorney. In 1946, Zikeyev[73] was convinced that the thalamus was somehow involved. He reported complete relief of pain in 31 of 32 patients treated with surgery followed by narcotic sleep for 5–6 days. His "sleeping mixture" contained sodium bromide, chloral hydrate, tinct. volarian, luminal, and pantopon. Various surgical techniques were used. It would have been interesting if Zikeyev had done a controlled study in which he used only the sleeping mixture, without no surgical intervention. In 1959, Adler[74] suggested that patients may be predisposed to RSD by certain personality traits, such as decreased ego strength and decreased skills for coping with tension and stress. Polack, Houdenhove, and Geertzen noted that the onset of RSD was often associated with a recent predisposing life event.[75–77] In the author's experience, patients often report multiple significant life stressors that precede development of the symptom complex.

Numerous other medical conditions have been associated with stress. Acting through the sympathetic nervous system, stress may result in hyperactivity of the end organ, as in hypertension, peptic ulcer disease, eczema, irritable bowel, migraine headaches, myofascial pain syndrome, and fibromyalgia. It is no longer considered appropriate, however, to treat peptic ulcer disease with sympathectomy. Studies have shown that with biofeedback and relaxation training hypertensive patients may lower their medication dosage or even discontinue medication altogether. The 1990 Consensus Report of an Ad Hoc Committee of the American Association for Hand Surgery on the Definition of RSD[78] noted a psychologic predisposition in most, if not all, patients with RSD. Predisposing factors include difficulty with open expression of anger as well as anxiety, depression, increased interpersonal sensitivity, increased somatization, and decreased body satisfaction. Citing reports by Fishbain et al., Reuler et al., Taenzer et al., Hardy et al., and Chaplin et al., the committee also noted that the severity of disease may diminish with time or even gradually burn out. Psychiatric features tend to increase steadily over time, whereas legal problems are rarely present at the time of injury, increase with time, and diminish after the legal case is settled (Figs. 1 and 2).

The classic staging system has not been verified by recent authors.[29,79] The origin of the staging system is lost—or at least rarely reviewed. In 1947,[13] Steinbrocker reported a staging system based on review of 6 patients, 5 of whom were under great emotional strain. It is difficult to understand how a system based on 6 patients could be maintained for over 50 years. If this is indeed the case, a major historical oversight has obviously occurred. Atrophy (defined as stage III) is a universal consequence of disuse and is not endemic to one disease process.

Some authors suggest that movement disorders may result from RSD, whereas other authors interpret movement disorders simply as additional symptoms of psychogenic

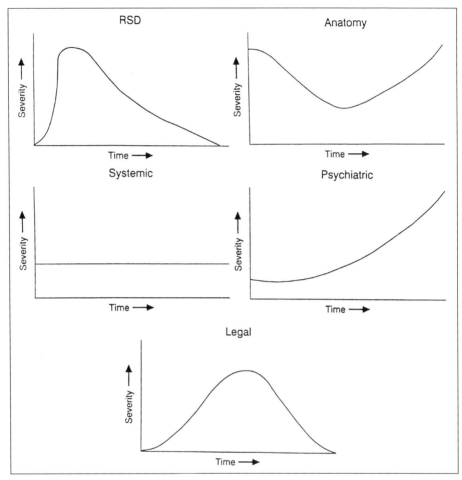

**FIGURE 1.**
In general, reflex sympathetic dystrophy (RSD) and its clinically relevant factors follow typical trends over time. *Above left,* RSD tends to peak early and then gradually burn out. *Above right,* Anatomic factors show an early peak for acute injury and a second peak for the sequelae of disuse. *Center left,* Systemic factors usually remain the same over time. *Center right,* Psychiatric factors tend to show a steady increase over time. *Below,* Legal problems are rare at the time of injury, peak later, and eventually resolve as the legal case is settled. (From Amadio PC, MacKinnon SES, Merritt WH, et al: Reflex Sympathetic Dystrophy Syndrome: Consensus Report of an Ad Hoc Committee of the American Association for Hand Surgery on the Definition of Reflex Sympathetic Dystrophy Syndrome. Plast Reconstr Surg 87:371–375, 1991, with permission.)

origin.[80–82] Psychologic support, as part of the overall rehabilitation effort, has been extremely beneficial in patient management. Depression, anxiety, and other psychologic disorders need to be addressed. In patients with few physical findings, the psychologic differential diagnosis also should include malingering and somatization disorder, in which the patient seeks medical attention for multiple recurring somatic complaints (some of which may be pain-related) that have no physical cause. The hallmark of somatization disorder is multiple physical symptoms. As described in the fourth edition of the *Diagnostic and Statistical Manual of Mental Disorders* (DSM-IV), patients should have a history of pain in at least four different sites, two different gastrointestinal symptoms other than pain, at least one sexual symptom, and one neurologic symptom.

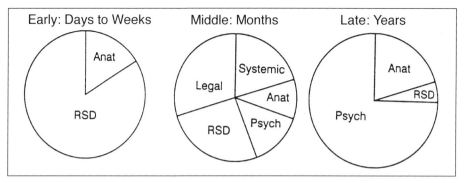

**FIGURE 2.**
Early and late stages tend to have fewer significant factors that may maintain the pain syndrome than the middle stages. *Left,* In the early stages (days to weeks), prognosis is generally good. Evaluation often finds treatable anatomic problems. *Center,* In the middle stages (months), prognosis is guarded. Usually multiple problems are evident; this stage offers the main challenge. Evaluation may find a treatable problem. *Right,* The late stages occur after years of impairment. Prognosis is poor. Evaluation rarely finds a treatable problem; if a treatable problem is found, treatment rarely results in "cure." The late stage may have little or no RSD but represents an end stage of disuse fibrosis, ankylosis, atrophy, and, often, psychiatric impairment. (From Amadio PC, MacKinnon SES, Merritt WH, et al: Reflex Sympathetic Dystrophy Syndrome: Consensus Report of an Ad Hoc Committee of the American Association for Hand Surgery on the Definition of Reflex Sympathetic Dystrophy Syndrome. Plast Reconstr Surg 87:371–375, 1991, with permission.)

Somatoform pain disorder, defined as preoccupation with pain, also may account for symptoms in patients with no or inadequate physical findings. The diagnostic criteria are preoccupation with pain for at least 6 months and absence of a pathophysiologic mechanism to explain symptoms or degree of physical impairment. Conversion disorder is yet another possibility. The author has seen several patients who were diagnosed with RSD but in fact suffered from conversion disorder. Longstanding duration of symptoms and many failed treatment interventions were typical. Since the publication of Charcot's work, with its detailed illustrations, physical manifestations of psychologic disorders have been nothing new (Fig. 3).

The basis of the initial assessment is exclusion of another condition that may explain symptoms, such as thromboembolism, Raynaud's phenomenon, peripheral vascular disease, or direct neural injury (Figs. 4–7). Rehabilitation should be team-oriented. Omohundro[83] recommends the involvement of a physiatrist in every case. Specialists such as neurologists, internists, and rheumatologists are invaluable in the exclusion process. Pain may be controlled from pharmacologic and psychologic perspectives. All patients with chronic pain syndromes complain of more pain when their psyche is disturbed. Effective communication among the treating physician, assisting specialist, psychologic support, physical therapist, occupational therapist, and other team members includes sharing of concise information and reiteration of the same message to the patient. Misinformation or conflicting information among various providers who are not aware of state-of-the-art research only confuses the patient and plants the seed of despair. Depriving the patient of hope is the first step in failure.

## DIAGNOSTIC CRITERIA

The most important feature of diagnosing CRPS is adherence to the 1994 IASP guidelines:

1. Initiating noxious event
2. Continued pain, allodynia, or hyperalgesia

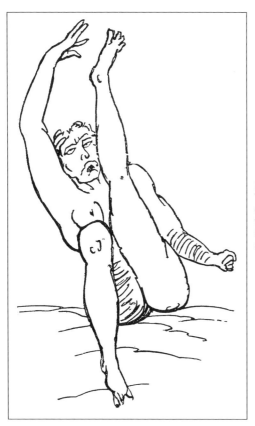

**FIGURE 3.**
The attitude of Ler during the period of contortion. (From Charcot JMN: Lectures on the Diseases of the Nervous System. Edited by Critchley M. London, New Sydenham Society, 1877, with permission.)

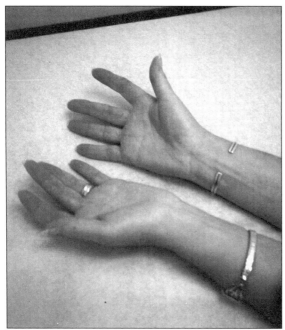

**FIGURE 4.**
Raynaud's phenomenon misdiagnosed as RSD.

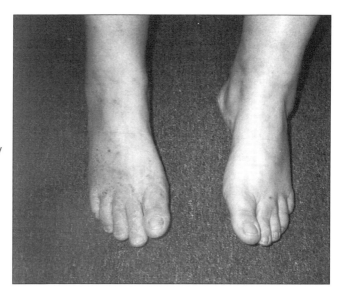

**FIGURE 5.**
Herpetic zoster mistakenly diagnosed as RSD.

3. Evidence of edema, vasomotor changes, or temperature changes
4. Exclusion of other conditions that would explain the symptoms.

Subjective complaints or a single finding or complaint of a cold limb is not diagnostic of CRPS and should be not viewed as a disease process. Of note, no diagnostic tests are included among the IASP criteria, and positive response to sympathetic blockade has been deleted. Based on these criteria, the history and physical examination are the most sensitive and accurate assessment tools.

Numerous additional studies have been used in the past. Radiographic studies have been advocated since the time of Sudeck and in some cases show a patchy demineralization after 3–6 weeks; this finding, however, is nonspecific[84–86] and also has been found

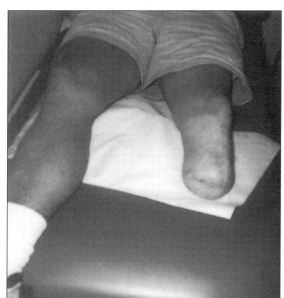

**FIGURE 6.**
Below-knee amputation for refractory "RSD." This case was successful by the patient's own testimony. The original mechanism of injury was a crush injury to the foot with damage to the distal tibial and calcaneal nerves. When symptoms fail to resolve despite numerous invasive procedures, patients may frequently ask for amputation and success or failure may be misinterpreted by an incorrect diagnosis or lack of a clear understanding of a pathophysiologic disease process.[25]

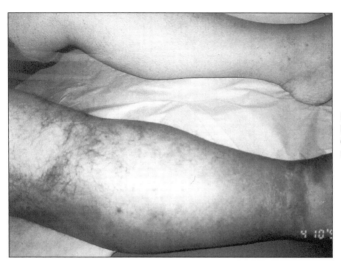

**FIGURE 7.**
Misdiagnosis of RSD after
envenomation by a brown
recluse spider.

in asymptomatic diabetic patients. In advanced cases of RSD, a more generalized osteo-porosis is noted in the affected extremity, but this finding is also nonspecific. Bone scanning with images obtained 3 hours after injection has shown increased uptake in the distal aspect of the affected and contralateral extremities[84,87,88]; this finding has been useful in 49–92% of cases. More recent studies have used triple-phase bone scanning. Holder and MacKinnon reported a sensitivity of 96% and a specificity of 97% for RSD.[89] Lee and Weeks' recent review of the literature related to triple-phase bone scan-ning for diagnosis of RSD found wide variability in correlation with clinical diagnosis.[90] The yield appeared to be greater within the first 26 weeks, but even then it was only 50% accurate. Lee and Weeks concluded that RSD was a clinical diagnosis and that triple-phase bone scanning should not be used as a diagnostic criterion. In the author's expe-rience, patients referred for postoperative bone scans have been diagnosed initially with osteomyelitis and later, by other clinicians, with RSD. More recently, radiologists have recognized that immobility may affect the results of the bone scan. In essence, positive changes on a bone scan do not necessarily reflect disease; they may reflect instead a local reaction to some phenomenon. Without further investigation, bone scans cannot lead to a diagnosis.

Thermography has been a controversial diagnostic test for some time. The proce-dure is based on assessing changes in skin temperature with an infrared camera. Some have found thermography quite useful in assessing RSD,[91–93] but the test is by nature nonspecific. Controlled studies to evaluate critically the role of thermography in assess-ing RSD have yet to be performed, but two controlled studies of thermography in pa-tients with entrapment neuropathies and radiculopathies of the lumbosacral spine concluded that thermograms had little diagnostic or prognostic value.[94,95] The finding by Perelman et al.[121] that 25% of normal controls had an abnormal thermogram sug-gests lack of specificity and sensitivity. It has been suggested that temperature changes of more than 2–3° may indicate RSD, but this finding must be interpreted in the overall clinical context. Such changes are not synonymous with a disorder of the sympathetic nervous system. For example, symptomatic patients with Raynaud's phenomenon cer-tainly have abnormal thermograms. Perelman suggested that lumbar conditions such as disc herniation, anular tears, encroachment of the neuroforamen, spondylolisthesis, and spinal stenosis may result in positive thermograms. He hypothesized that pressure on the nerve root stimulates the sympathetic system, which causes constriction of small arterial vessels in the skin and produces an area of diminished temperature within the particular dermatome. He further hypothesized that a positive thermogram with a negative diagnostic imaging study may reflect injury to the vertebral nerve.

Because controlled studies have not been performed with either triple-phase bone scans or thermography, interpreter reliability is a crucial factor when the presumptive diagnosis is provided and no other objective data are available. For this reason, the IASP no longer includes the triple-phase bone scan, thermography, or positive response to sympathetic blockade among its diagnostic criteria. Electrodiagnostic tests produce normal results in patients with CRPS unless a classic neural injury is present. If neural injury is present, abnormal results reflect merely the changes associated with the injury (as in the original description of causalgia) and are not diagnostic of CRPS.

Skin temperature and blood flow tests have been advocated to assess RSD syndrome; however, controlled studies to evaluate specificity of results are limited by diagnostic criteria.[97] Sweat testing with chemical substances such as cobalt blue, Ninhydrin, or starch iodine for sweat testing shows some alteration in response in patients with RSD, but the results are neither sensitive nor specific. Veldman found that sweat testing is subject to the same problems as bone scanning and thermography, which are more popular diagnostic methods. In essence, a patient with an immobilized, swollen extremity may or may not have a positive bone scan or thermogram, but a positive result in no way implicates the sympathetic nervous system as a pathophysiologic mechanism.

Many authors have considered sympathetic blockade of paramount importance in the diagnosis of RSD, although the rate of positive response varies. This method, however, was challenged in 1994 by the IASP, which omitted a positive response to sympathetic blockade from its list of diagnostic criteria.

## TREATMENT

Sympathetic blockade is outdated as a diagnostic tool, but it has been shown to benefit various other conditions and has a strong placebo effect. In a controlled study,[98] Verdugo and Ochoa found no statistical difference in the effects of sympathetic blockade and placebo. Their research is an important contribution to the advancement of medical treatment and currently is being reproduced around the world. From a physiologic standpoint, sympathetic blockade may have a transient effect on pain or temperature changes. However, if the problem originates outside the sympathetic system, symptoms obviously will recur (i.e., vasomotor changes due to cortical disorders or mechanical inflammatory effects on the sinuvertebral or vertebral nerve, which indirectly affect the sympathetic ganglia).

The literature reflects variable responses to sympathetic blockade. In 1992 Bonica reported success rates that ranged from 18–50%.[99] The findings of radiographic studies and bone scans are nonspecific.[100–101] In his 1993 prospective study of 829 patients with RSD, Veldman found a lasting success rate of 7% with sympathetic block or sympathectomy. He concluded that "the results clearly show that interruption of the sympathetic system is not a panacea in RSD."[29]

Intravenous regional blocks also have been advocated. In a small study in 1974, Hannington-Kiff,[67] the father of intravenous regional blockade, used guanethidine to prevent the release of norephedrine at the postganglionic neurons. Subsequently he abandoned his original concept and now favors the concept of opioid deprivation.[102] In 1991, Raja et al.[103] used phentolamine (Regitine), which blocks the alpha receptors and theoretically depresses sympathetic activity. In 1994, Verdugo and Ochoa reported that phentolamine was no better than placebo,[98] and in the same year Geertzen reported that that dimethyl sulfoxide (DMSO), a toxic oxygen radical scavenger, was more effective than guanethidine and intravenous regional block.[77] In 1992, Vanos, Ramamurthy, and

Hoffman noted that all 7 patients treated with ketorolac (Toradol) experienced significant relief.[104] The authors concluded that ketorolac may be effective in treating RSD by intravenous regional block in a manner similar to corticosteroids, but with relatively fewer side effects. In a double-blind comparison of intravenous regional blockade with guanethidine, reserpine (an antihypertensive medication that depletes stores of norepinephrine and inhibits its release), and normal saline, Blanchard et al.[105] found no difference among the three agents. Ramamurthy et al.[106] found that in patients with RSD a 20-minute tourniquet time was as effective as saline or intravenous regional block with guanethidine or reserpine—and, one suspects, less costly. The same group[106] found no differences in comparing guanethidine with saline or simple inflation of a blood pressure cuff.

Clearly the history of RSD therapy is chaotic. Nearly every medication and form of treatment has used in the past, including both injectable and oral alpha and beta receptor antagonists. Alpha-methyldopa (Catapres) is a false transmitter at the ending of postganglionic neurons. Phenoxybenzamine (Dibenzyline) blocks alpha receptors, whereas propranolol (Inderal) blocks beta receptors. In 1993 Rauck[107] assessed the use of epidural clonidine (an alpha$_2$ agonist) in cases of RSD refractory to treatment with opiates, based on the assumption that spinal alpha$_2$ receptors may regulate nociceptive processing. This approach directly contradicts the concept of blocking alpha receptors with phentolamine. In addition, other physicians have used the alpha$_2$ antagonist yohimbine (an agent for treatment of impotence) to block alpha$_2$ receptors—another direct contradiction of the clonidine approach. In brief, both alpha and beta blockers have been used with varying degrees of success.

Several authors have advocated the use of corticosteroids.[84,108–110] Davis[109] claimed a success rate of 100%, whereas Kozin[84] found corticosteroids comparable to sympathetic blockade.

The rationale for using many medications is questionable because of general confusion about the symptom complex. Calcitonin,[111] antiinflammatory agents, calcium channel blockers, anticonvulsants (e.g., Dilantin and Tegretol), and gabapentin (Neurontin) have been tried recently. In a review of 5 patients with persistent RSD, gabapentin was believed to be of some benefit.[112] No comparisons were made with placebo or any other agent. The fact remains that appropriate and thorough research has not been done and cannot be done until physicians arrive at consistent criteria for diagnosis and treatment.

Conservative management has been used since 1864, when Mitchell used wet dressings for blistering and local injections of morphine.[113] Numerous physicians have advocated the use of physical therapy.[1–35,114–118] In 1966 Johnson recommended exercise in response to various stimuli.[113] Plewes[119] obtained good results with physical treatment that included periods of exposure to hot air (105° F) with the extremity elevated. He also recommended paraffin baths and exercise twice daily. Plewes maintained that his regimen was superior to sympathetic blockade and corticosteroid therapy. Buker believed that patients should be managed with physical therapy alone.[120] The rationale behind physical therapy is the basic principle of rehabilitation: to prevent immobility, loss of range of motion, and atrophy and to control pain.

Often progression or lack of progression is due to the patient's perception of pain control. Negative attitudes are often perpetuated by poor education and promotion of hysteria. Psychologic assessment, biofeedback, relaxation training, and additional psychologic tools are paramount.

## CONCLUSION

Progress demands recognition of past successes and failures. Recent advances must be understood within the context of the origins and progression of the symptom complex. Unfortunately, clinicians may embrace outdated literature from the past decade and current literature that is reminiscent of the past century. All patients should be analyzed individually with a thorough history, physical examination, and psychologic assessment. In addition, all patients should receive proper education to prevent hysteria and heightened anxiety as well as a supportive rehabilitation team with all members speaking a common language. Over the past century, many treatment modalities have been used, from conservative to invasive, including amputation. As outdated literature is replaced with more current reasoning—and in particular, as terms implying a specific pathophysiologic mechanism are replaced by descriptive terms—we must remember that first we should do no harm.

## REFERENCES

1. Racz GB, Heavener JE, Noe CE: Definitions, classifications and taxonomy: An overview. Phys Med Rehabil State Art Rev 10:2, 1996.
2. Mitchell SW: On the diseases of nerves resulting from injuries. In Flict SA (ed): Contributions Relating to the Causation and Prevention of Disease, and to Camp Diseases. New York, U.S. Sanitary Commission Memoirs, 1867.
3. Evans JA: Reflex sympathetic dystrophy: Report on fifty-seven cases. Ann Intern Med 26:417–426, 1947.
4. De Takats G: Reflex dystrophy of the extremities. Arch Surg 34:939–956, 1937.
5. Roberts WJ: A hypothesis on the physiologic basis for causalgia and related pains. Pain 24:297–311, 1986.
6. Sudeck KP: Uber die akute entzundilicephap Knochenatrophie. Arch Klin Chir 62:147, 1900.
7. Glick EN: Reflex dystrophy (algoneurodystrophy): Results of treatment by corticosteroids. Rheumatol Phys Med 12:84–88, 1973.
8. Zur veth M: Periphere akute Trophoneurose der Hand. Monatschr Unfalkheillkd 30:309, 1929.
9. Morton JJ, Scott WJM: Some angioplastic syndromes in the extremities. Ann Surg 94:839–859, 1931.
10. Fontaine R, Hermann LG: Post-traumatic osteoporosis. Ann Surg 97:26–61, 1933.
11. Lehman EP: Traumatic vasospasm: A study of four cases of vasospasm in the upper extremities. Arch Surg 29:92–107, 1934.
12. Homans J: Minor causalgia: A hyperesthetic neurovascular syndrome. N Engl J Med 222:870–874, 1940.
13. Steinbrocker O: The shoulder-hand syndrome. Am J Med 3:402–407, 1947.
14. Patman RD, Veldman P, Reynen HN, et al: Management of post-traumatic pain syndrome: A report of 113 cases. Ann Surg 177:780–787, 1973.
15. Ochoa J: The newly recognized painful ABC syndrome: Thermographic aspects. Thermology 2:65, 1986.
16. Ochoa JL: Essence investigations and management of "neuropathic" pains: Hopes from acknowledgement of chaos [guest editorial]. Muscle Nerve 16:997–1062, 1993.
17. Paget J: Clinical lectures on some cases of local paralysis. Med Times Hosp Gaz 1:331, 1864.
18. Mitchell SW, Morehouse GR, Keen WW: Gunshot Wounds and Other Injuries of Nerves. Philadelphia, J.B. Lippincott, 1864.
19. Mitchell SW: Injuries of Nerves and Their Consequences. London, Smith & Elder, 1872.
20. Charcot JMN: Lectures on the Diseases of the Nervous System. Edited by Chritchley M. London, New Syndenham Society, 1877.
21. Webb EM, Davis EW: Causalgia: A review. Calif Med 69(6), 1948.
22. Pott P: The Chirurgical Works of Percival Pott. Dublin, James Williams, 1778.
23. Bonica JJ: The Management of Pain with Special Emphasis on the Use of Analgesic Block: Diagnosis, Prognosis, and Therapy. Philadelphia, Lea & Febiger, 1953.
24. Abernathy J: The Surgical and Physiologic Works of John Abernathy, vol. 2, 2nd ed. 1819.
25. Denmark A: Examples of symptoms resembling tic douloureux, produced by a wound in the radial nerve. Med Chir Tr 4:48, 1813.
26. Dielssen PC, Veldman A, Goris PR: Amputation for reflex sympathetic dystrophy. J Bone Joint Surg 77B:270–388, 1995.
27. Ochoa J, Yarnitsky D: Triple cold ("CCC") pain syndrome [abstract]. Pain (Suppl 5):S278, 1990.
28. Frost SA, et al: Does hyperalgesia to cooling stimuli characterize patients with sympathetically maintained pain (reflex sympathetic dystrophy)? In Webner R, Gebhert GF, Bond MR (eds): Proceedings of the Fifth World Congress on Pain: Pain Research and Clinical Management. Amsterdam, Elsevier, 1988, pp 151–156.
29. Veldman P, Reynen HJM, Han M, et al: Signs and symptoms of reflex sympathetic dystrophy: Prospective study of eight-hundred and twenty-nine patients. Lancet 342:1012–1016, 1993.

30. Leriche LR: De la causalgie: Envisagée comme une nevrite du sympathique et de son traitement par la de nudation et l'excision des plexus nerveux peri-arteriels. Presse Med 24:178–180, 1916.
31. Spurling RG: Causalgia of the upper extremity. Treatment by dorsal sympathetic ganglionectomy. Arch Neurol Psychiatry 23:784, 1930.
32. Livingston WK: Pain Mechanisms: A Physiologic Interpretation of Causalgia and Its Related States. New York, Macmillan, 1943.
33. de No L: Analysis of activity of chains of internuncial neurons. J Neurophysiol 1:207–244, 1938.
34. Mitchell SW: The Medical Department in the Civil War. JAMA 62:1445–1450, 1914.
35. Omer G, Thomas S: Treatment of causalgia: A review of cases at Brook General Hospital. Texas Med 67:93, 1971.
36. Johnson EW, Pannozzo AN: Management of shoulder-hand syndrome. JAMA 195, 1966.
37. De Takats G: Causalgic states in peace and war. JAMA 128:699–704, 1945.
38. Freeman NE: Treatment of causalgia arising from gunshot wounds of peripheral nerves. Surgery 22:62–82, 1947.
39. Fischer A, Personal communication, 1996.
40. Treede RD, et al: Evidence that alpha-adrenergic receptors mediate sympathetically maintained pain (reflex sympathetic dystrophy). Pain (Suppl 5):S487, 1990.
41. Casten D, Betcher A: Reflex sympathetic dystrophy. Surg Obstet Gynecol Jan:97–101, 1955.
42. Tahmoush AJ: Causalgia: Redefinition as a clinical pain syndrome. Pain 10:187, 1981.
43. Kozin F, Soin JS, Ryan LM, et al: Bone scintigraphy in the reflex sympathetic dystrophy syndrome. Radiology 130:437–443, 1981.
44. Pak TJ, Martin GM, Magness JL, Kavanaugh GJ: Reflex sympathetic dystrophy: Review of 140 cases. Minn Med 5:507–512, 1970.
45. Gibbons JJ, Wilson P: RSD score: Criteria for the diagnosis of reflex sympathetic dystrophy and causalgia. Clin J Pain 8:260–253, 1992.
46. Carter HW: On causalgia and applied painful conditions due to lesions of the peripheral nerves. J Neurol Psychopathol 3:1, 1922.
47. Lewis O, Gatewood W: Treatment of causalgia: Results of interneural injection of 60% alcohol. JAMA 74:1, 1920.
48. Kirklin JW, Henoweth AT, Murphy F: Causalgia: A review of its characteristics, diagnosis and treatment. Surgery 21:321, 1947.
49. Sunderland S, Kelly M: The painful sequelae of injuries to peripheral nerves. Aust N Z Surg 18:75, 1948.
50. Rothberg JM, Tahmoush AJ, Oldakowski RL The epidemiology of causalgia among soldiers wounded in Vietnam. Milit Med 148:347, 1983.
51. Plewes LW: Sudeck's atrophy in the hand. J Bone Joint Surg 38B:195–203, 1956.
52. Davis SW, Petrillo CR, Eichberg RD, Chu DS: Shoulder-hand syndrome in the hemiplegic population: A five-year retrospective study. Arch Phys Med Rehabil 58:353–356, 1977.
53. Etof Y, Hirais M, et al: Shoulder-hand syndrome associated with hemiplegia. Nippon Ronen Igakkai Zasshi 12(4):245–251, 1975.
54. Bacorn RW, Kurtzke JF: Colles' fracture: A study of two-thousand cases from the New York State Workman's Compensation Board. J Bone Joint Surg 35A:643–658, 1953.
55. Dunningham TH: The treatment of Sudeck's atrophy in the upper limb by sympathetic blockade. Injury 12:139–144, 1980.
56. Lankford LL: Reflex sympathetic dystrophy. In Green DP (ed): Operative Hand Surgery, vol. 1, 3rd ed. Edinburgh, Churchill Livingstone, 1993, pp 627–660.
57. De Takats G: Sympathetic reflex dystrophy. Med Clin North Am 49:117–129, 1965.
58. Kwan ST: The treatment of causalgia by thoracic sympathetic ganglionectomy. Ann Surg 101:222–227, 1935.
59. Doupe CCH, Chance GQ: Post-traumatic pain and causalgia syndrome. J Neurol Neurosurg Psychiatry 7:33–48, 1944.
60. Devor M: Nerve pathophysiology and mechanisms of pain and causalgia. J Auton Nerv Syst 7:731, 1983.
61. Lewis T: Pain. London, Macmillan, 1942.
62. Goris RJA: Conditions associated with impaired oxygen extraction. In Gutierez G, Vincent JL (eds): Tissue Oxygen Utilization. Berlin, Springer-Verlag, 1991, pp 350–369.
63. Oyen OWJG, Arntz IE, Claessens AMJ, et al: Reflex sympathetic dystrophy of the hand: An excessive inflammatory response? Pain 1993.
64. Heerschap A, den Hollander JA, Ryan RH, Goris RJA: Metabolic changes in reflex sympathetic dystrophy: A 31p NMR spectroscopy study. Muscle Nerve 16:367–373, 1993.
65. Tilman PBJ, Stadhouders AM, Jap PHK, Goris RJA: Histopathologic findings in skeletal muscle tissue with patients suffering from reflex sympathetic dystrophy. Micron Microscop Acta 21:272–272, 1990.

66. Melzack R, Wall PD: Pain mechanisms: A new theory. Science 150:971–979, 1965.
67. Hannington-Kiff JG: Intravenous regional sympathetic block with guanethidine. Lancet 1:1019–1020, 1974.
68. Bennett GJ, Nz Xie YK: A peripheral neuropathy in rats that produces disorders of pain sensation like those seen in man. Pain 33:87–107, 1988.
69. Bennett GJ: The role of the sympathetic nervous system in painful peripheral neuropathy. Pain 45:221–223, 1991.
70. Janig W: Experimental approach to reflex sympathetic dystrophy and related syndromes. Pain 46:241–245, 1991.
71. Janig W, et al: The reflex sympathetic dystrophy syndrome: Consensus statement and general recommendations for diagnosis and clinical research. In Bond MR, Charlton JE, Woolf CJ (eds): Proceedings of the Sixth World Congress on Pain. Amsterdam, Elsevier, 1991, pp 373–376.
72. Pillemer FG, Micheli LJ: Psychological considerations in youth sports. Clin Sports Med 7(3), 1988.
73. Zikeyev VV: Causalgia and its treatment. Am Rev Soviet Med 4:16, 1946.
74. Adler E, Weiss AA, Vonari DA: Psychosomatic approach to sympathetic reflex dystrophy. Psychiatry Neurol 138:256–271, 1959.
75. Pollack HJ, Neuman R, Pollack EM, Sudeck UND: Psyche Beitr Orthop U Traumatol 27(H8):463–468, 1978.
76. Van Houdenhove B: Neuro-algodystrophy: A psychiatrist's view. Clin Rheum 3:399–406, 1986.
77. Geertzen JHB, De Bruijn H, et al: Reflex sympathetic dystrophy: Early treatment and psychological aspects. Arch Phys Med Rehabil 75(Apr), 1994.
78. Amadio PC, et al: Reflex sympathetic dystrophy syndrome: Consensus Report of an Ad Hoc Committee of the American Association for Hand Surgery on the Definition of Reflex Sympathetic Dystrophy Syndrome. Plast Reconstr Surg 87:371–375, 1991.
79. Lox DM: Personal data to be published.
80. Schwartzman RJ, Kerrigan J: The movement disorder of reflex sympathetic dystrophy. Neurology 40:57–61, 1990.
81. Ecker A: Movement disorder of RSD. Neurology 40:1477, 1990.
82. Lang A, Fahn S: Movements disorder of RSD. Neurology 40:1476–1477, 1990.
83. Omohundro PH Payne R: Reflex sympathetic dystrophy. Spine State Art Rev 2:685–698, 1988.
84. Kozin F, McCarty DJ, Sims J, et al: The reflex sympathetic dystrophy syndrome. Clinical and histological studies: Evidence for bilaterality, response to cortical steroids and articular involvement. Am J Med 60:321–331, 1976.
85. Mailis A: In response to RSD editorial by Dr. Wilson [letter]. Clin J Pain 9:152–154, 1993.
86. Ochoa J, Verdugo R: Reflex sympathetic dystrophy: A common clinical avenue for somatoform expression. Neurol Clin 13(2), 1995.
87. Maurer AH, Holder LE, Espiniola DA, et al: Three-phase radionuclide scintigraphy of the hand. Radiology 146:761–775, 1983.
88. Genant HK, Kosin F, Bekerman C, et al: The reflex sympathetic dystrophy syndrome: A comprehensive analysis using fine detailed radiography, photon absorptiometry and bone and joint scintigraphy. Radiology 117:21–32, 1975.
89. Holder LE, MacKinnon SE: Reflex sympathetic dystrophy in the hands: Clinical and scintigraphic criteria. Radiology 152:517, 1984.
90. Lee GLW, Weeks PM: The role of bone scintigraphy in diagnosing reflex sympathetic dystrophy. J Hand Surg 20A:458–463, 1995.
91. Hendler N, et al: Thermographic validation of physical complaints in psychogenic pain patients. Psychosomatics 23:283, 1982.
92. Ochoa JL: The newly recognized painful ABC syndrome. Thermographic aspects. Thermology 2:65, 1986.
93. Lightman HI, et al: Thermography in childhood reflex sympathetic dystrophy. J Pediatr 111:551–555, 1987.
94. So YT, et al: Evaluation of thermography in the diagnosis of selected entrapment neuropathies. Neurology 39:1–5, 1989.
95. So YT, et al: The role of thermography in evaluation of lumbosacral radiculopathy. Neurology 39:1154–1158, 1989.
96. Perelman R, et al: A comparison of lumbosacral thermograms with CT scans. In Medical Thermology. Washington, DC, American Academy of Thermology, pp 127–133.
97. Tahmoush AJ, Malley J, Jennings JR: Skin conductants, temperature, and blood flow in causalgia. Neurology 33:1483–1486, 1983.
98. Verdugo RJ, Ochoa JL: Neurology 44:1003–1010, 1994.
99. Bonica JJ: The Management of Pain, vol. 1, 2nd ed. Philadelphia, Lea & Febiger, 1990, pp 226–227.
100. Slessor AJ: Causalgia: A review of twenty-two cases. Edinburgh Med J 44:563, 1948.
101. Rasmussen TB, Freedman H: Treatment of causalgia. J Neurosurg 3:165, 1946.

102. Hannington-Kiff JG: Does failed natural opioid modulation in regional sympathetic ganglia cause reflex sympathetic dystrophy? Lancet 338:1125–1127, 1991.

103. Raja SN, et al: Systemic alpha-adrenergic blockade with phentolamine: A diagnostic test for sympathetic maintained pain. Anesthesiology 74:691–698, 1991.

104. Vanos DN, Ramamurthy S, Hoffman J: Intravenous regional block using ketorolac: Preliminary results in the treatment of reflex sympathetic dystrophy. Anesth Analg 7:139–141, 1992.

105. Blanchard J, Ramamurthy S, Walsh N, et al: Intravenous regional sympatholysis: A double-blind comparison of guanethidine, reserpine and normal saline. J Pain Sympt Manage 5, 1990.

106. Ramamurthy S, Hoffman J, Walsh N, Schoenfeld L: Role of tourniquet-induced analgesia in I.V. regional sympatholysis. Anesthesiology 65, 1986.

107. Rauck R, et al: Epidural clonidine treatment for refractory reflex sympathetic dystrophy. Anesthesiology 79(6), 1993.

108. Glick EN: Reflex dystrophy (algoneurodystrophy): Results of treatment by corticosteroids. Rheumatol Rehabil 12:84–88, 1973.

109. Davis, Sanders, Petrillo, et al: Shoulder-hand syndrome in a hemiplegic population: A five-year retrospective study. Arch Phys Med Rehabil 58:353–356, 1977.

110. Gobelet C, et al: The effect of adding calcitonin to physical treatment of reflex sympathetic dystrophy. Pain 48:171–175, 1992.

111. Rosen PS, Graham W: The shoulder hand syndrome: Historical view with observation of seventy-three patients. Can Med Assoc J 77:86, 91, 1957.

112. Gobelet C, Waldburger M, Meier JL: The effect of adding calcitonin to physical treatment of reflex sympathetic dystrophy. Pain 48:171–175, 1992.

113. Mellick L, Mellick G: Successful treatment of reflex sympathetic dystrophy with gabapentin. Am J Emerg Med 13:96, 1995.

114. Johnson EM, Pannozzo AM: Management of shoulder-hand syndrome. JAMA 195:108–110, 1966.

115. Cailliet R: Shoulder Pain. Philadelphia, F.A. Davis, 1966.

116. Escobar P: Reflex sympathetic dystrophy. Orthop Rev 15:41–46, 1986.

117. Howard T: Cardiac pain and periarthritis of the shoulder. Med J Rec 131:364–365, 1930.

118. Oppenheimer A: The swollen atrophic hand. Surg Gynecol Obstet 67:446–453, 1938.

119. Plewes LW: Sudeck's atrophy in the hand. J Bone Joint Surg 38B:195–203, 1956.

120. Buker RH, et al: Causalgia and transthoracic sympathectomy. Am J Surg 124:724, 1972.

121. Perelman RB, Adler D, Humphrey M: A comparison of lumbosacral thermograms with CT scans. In Abernathy M, Uematsu S (eds): Medical Thermology. Vienna, VA, American Academy of Thermology, 1986, pp 127–133.

# 11

# Posttraumatic Headache

ROGER K. CADY, MD
KATHLEEN FARMER, PsyD

Injury to the head and neck is commonly associated with the symptom of headache. Trauma may be the initiating event of a headache syndrome or exacerbate preexisting headache pathology. Although headache is the most common symptom after injury to the head and upper cervical spine, it often occurs amid a constellation of other symptoms, such as fatigue, vertigo, tinnitus, dizziness, or changes in cognition. This symptom complex appears fairly consistent from patient to patient and constitutes the posttraumatic headache syndrome.[1]

Headache due to head trauma may be considered as postconcussive after a period of unconsciousness or as posttraumatic when there is no associated loss of consciousness. The clinical value of this differentiation is arguable. Of interest is the observation that mild head trauma, not associated with loss of consciousness, may follow a more intractable clinical course.[2]

Mild head injury (MHI) or mild traumatic brain injury is difficult to define because most evaluations of head trauma are based on structural damage. The American College of Rehabilitation Medicine defines mild brain injury as "traumatically induced physiologic disruption of brain function, indicated by at least one of the following: a loss of consciousness, a period of post-traumatic amnesia, an alteration of mental function following head trauma, presence of focal, transient neurologic deficits, or a Glasgow Coma Scale score of less than 13."[3] Although helpful, these criteria do not account fully for incidents of cervical spine injury (whiplash injury) with no observed head trauma or alteration of brain function.

## HISTORICAL PERSPECTIVE

As early as 1882, J. E. Ericksen noted that severe symptoms could evolve from seemingly minor head trauma.[4] However, his assertion was challenged by H. Page, who proposed that symptoms of the nervous system following head trauma were unlikely without clear evidence of physical damage.[5] Page laid the foundation for the notion that the syndrome following head trauma was a functional disorder. This debate about the relationship between head injury and posttraumatic headache syndrome persists today. Fueled by litigation concerns, coupled with the lack of objective confirmation of central nervous system injury after mild head trauma, many physicians regard malingering, secondary gain, and compensation neurosis as reasonable explanations for the symptoms observed after mild head trauma. This debate was delineated in a 1981 monograph by Trimble entitled "Post-traumatic Neurosis."[6]

A clearer understanding of a pathologic basis for posttraumatic headache is now emerging. Modern neuroimaging scans detect anatomic and biochemical changes in the brains of many patients with head injury.[7] Pathophysiologic and anatomic mechanisms are being delineated, providing a more biologic basis for the syndrome.

The lack of validation of such patients by sophisticated legal, medical, and third-party reimbursement systems fails to eliminate their existence in clinical practice. In an interesting study by Strauss and Savitsky, physicians discounted posttraumatic headache syndrome until they found themselves afflicted.[8] As with many chronic pain conditions, history suggests that as scientific understanding advances, many conditions once believed functional become understandable on a pathophysiologic basis.

## CLINICAL BASIS OF THE POSTTRAUMATIC HEADACHE

The modern basis for understanding the posttraumatic headache syndrome began during the 1940s when observers associated posttraumatic headache with a combination of the specifics of head injury, premorbid personality, and psychosocial determinants, including compensation. In 1946, Simons and Wolff investigated patients with posttraumatic headache and concluded that after head trauma, persistent headache can be explained by excessive muscle contraction, scarring, and entrapment of vascular and nerve structures.[9]

These observations may explain posttraumatic headache in some, but many patients afflicted with significant symptoms have no documentable permanent injury. However, modern studies with magnetic resonance imaging (MRI) and single photon emission computed tomography (SPECT) as well as histologic studies have confirmed brainstem and central metabolic abnormalities in patients with minimal brain injuries, thus expanding the mechanisms postulated by Simons and Wolff.[10–12]

## CLINICAL PRESENTATION

Headache is frequently one of several symptoms observed in patients after head injury. The ten most common symptoms associated with head injury were described by Levin (Table 1).[13]

Headache associated with posttraumatic syndrome is generally diffuse and classifiable as chronic tension-type headache, according to criteria of the International Headache Society (IHS).[14] However, trauma has been reported to initiate migraine-like headache and, more rarely, cluster headache.[15,16] In addition, trauma may exacerbate any preexisting headache disorder.[1] The onset of headache after trauma may be variable. Headache commonly begins within 24 hours of the traumatic event but may occur days or weeks later.

Neck pain associated with posttraumatic headache syndrome, especially after a whiplash injury, is generally suboccipital and resembles pain associated with tension-type headache. Pain may be referred to the temporal or frontal area of the head from cervical injury. Other pain-sensitive structures in the cervical spine associated with referred pain include upper cervical facet joints, muscles (sternocleidomastoid, trapezius, splenius capitis and cervicis, and suboccipital muscles), ligamentous structures, and the greater occipital nerve.[17]

Associated symptoms of posttraumatic headache syndrome include dizziness, vertigo, tinnitus, light-headedness, and hyperacusis. These symptoms suggest brainstem involvement. Anatomically, the brainstem is particularly vulnerable to closed head injury or flexion-extension injury of the spine.

**TABLE 1.**
Ten Most Common Postconcussive Symptoms

| | |
|---|---|
| Headache | Depression |
| Fatigability | Anxiety |
| Dizziness | Cognitive impairment |
| Sleep disorder | Change in appetite |
| Disruption of recent memory | Blurred vision |

Cognitive dysfunction is common after minor head trauma. Such symptoms are often overlooked or may not surface clinically until a patient has physically recovered and begins to face the demands of normal living. Common complaints include disturbances of recent memory, counting change, and concentration. A neuropsychologic evaluation measures the level of impairment and forecasts rehabilitation possibilities. Medication may exacerbate these symptoms. Psychologic dysfunction is common, particularly as the condition becomes more chronic. Depression, anxiety, panic disorder, and posttraumatic stress disorder may develop. Although such negative reactions may be secondary to fear and loss of physical function, they also may be related more directly to injury. Constitutional symptoms of easy fatigability, loss of libido, malaise, sleep disturbance, appetite changes, and weight gain or loss often emerge without being organized into a recognizable psychiatric diagnosis.

## MEDICAL EVALUATION

Evaluation of the patient with traumatic head injury includes a detailed history, physical and neurologic examination, and often laboratory, imaging, and neuropsychologic testing. Because litigation may be pending, documentation needs to be detailed, including medical findings, medications, and telephone follow-up.

### History

An accurate history is paramount. In the period after acute trauma, history more than physical examination or neurodiagnostic studies is the cornerstone of diagnosis. History should record major medical conditions, past headache or spinal trauma, preexisting headache disorder, reconstruction of the dynamics of injury, and present or past workers' compensation claim. A description of the headache should include location, intensity, duration, exacerbating and alleviating factors, frequency, associated symptoms (e.g., photophobia, phonophobia, nausea, vertigo, tinnitus, muscle pain), and medication usage.

The use of medication needs to be explored in detail, specifying quantity and frequency, including over-the-counter preparations. If a patient has a family history or personal history of migraine, use of medications that may produce rebound or pharmacologically maintained headache should be considered.

During a history-taking session, the physician should explore the efficiency of short-term and long-term memory as well as other cognitive functions. The patient's current level of mental activity should be compared with the level of activity before injury. Often patients notice cognitive changes only after being placed in situations that adequately test such functions. Direct questioning and discussion with family members may help to pinpoint a person's level of cognitive function.

Evaluation of psychiatric and psychologic status is also necessary. The physician should screen for depression, sleep disturbance, sexual dysfunction, weight or appetite change, mood swings, and changes in basic personality. In addition, level of motivation, interactions with family, work performance, and reliance on a support system should be explored.

## Physical Examination

A complete physical examination provides diagnostic information as well as reassurance to the patient. Special attention to areas of head and cervical injury helps to formulate an immediate treatment plan. Remote injury also needs to be included in the overall assessment. The patient with head trauma should be given a complete neurologic screening, postural examination, and evaluation of the head and neck. The patient should be positioned supine on a table, and the head and neck area should be carefully palpated. Tender points, trigger points, ligamentous restrictions, and pain should be documented, and range of motion, which is frequently normal, should be tested.

## Laboratory Evaluation and Testing

Unless preexisting or concomitant medical conditions warrant exclusion, standard laboratory screening has little benefit beyond the acute injury phase. Exceptions include screening for medication compliance or complications, such as renal, hepatic, or colorectal screening.

The role of thermography is under investigation, but at present it is controversial enough to provide little clinical relevance to the evaluation of the posttraumatic patient. More objective criteria may enhance its future.

Electroencephalography is useful if seizure disorders are suspected or if headache is associated with loss of consciousness, but it is not recommended as routine screening. Many clinicians prefer topographic electroencephalographic (EEG) brain mapping and auditory and visual evoked potentials. Cognitive evoked potentials may be useful with complaints of disturbance of memory, concentration, or thinking.[18]

Electromyelographic studies are useful to rule out cervical pathology. However, patients with traumatic head injury frequently demonstrate nondermatomal patterns of pain and increased muscle tension, suggesting aberrancy at levels other than the spinal cord.

## Neuroimaging

The use of CT and MRI is vital in the acute phase but unlikely to benefit clinical decision making in the later rehabilitation phase. Newer scanning methods such as MRI, SPECT, and positron emission tomography (PET) demonstrate structural and metabolic abnormalities and may be useful as documentation of injury but have little bearing on rehabilitation.[7] In patients with minimal brain injury, neurodiagnostic studies are typically normal. However, this does not imply lack of significant injury, as witnessed by the frequency of normal CT scans in fatal head injuries.

## Neuropsychologic Testing

The Halstead-Reitan Neuropsychological Battery[19] had been studied, tested, and honed over the past 40 years into an instrument that differentiates cognitive deficits and predicts the location of the injury or lesion. Based on a six-factor theory of brain-behavior relationships, the battery measures the functioning of the brain in six different capacities: (1) sensory input, (2) response, (3) attention/concentration, (4) language skills, (5) visuospatial skills, and (6) concept formation, reasoning, and logical analysis. The resulting scores measure the level of performance, pattern of performance, differences between the right and left hemisphere of the brain, and pathognomonic signs.[20]

Neuropsychologic testing is essential when clinical neurologic examination uncovers no objective evidence. Whereas imaging exposes structural problems and a neurologic examination indicates gross abnormalities, a neuropsychologic battery locates subtle functional deficits. Standardization provides clear guidelines that classify scores as normal or mildly, moderately, or severely impaired.

Whiplash injuries may produce microtrauma,[21] which is measured by neuro-psychologic tests as functional lapses in the integrity of the cerebral cortex. From a subjective viewpoint, the injured person recognizes that thinking is not clear, memory is fuzzy, or simple tasks such as balancing a checkbook seem impossible. Neuro-psychologic testing lends objective evidence to these amorphous beliefs. Cognitive re-training helps the individual to regain what has been lost by relearning the integration of fundamentals of the skill that seems to be missing.[22]

### Head Trauma Scoring

The Glasgow Coma Scale (GCS) is a well-accepted measure of brain injury, par-ticularly in the emergency setting. Its relevance in mild brain injury is becoming readily apparent. The GCS is a 15-point scale that evaluates three measures of brain injury: eye opening, verbal response, and motor response. A score of 15 indicates normal alertness. Scores for severe brain injury are well documented. Mild brain injury is defined as GCS scores of 13 or greater.[3]

## CLASSIFICATION OF POSTTRAUMATIC HEADACHE DISORDERS

The IHS criteria for classification and diagnosis of headache disorders, cranial neuralgias, and facial pain classify headache associated with head trauma as acute or chronic posttraumatic headache (PTH). Preexisting headache disorders that worsen after injury are classified according to the underlying headache pattern.

Acute headache disorders resolve within 8 weeks after injury and chronic disorders last longer than 8 weeks. Both acute and chronic posttraumatic headache disorders are divided into disorders associated with (1) significant head trauma and/or confirmatory signs or (2) minor head trauma with no confirmatory signs. The significance of trauma is defined by loss of consciousness, posttraumatic amnesia lasting more than 10 min-utes, or abnormal results on at least two of the following evaluations: neurologic exam-ination, skull radiograph, neuroimaging, evoked potential, spinal fluid examination, vestibular function testing, or neuropsychologic testing. Headache must occur less than 14 days after injury or after regaining consciousness.[14]

These criteria do not adequately account for the role of cervical injury in posttrau-matic headache syndrome or for the complexity of presentations often encountered clinically. From a practical and therapeutic standpoint, it may assist physicians to view headache symptoms on a spectrum, with tension-type symptoms at one end and mi-graine at the other. This pathophysiologic model[23–25] offers several advantages over a more compartmentalized schema in understanding PTH.

## ANATOMIC AND PHYSIOLOGIC CONSIDERATIONS

The pathophysiology of posttraumatic headache disorders is not completely un-derstood. Recent advances in anatomic understanding of referred head pain, the physio-logic and anatomic interconnections of the cervical and cranial nerves, and mechanisms of trigeminally mediated pain have produced significant advances.

### Trigeminal Nerve and Sympathetic Nervous System

The trigeminal nerve provides sensory innervation to the face, muscles of masti-cation, mouth, and cranial vault and has motor connections with cranial nerves III, VII, and XI. The three major divisions—ophthalmic, maxillary, and mandibular—converge into a group of loosely defined nuclei termed the caudate nuclei of the trigeminal nerve. Of importance is the fact that these nuclei extend from the level of the pons caudally into the cervical spine at least to the level of C2. Rich interneuronal connections allow activation of the trigeminal system from cervical levels at least as low as C8.[17]

In addition, the sympathetic nervous system has the potential for significant activation of the trigeminal system. Sympathetic fibers innervating the cranial and cervical structures of the head and neck originate at T1 and T2 forming the stellate ganglia. Fibers extend cephalad, forming interiorly a second large plexus (cervical and cranial plexus) behind the origin of the vertebral artery and superiorly the cervical ganglia lying on the capitus longus muscle at the base of the skull behind the carotid sheath. Sympathetic fibers follow the carotid arteries, supplying carotid, basilar, and cerebellar circulatory trees. Interconnections from the sympathetic fibers in the carotid sheath to the caudate nucleus of the trigeminal nerve provide significant potential for cross-activation of the two systems.[17]

Centrally, the caudate nucleus of the trigeminal nerve forms the ascending pain pathway to the thalamus and ultimately to the cortex. Pain perception occurs at the thalamic level, but interpretation of painful events requires cortical interpretation. This ascending pain pathway has rich interconnections to the autonomic nervous system, hypothalamus, limbic brain, and cortex that may provide facilitory or inhibitory influence on pain transmission and perception.[17]

### Neurogenic Inflammation

Recent work by Moskowitz has demonstrated that antidromic stimulation of the trigeminal nerve can release several vasoactive peptides,[26] such as substance P, bradykinin, neurokinin A, neuropeptide Y, vasoactive intestinal peptide (VIP), and calcitonin-gene-related peptide (CGRP) from trigeminal afferents innervating cranial vessels. This release initiates a sterile inflammatory process around vascular structures, lowering the pain perception threshold. When activated, stimuli such as head movement or vascular distention, which normally do not produce pain, may become painful. Although these mechanisms may have their greatest relevance in migraine, disruption of the trigeminal system conceivably may explain neurogenic pain in some patients with posttraumatic headache, especially for the segment of the population genetically susceptible to migraine. Posttraumatic cervicogenic headache, although somewhat controversial, may present with vascular features.

### Cervical Factors

The occipital nerve arises from the C2–C3 level, providing sensory innervation to the suboccipital, occipital, and parietal areas of the head. Terminal fibers of the occipital nerve interdigitate with those of the trigeminal system, and pain referral patterns between these two systems have been delineated. Upper cervical dermatomes have been delineated, suggesting rich overlap of trigeminal and occipital innervation.[17]

### REFERRED PAIN AND TRIGGER POINTS

Seminal work by Travel and Rinzler delineated five cervical muscles that refer pain to the head.[27,28] Other referral patterns of head and cervical pain also have been elucidated. The anatomic and physiologic basis for these pain referral patterns remains incompletely understood, but their presence has important therapeutic implications.

Trigger points are defined as areas of sensory hypersensitivity in a muscle that, when palpated, may produce localized pain which may be referred to a distant site. Trigger points of the head and neck also may produce tinnitus, vertigo, and lacrimation.[29] Trigger points may be active or latent. Active trigger points are painful and reproduce pain on palpation to a definable and reproducible distant area. Latent trigger points, not clinically associated with pain, are tender with palpation and may produce muscle dysfunction.

Trigger points often develop after trauma. It is presumed that muscle injury leads to reflex vasoconstriction and release of noxious peptides from injured tissue, such as bradykinins, histamine, and prostaglandins. These sensitize nociceptive fibers, producing localized areas of increased muscle tension and impairment of vascular dynamics. Over time, accompanying metabolic changes at a cellular level include decreased levels of adenosine triphosphate. Ultimately there is an "energy crisis" within the muscle tissue.[30,31] Such altered biochemical conditions sensitize afferent nerves innervating the tissues and lead to a state of facilitation (activation by stimuli at lower thresholds than in undamaged tissue). Sensitization to sympathetic tone is also noted.

The development and sustenance of trigger points also may be complicated by abnormal postural dynamics that may occur with pain and/or injury.[32] Numerous studies have demonstrated that postural imbalance plays an important role in maintaining and unmasking latent trigger areas.[17,32]

Work by Massey has suggested that tissue injury may unmask latent intraspinal pathways, resulting in facilitated pain at a site distant from the injury.[33] Massey found that injection of noxious substances into the muscle of a dog lowered the threshold of pain activation at distant sites within the muscle. This finding has obvious implications for the clinical pain patterns seen after injury.

Central regulation of muscle tone also may be a factor in the genesis of posttraumatic and primary head pain syndromes. As indicated by spasm associated with spinal cord injury, the predominant influence of the central nervous system on muscle tone is inhibitory. Disruption of this inhibitory influence through injury or neurochemical perturbations in the brain may result in sustained muscle tension, pain, and tenderness of muscles of the head and neck. That these mechanisms play a role in the muscle pain of conditions such as migraine and chronic tension-type headache has been proposed by Schoenen, who reported diminished or absent extroceptive silent period in the masseter and temporal muscles of patients with chronic tension-type headache.[34]

Obviously a complex web of autonomic, neurovascular, peripheral, and central factors is involved in the genesis of head pain. No one mechanism explains the phenomenon thoroughly. Headache may be a final common pathway for many physiologic disruptions. With time and persistent pain, changes in the central nervous system may perpetuate the pain-spasm cycle. Patients with chronic neuropathic pain have decreased levels of B-endorphin and lower pain thresholds to pain stimuli, suggesting that exhaustion of the endogenous opiate system may be a factor in chronic pain syndromes.[35,36] It is likely that over time pain mechanisms move from the periphery and become maintained by central factors.

## VASCULAR-CENTRAL-MYOGENIC MODEL FOR HEAD PAIN

Olesen has integrated the myogenic and vascular components of headache into what is termed the vascular-central-myogenic model.[25] According to this hypothesis, head pain is determined ultimately by the sum of nociceptive input from vascular and myogenic factors converging in the caudate nucleus of the trigeminal nerve. Modulating influences from endocrine, limbic, autonomic, and central factors may further influence this system. Long-term activation, as with injury or poorly controlled primary headaches, may result in secondary changes of central pain mechanisms (serotonin and endogenous opiates) and aggravate the chronicity of headache.

It is likely that many factors yet to be described are involved in posttraumatic headache. However, a significant anatomic and physiologic basis exists from which the physician can make rational therapeutic decisions.

## MECHANISM OF INJURY

Various mechanisms of injury are possible with trauma to the head. By understanding the mechanism of injury, the physician can correlate and anticipate clinical symptoms. Important points of consideration include site of injury, mechanism of injury, loss of consciousness, posttraumatic amnesia, rotational component of injury, and premorbid psychologic and neurologic function of the patient.

### Coup-Contrecoup Injury

Coup refers to the point of direct impact from an injury force. Contrecoup refers to the force of injury directed through brain tissue and affecting brain tissue opposite to the point of the impact. The brain tissue literally bounces off the bony skull opposite the site of injury. Coup injuries are fairly straightforward, with damage to scalp (including skin, support tissue, vascular tissue, and nervous structures), bony structures, intracranial vascular structures, meninges, and brain tissue. Contrecoup injuries, although remote, are not uncommon. Smith estimated that nearly 50% of all focal injuries involving direct impact are due to contrecoup mechanisms.[37] Roberts[38] suggested a higher figure of 80%. Obviously, the role of coup-contrecoup injury associated with head trauma is significant.

### Acceleration/Deceleration (Whiplash) Injury

Whiplash injury refers to neck hyperextension followed by flexion. This mechanism of injury typically is associated with motor vehicle accidents in which a motorist is struck from behind by another vehicle. Headache is noted in over 80% of individuals immediately after such an injury and is usually of a tension-type variety.[39] Such headaches have been attributed to injury of cervical muscles, the greater occipital nerve, or temporomandibular joint.[40] However, in an animal study, hippocampal spiking of the EEG was found after whiplash injury, indicating that whiplash may injure the brain.[41] Despite the frequency of such injury, whiplash injuries remain controversial and are poorly defined.

In a study by Sturzenegger, more symptoms and severe headaches occurred in occupants of motor vehicles who were unprepared with the head rotated at the time of the accident.[42] Of interest, use of seat belts, speed of the vehicle, and amount of damage to the vehicle had little influence on the severity of clinical symptoms.[42,43] Nonetheless, the force of impact to an occupant involved in a whiplash injury is important to consider in assessing the potential for damage.

Watkinson et al.[44] followed a group of 35 patients with whiplash injury over 10.8 years. Findings indicated that complaints at the time of the accident underestimated the true effect of soft tissue injuries of the cervical spine. Objective radiographic findings showed that degenerative changes of the cervical spine occurred in 68% of patients; 87% were symptomatic. The authors concluded that the complaints of patients with whiplash injuries were organic and that the condition did not recover with time without treatment.

Rotational force is important to understand in the whiplash patient and as a mechanism whenever loss of consciousness is observed. Movement of the brain within the bony confines of the skull, as occurs with trauma, may stretch and shear many small vessels, nerves, and support structures of the brainstem. Microscopic evidence for shearing of these structures has been noted[10] and tends to be concentrated in the frontal and temporal lobes.[45] Rotational velocity seems to be important in producing concussion and loss of consciousness. The brainstem with the reticular activating system appears anatomically vulnerable to injury. Head trauma involving this area may result in loss of consciousness. In addition, many of the caudate nuclei of the trigeminal nerve traverse through brainstem structures. Injury to these structures may play a critical role in posttraumatic head injury syndrome.

Several paradoxes are found between the severity and disability of posttraumatic headache syndrome and the extent of head and cervical injury. For instance, a severe head injury involving a cranial fracture or amnesia is less likely to result in long-term posttraumatic symptoms.[46] Mechanisms underlying MHI do not adequately explain this observation, but it may be that injury without fracture of the skull does not accommodate swelling of brain tissue or space-occupying pathology such as hematomas as well as injury with associated cranial fractures. Furthermore, MHI may not receive the aggressive early intervention given to more severe brain injury. As a result, posttraumatic headaches often are considered an overreaction to mild injury.

## CHRONIC HEADACHE PATTERNS FOLLOWING TRAUMA

### Episodic Migraine

Head trauma can exacerbate migraine symptoms or be the precipitating factor of a biochemical predisposition to migraine. After injury, migraine may occur for the first time or become more severe or more frequent. Such attacks typically fulfill IHS migraine criteria and are generally treatable by standard migraine therapy. Medications frequently used to treat episodic migraines include various nonsteroidal combinations such as acetaminophen, dichloralphenazone, and isometheptene (Midrin); ergotamines; and the 5-HT-1 agonist, sumatriptan. Treatment should be based on effectiveness and ability to minimize disability.

### Transformed Migraine

Matthew suggests that as migraine attacks become more frequent, a transformation often occurs from more neurovascular and gastrointestinal symptoms to more myogenic and psychogenic complaints.[47] This transformation seems to parallel a headache pattern that consists of comorbid tension-type headache with superimposed episodes of migraine. In this population of headache patients, it is important to understand the role of drugs in expediting the transformational process. Numerous drugs have been implicated as catalysts for migraine transformation, including over-the-counter analgesics, prescription analgesics, narcotics, ergotamines, and benzodiazepines.

If headache patterns are pharmacologically maintained, prophylactic drugs are ineffective and other acute-treatment drugs are less effective. Over time there is often a pattern of escalating usage of the offending drug.[48] It is essential to discontinue use of the daily acute-treatment medication to assess its role in the maintenance of the chronic headache pattern. Of patients caught in the transformed migraine spiral, a majority also suffer from comorbid conditions, such as depression, anxiety, sleep disturbance, and muscle pain syndromes. Treatment of such patients needs to focus on appropriate prophylactic medication.

The choice of prophylactic drugs is largely the same as that for migraine; when possible, it should be based on underlying comorbid factors such as depression or sleep disturbance. Significant muscle tension may be treated with muscle relaxants such as baclofen or cyclobenzaprine. When the overly used acute-treatment medications are withdrawn, many patients revert to episodic headache patterns.[49] This pattern may not be as characteristic for patients with posttraumatic transformed migraine but should be taken into account initially.

### Chronic Tension-type Headache

As stated earlier, the most common pattern of chronic headache after trauma is the chronic tension-type headache. Because this pattern involves a daily or near-daily headache, acute-treatment medications must be used judiciously; prophylactic medications are the mainstay of therapy. Comorbid disorders such as depression, anxiety, panic, sleep disturbance, and fibromyalgia also should be considered. The choice of appropriate pharmacologic therapy should address comorbid factors. Less severe headaches are best treated with nonsteroidal antiinflammatory drugs (NSAIDs). Headaches with vascular symptoms should be treated with ergotamines or 5-HT-1 agonists.

### Cluster-type Headaches

Cluster headaches after head trauma are uncommon.[15] Cluster headache may present in an episodic form, with daily or near-daily cluster attacks for weeks to months that resolve spontaneously or as a chronic unremitting disorder. Cluster attacks are characterized by abrupt onset of severe unilateral pain lasting 15 minutes to 3 hours. Associated with the attack are ipsilateral autonomic disruptions, such as lacrimation, rhinorrhea, sweating, or ptosis.

### Other Headache Patterns

Although other headache patterns are seen after trauma, the components of the headache syndrome should be organized into categories that have been proved to be responsive to treatment. For example, if headaches appear to be associated with neurovascular inflammation with severe pounding, throbbing pain that is aggravated by activity and associated with nausea, photophobia, and phonophobia, treatment with ergotamines, ergotamine tartrate, dihydroergotamine, or sumatriptan should be considered. Ideally these drugs should not be used more than two days per week.

When myofascial symptoms are evident, muscle relaxants such as baclofen or cyclobenzaprine should be considered. Other symptoms, such as vertigo, can be treated by pharmacologic and/or nonpharmacologic means. Of particular note is a rare headache, dysautonomic cephalalgia, described by Vijayan. Severe unilateral frontotemporal pain associated with ipsilateral sweating of the face and pupillary dilatation on the affected side responds to prophylactic propranolol.[50]

## MANAGEMENT OF POSTTRAUMATIC HEADACHE SYNDROME

### Acute Phase

Management of the acute head injury is beyond the scope of this chapter. However, adequate management of acute injury often minimizes the development of more chronic symptoms, particularly chronic pain. Clearly, adequate control of acute pain reassures the patient and prevents exhaustion of central pain mechanisms and development of learned pain. Reassurance and realistic goal assessment are also beneficial.

### Subacute Phase

The subacute phase of head injury is defined as the phase after resolution of serious or life-threatening medical conditions due to head injury. Often concomitant medical problems continue to require management, but aggressive rehabilitation efforts need to be initiated. Adequate pain control, aggressive modality-oriented physical therapy, and/or occupational therapy may be useful. Neuropsychologic testing and retraining also should be initiated if abnormalities are noted. Most patients with head injury move through the subacute phase, with resolution of sequelae of head trauma.

### Chronic Phase

Management of patients with chronic posttraumatic headache disorders may be difficult because of the wide range of underlying physical, vascular, neurochemical, and psychologic factors involved. Clinical presentations are numerous and varied. A physician's ability to dissect the components of a headache problem is the cornerstone for designing rational therapy.

The ideal treatment would relieve headache, associated symptoms, and psychologic effects permanently and safely and facilitate return to normal function. No such therapy exists, but therapy addressing many components of posttraumatic headache are available and can assist the majority of patients with posttraumatic headache syndromes.

Several components of therapy are essential to the treatment plan, including education, goal setting, psychologic support, and rational selection of pharmacologic, surgical, and nonpharmacologic interventions. Therapy that elicits participation of the patient is encouraged.

### Education

Patients suffering with posttraumatic headache and mild head injury are often faced with the same dilemma as the health care provider: how can trauma with little physical evidence result in such disability? Therefore, it is paramount that the physician validates the physical basis of the patient's symptoms. Patients welcome explanations that normal imaging studies and tests do not imply lack of injury. Providing understandable explanations of how mild brain injury can result in significant impairment of brain function helps patients and families to understand and accept the often confusing array of symptoms after trauma.

Patients experiencing posttraumatic headache probably have had multiple diagnostic evaluations and repeated trials of failed therapy. Support from family, friends, and coworkers has often eroded. Third-party payers are frequently hostile and confrontive, and litigation is often pending. There remains a considerable bias that PTH is a psychologic condition or, even worse, malingering. However, studies suggest that only 10% of head-injured patients exploit injury for financial gain.[51] Furthermore, several studies show that legal settlement does not terminate symptoms or disability of PTH.[52–54] In this environment, the physician's role is to provide compassionate care and understanding, which often are the most important services offered.

### Goal Setting

Goal setting is another essential component of treatment that is a collaborative effort between patient and health care provider. Initially, goals may revolve around wishful thinking, such as "I want to be like I used to be" or "I want my life back." Goals need to be realistic, concrete, and simple. Physicians need to provide short- and long-term goals that are measurable and emphasize function rather than pain relief. When PTH has evolved into a complex chronic condition, interdisciplinary care models are indicated. Involvement and coordination of various medical specialties, such as psychology, physical therapy, and occupational therapy, can be critical.

### Lifestyle Modification

A critical component to successful treatment is engaging the patient to share responsibility in managing pain. This process begins with providing a model of care that is understandable and not overwhelming in scope. Instead of focusing on cause and effect, the physician should define components of the problem. A management task is then assigned to each component. Treatment is based on common sense rather than magical cure. An ominous problem is dissected into manageable segments. Whenever possible, the patient's input and active participation in the solution should be encouraged. In the chronic phase of recovery it is often beneficial to explain rehabilitation as a proactive process that succeeds by resolving pieces of the problem rather than "fixing" tissue damage. Discussing blocks to healing with patients allows their participation in the rehabilitation process. Important blocks to healing are discussed below.

**Physical Inactivity.**    Beyond the acute injury phase, physical inactivity is often detrimental to recovery. Evidence suggests that bed rest hinders the healing process of chronic back pain by immobilizing the body and thereby promoting physical deconditioning, bone demineralization, depression, helplessness, and dependency.[55] Although strenuous exercise that jars the head and neck may produce headache, programs such as swimming or water aerobics may be well tolerated. Active exercise promotes a sense of well-being and release of endorphins.

**Nutrition.**    Deficiencies in amino acids, minerals such as magnesium, and vitamins have been reported in patients with chronic pain. The exact role of these abnormalities is not yet clearly defined, but on an intuitive basis proper nutrition is the foundation for a healthy body. Eating ample fresh vegetables, fruits, and protein should be encouraged. Recommending a high-quality vitamin supplement carries little risk and encourages the patient to pay attention to nutritional intake. Magnesium supplementation has been suggested as beneficial in acute migraine and menstrual migraine.[56] Because magnesium levels may be low in patients with chronic headache and depression,[57,58] magnesium supplementation (500 mg daily) is a helpful step that patients can do on their own. If the patient has endured prolonged periods of bed rest or physical inactivity, calcium supplementation (1.2–1.5 gm daily) should be considered.

**Mental Attitude.**    Negative emotions are often understandable given the emotional dynamics that may evolve after injury. Blame, self-doubt, anger, fear, and depression are common. Although it is important to validate the patient's feelings, it is equally important to point out that such feelings erode motivation and are useful only if they have a positive outlet. Often a firm compassionate approach that reassures the patient of the physician's role as advocate can help to improve mental outlook.

**Habit Regulation.**    **Tobacco** cessation is an important goal in managing posttraumatic headache. Numerous vasoactive compounds are found in tobacco, and vasodilators such as carbon monoxide are significant in cigarettes. If patients are unwilling or unable to stop smoking on their own, nicotine patches may be a worthwhile compromise. **Alcohol** provokes headaches of many types but is often used by patients in the belief that it helps to relieve pain or dulls unwanted emotions. Alcohol, however, has a depressant effect on the central nervous system and should be minimized. Chronic alcohol use can also disrupt sleep. **Caffeine** is often overused in the chronic headache population. As a methylxanthine, it elevates circulating levels of catecholamines, which may increase anxiety and disrupt sleep. Caffeine intake should be limited to < 300 mg/per day and not be used after 3 PM.

**Sleep.**    Sleep is one of the most restorative processes for the central nervous system and benefits almost all types of headaches. Sleep disruption, however, is commonly encountered in the chronic headache population. Although medications such as tricyclics and selective serotonin reuptake inhibitors may be useful, it is often worth counseling patients about developing sleep habits, such as restful activity before bed, a set bedtime and awake time, and contingency plans for night wakening (e.g., relaxation tapes).

**Recreation.**    The belief that if one is hurting, life cannot be enjoyed is often encountered in the chronic headache population. A rational discussion brings this misperception into awareness and gives the patient permission to engage in enjoyable activities. Involving family members in discussions and planning of recreational activities may be worthwhile.

### Pharmacologic Interventions
Choice of pharmacologic intervention is based largely on symptoms and premorbid headache pattern. For example, if trauma has exacerbated preexisting migraine, migraine therapy is indicated. However, if a migraine pattern has changed with evidence of more myofascial involvement, treatment options may need to be expanded.

A convenient model for organizing a therapeutic approach is the vascular-myofascial-supraspinal model proposed by Olesen (see discussion of pathophysiology). This model suggests that the expression of headache is the sum of input into the trigeminal system with vascular, sympathetic, myofascial, and central factors potentially contributing to the clinical picture. Consideration of the degree to which each of these components may contribute to the clinical picture organizes a treatment approach and allows a more comprehensive strategy.

Almost all drugs can potentiate the symptom of headache, and many impair cognitive function or exacerbate other symptoms associated with posttraumatic headache, such as vertigo. Therefore, it is paramount that physicians carefully review all medications used by the patient, including over-the-counter preparations. Many acute-treatment medications, when used by patients genetically predisposed to migraine on a daily or near-daily basis, can transform episodic migraine into chronic daily headache.[73,74] If transformation is suspected, withdrawal of offending medication is necessary before the underlying headache pattern can be adequately diagnosed or treated. In pursuit of relief, patients often have a pharmacy of medications and home remedies at hand. A good rule of thumb is to consider a drug holiday from all nonessential medications.

For many patients with posttraumatic headache, drug therapy is a balance of rational decision making and trial and error. Patients may respond to simple interventions or require complicated medication regimens. Typically pharmacologic treatment is divided into acute and prophylactic and is similar to that used to treat primary headache disorders. Appendices I-V provide recommendations for pharmacologic therapy for various types of headache patterns in patients with posttraumatic headache. They serve only as guidelines for primary care management. Obviously, each pharmacologic regimen must be individualized to the patient's specific needs and tailored for sound management of headache. At times, combinations of therapies are used.

### Nonpharmacologic Intervention

Numerous nonpharmacologic therapies have been useful in the treatment of posttraumatic headache: psychologic intervention, manual therapy, trigger point injections, electrical stimulation, photostimulation, nutrition counseling, exercise guidelines, and a caring attitude.

**Psychologic Intervention.**    The psychologist working with patients with posttraumatic headache should have knowledge, training, and experience with pain as the chief clinical complaint. The psychologist validates the person's problems through neuropsychologic testing and teaches self-management plans through cognitive retraining and biofeedback.

Thermal biofeedback assists 85% of patients to manage the frequency, intensity, and duration of headaches. An overall pain rating can be reduced by 50% or more simply by retraining the body through biofeedback to alter the internal physiology from stress to relaxation. The reprogramming takes about 6 weeks, with the patient practicing at home at least twice a day.

Education is vital. The person needs to know what is happening to the body and what to do to reverse the spiraling process of pain, fear, immobility, sense of uselessness, and despair. Given the tools, a person can turn his or her life around. But the procedure takes time. Eventually, the person develops an understanding of the disease and an internal locus of control for headache symptoms. Many patients learn for the first time effective techniques for managing headaches other than taking medicine.

The road to recovery is always dynamic. The psychologist forms a trusting relationship with the headache sufferer that encourages a return for a refresher course when needed.

**Manual Therapy.**    Manual therapy such as osteopathic manipulation or physical therapy also may be useful when myofascial complaints predominate.[61] Massage helps the patient to feel positive about the body as other than a source of pain.

**Trigger Point Injections.**    Trigger point injections with local anesthetic agents are often beneficial to relieve acutely exacerbated symptoms of headache or muscle pain. Selected nerve blocks of the occipital nerve, upper cervical facet nerve, or sphenopalatine ganglia may produce dramatic results, although are rarely curative. Facet nerve blocks and facet denervation are important considerations in selected cases.[62]

**Electrical Stimulation.**    Electrical stimulation and various forms of electrical therapy may be useful as well as transcranial electrical stimulation. Transcutaneous electrical stimulation, if used properly, also has been shown to be effective.[17] Bioelectric treatment of 342 chronic headache sufferers produced "significant improvement or no headache pain" after 14 15-minute treatments in 30 days. Patients without significant improvement in pain ratings after treatment resumed pharmacologic treatment in combination with bioelectric treatment for 5–10 additional treatments. Treatment success then increased to 93%.[63]

**Acupuncture.**    Acupuncture may play a role in selected cases and has demonstrated value in reducing headache intensity as well as medication usage.

### Consultation and Referral

As posttraumatic headaches become more chronic and refractory to standard interventions, management needs of individual patients often exceed the resources of the primary care physician. Occasionally diagnostic needs arise, and appropriate specialty consultation is warranted. However, in most cases, as diagnostic questions are answered, intense management is required. At this point, interdisciplinary treatment programs should be considered. Important components of such programs should include behavioral approaches to pain management. The role of medication and procedures generally decreases with duration of symptoms. Conversely, it is important to recognize early patients with problems beyond the scope of one's practice. Early detection of the need for interdisciplinary care minimizes repeated treatment failures and development of chronic pain dynamics.

Treatment for posttraumatic headache is often complex, requiring an interdisciplinary approach. While reviewing the patient's history, when straightforward interventions have failed to bring symptoms under control, referral to an intradisciplinary headache clinic may be appropriate. Many headache centers have demonstrated success with this model.

### CONCLUSION

Posttraumatic headache is a significant and poorly understood disorder. Over 2 million Americans each year suffer from posttraumatic headache disorders. These disorders need to be validated and explored carefully. Individualized treatment needs to be devised and researched.

## APPENDIX I.
### Treatment of Acute Migraine

1. Early symptoms, including prodromes without nausea:*

| | |
|---|---|
| Ibuprofen | 400–800 mg/every 6–8 hr as needed |
| Ketoprofen | 50–100 mg/every 8 hr as needed |
| Naprosyn | 375–750 mg/every 12 hr |
| Flurbiprofen | 200–300 mg/day |
| Misein | 2 capsules and 1 every hr up to 5/24 hr |

   * Most NSAIDs are useful. Physicians should choose those they are most familiar with.

2. Moderate symptoms without severe nausea or vomiting

| | |
|---|---|
| Sumatriptan | 25–50 mg orally; may repeat for nonresponse after 2 hr or if migraine recurs. |
| Ergotamine tartrate | 2 mg orally; repeat after 1 hr |
| NSAID as above in selected cases | |
| Combination analgesic in selected instances | |

3. Severe migraine with nausea or vomiting:*

| | |
|---|---|
| Sumatriptan | 6 mg SC |
| DHE and metoclopramide | 0.5 1 mg IV, IM, or SC plus 10 mg IM or IV |
| Prochlorperazine | 10 mg IV |
| Chlorpromazine | 12.5 mg IV |

   * Consider fluid replacement if patient volume depleted.

IV = intravenously, IM = intramuscularly, SC = subcutaneously, NSAIDs = nonsteroidal antiinflammatory drugs.

## APPENDIX II.
### Pharmacologic Treatment of Frequent Migraine or Transformed Migraine

1. Treatment of daily or near daily headache associated with sleep disruption or depression:

| | *Sleep Disruption* | *Depression* |
|---|---|---|
| Nortriptyline | 10–50 mg at bedtime | 7.5–150 mg/day |
| Amitriptyline | 10–50 mg at bedtime | 7.5–150 mg/day |
| Trazodone | 25–75 mg | 100–300 mg/day |
| SSRIs | per PI as below | per PI |

2. Treatment of daily component of headache without associated sleep disruption:

| | |
|---|---|
| Protriptyline (Vivactil) | 5–40 mg/day |
| Paroxetine (Paxil) | 10–40 mg/day |
| Sertraline (Zoloft) | 50–150 mg/day |
| Fluoxetine (Prozac) | 10–40 mg/day |
| Nefazodone (Serzone) | 100–300 mg/day |

3. Treatment of acute migraine attack in transformed migraine:

| | |
|---|---|
| Sumatriptan | 25–50 mg orally or 6 mg SC |
| Ergotamine tartrate and metoclopramide | 2 mg and 10 mg orally |
| DHE | 0.5–1 mg IV or IM |
| Metoclopramide* | 10 mg orally or IV |

   * Monitor frequency of these medications. If possible, limit their use to less than 2 days/wk.

SSRIs = selective serotonin reuptake inhibitors, PI = product information, SC = subcutaneously, IV = intravenously, IM = intramuscularly.

## APPENDIX III.
### Therapy for Acute Attacks of Posttraumatic Cluster Headache

1. Acute episodes

| | |
|---|---|
| Oxygen | 100% per face mask for 10–15 minutes with |
| Sumatriptan | 6 mg SC |
| DHE | 0.5–1 mg IV or IM |

2. For frequent attacks requiring prophylaxis:
   Prednisone in tapering schedule, 60 to 0 mg over 7–10 days with verapamil, 80–120 mg 3 times/day or lithium carbonate 300 mg 3 times/day for duration of the cluster
   Ergotamine tartrate, 2 mg at bedtime if nighttime breakthrough is noted

IV = intravenously, IM = intramuscularly.

## APPENDIX IV.
Treatment of Chronic Tension-type Headache

1. Treatment of daily headache component associated with anxiety, mood disability, bipolar disorder, or medication withdrawal.

| | |
|---|---|
| Disodium valproate | 250–1,000 mg/day |
| Beta blockers | |
| Atenolol | 50–100 mg/day |
| Corgard | 20–40 mg/day |
| Propranolol | 20–320 mg/day |

2. Treatment of daily headache with significant myofascial involvement

| | |
|---|---|
| Baclofen | 5–20 q |
| Cyclobenzeprine | 10 mg 3 times/day |
| Trigger point injections with 0.25% bupivacaine | |
| Transcutaneous electrical nerve stimulation | |

3. Other common pharmacologic interventions*

| | |
|---|---|
| Verapamil | up to 480 mg/day |
| Cyproheptadine | 4–16 mg/day |
| Methysergide | 4–8 mg/day |
| Methylergonovine | 0.2 mg 2–3 k/day |

\* Many specialists report success with monoamine oxidase inhibitors, but in general they are not recommended unless experience with these drugs is obtained.

4. Sleep disruption with depression*

| | Sleep Disruption | Depression |
|---|---|---|
| Nortriptyline | 10–50 mg/day | 75–150 mg |
| Amitriptyline | 10–50 mg/day | 75–150 mg |
| Trazodone | 25–75 mg/day | 100–300 mg |
| SSRIs | per PI | per PI |

\* Often a combination of SSRI and low-dose TCA at bedtime will assist patient with depression and sleep disruption.

5. Without sleep disruption, excessive sedation, or in elderly patients

| | | |
|---|---|---|
| Vivactil | | 5–40 mg/day |
| or | | |
| | Paxil | 10–40 mg |
| SSRI | Zoloft | 50–150 mg |
| | Prozac | 20–40 mg |
| | Serazone | 100–300 mg |

6. With anxiety, mood disruption, or medication withdrawal

| | |
|---|---|
| Disodium valproate | 250–1000 mg/day |
| Gabapentin | 300–1500 mg/day |
| Beta blockers | |
| Atenolol | 50–100 mg/day |
| Nadolol | 80–160 mg/day |

7. With myofascial involvement

| | |
|---|---|
| Baclofen | 10–20 mg 3 times/day |
| Cyclobenzaprine | 10 mg 3 times/day |
| Trigger point injection 0.25% bupivacaine | |
| Appropriate nerve blocks | |
| Transcutaneous electrical nerve stimulation | |
| Acupuncture | |

SSRI = selective serotonin reuptake inhibitor, PI = product information.

# REFERENCES

1. Elkind AH: Posttraumatic headache. In Diamond S, Dalessio DJ (eds): The Practicing Physician's Approach to Headache, 5th ed. Baltimore, Williams & Wilkins, 1992, pp 146–161.
2. Yagamuchi M: Incidence of headache and severity of head injury. Headache 32:427–431, 1992.
3. Rimel RW, Giordani B, Barth JT, et al: Disability caused by minor head injury. Neurosurgery 9:221–228, 1981.
4. Erichsen JE: On Concussion of the Spine: Nervous Shock and Other Obscure Injuries of the Nervous System in their Clinical and Medicolegal Aspects. London, Longmans, Green, 1982.
5. Page H: Injuries of the Spine and Spinal Cord without Apparent Mechanical Lesion. London, J & A Churchill, 1985.
6. Trimble MR: Post-traumatic Neurosis. Chichester, John Wiley & Sons, 1981.
7. Gean AD: White matter shearing injury and brain stem injury. In Imaging of Head Trauma. New York, Raven Press, 1994, pp 217–248.
8. Strauss I, Savitsky N: Head injury. Arch Neurol Psychol 31:893, 1934.
9. Simons DJ, Wolff HG: Studies on headache: Mechanisms of chronic post-traumatic headache. Psychosom Med 8:227–242, 1946.
10. Oppenheimer DR: Microscopic lesions in the brain following head injury. J Neurol Neurosurg Psychiatry 31:299, 1968.
11. Povlishock JT, et al: Axonal changes in minor head injury. J Neuropathol Exp Neurol 42:225–242, 1983.
12. Packard RC: Post-traumatic. Semin Neurol 14:40–45, 1994.
13. Levin HS, Gary HE Jr, High Wm Jr, et al: Minor head injury and the post concussion syndrome: Methodological issues in outcome studies. In Levin HS (ed): Neurobehavioral Recovery from Head Injury. New York, Oxford University Press, 1987, pp 267–275.
14. Headache Classification Committee of the International Headache Society: Classification and diagnostic criteria for headache disorders, cranial neuralgias, and facial pain. Cephalalgia 8(Suppl 7):1–96, 1988.
15. Evans RW: The postconcussive syndrome and the sequelae of mild head injury. Neurol Clin 10:815–847, 1992.
16. Duckro PN, Greenberg M, Schultz KT, et al: Clinical features of chronic post-traumatic headache. Headache Q 3:295–308, 1992.
17. Shealy CN: Spinally mediated headache. In Cady RK, Fox AW (eds): Treating the Headache Patient. New York, Marcel Dekker, 1995, pp 235–256.
18. Packard RC, Ham LP: Promising techniques in the assessment of mild head injury. Semin Neurol, in press.
19. Reitan R, Wolfson D: The Halstead-Reitan Neuropsychological Test Battery. Tucson, AZ, Neuropsychology Press, 1985.
20. Reitan R, Wolfson D: Traumatic Brain Injury, vol. I. Tucson, AZ, Neuropsychology Press, 1986, pp 63–72.
21. Ommaya AK: Mechanisms of cerebral concussion, contusion, and other effects of head injury. In JR Youmans (ed): Neurological Surgery. Philadelphia, W.B. Saunders, 1982.
22. Reitan R, Wolfson D: Traumatic Brain Injury, vol. II. Tucson, AZ, Neuropsychology Press, 1986, pp 185–225.
23. Featherstone HJ: Migraine and muscle contraction headaches: A continuum. Headache 25:194, 1985.
24. Wilkerson M, Blau JN: Are classical and common migraine different entities? Headache 25:211, 1985.
25. Olesen J: Clinical and pathophysiologic observations in migraine and tension-type headache explained by integration of vascular, supraspinal, and myofascial inputs. Pain 46:125–132, 1991.
26. Moskowitz MA: The trigeminovascular system. In Olesen J, Tfely-Hansen P, Welch KMA (eds): The Headaches. New York, Raven Press, 1993, pp 97–104.
27. Travell J, Rinzler SH: The myofascial genesis of pain. Postgrad Med 11:425–434, 1952.
28. Travell J, Simons D: Myofascial Pain and Dysfunction: The Trigger Point Manual. Baltimore, Williams & Wilkins, 1983.
29. Fricton DA, Kroening R, Haley D, Siegart R: Myofascial pain syndrome of the head and neck: A review of clinical characteristics of 164 patients. Oral Surg 60:615–623, 1985.
30. Bengtsson A, Hendriksson KG, Larsson J: Reduced high-energy phosphate levels in painful muscles in patients with primary fibromyalgia. Arthritis Rheum 29:817–821, 1986.
31. Lund N, Bengtssen A, Thorborg P: Muscle tissue oxygen pressure in primary fibromyalgia. Scand Rheumatol 15:165–173, 1986.
32. Fricton JR: Myofascial pain syndrome. In Fricton JR, Awad E (eds): Advances in Pain Research and Therapy, vol. 17. New York, Raven Press, 1990, pp 107–127.
33. Massey EW, Massey J: Elongated styloid process (Eagles' syndrome) causing hemicrania. Headache 19:339, 1979.
34. Schoenen J: Tension-type headache: Pathophysiologic evidence for a disturbance of "limbic" pathways to the brain stem. Headache 30:314–315, 1990.
35. Terenius L: Endorphins and modulation of pain. In Critchley M, et al (eds): Advances in Neurology, vol. 33. New York, Raven Press, 1982, pp 59–64.

36. von Knorring L, Almay BGL, Johnasson F, Terenius L: Pain perception and endorphin levels in the cerebralspinal fluid. Pain 5:359–365, 1978.
37. Smith E: Influence of site of impact on cognitive impairment persisting long after severe closed head injury. J Neurol Neurosurg Psychiatry 37:719–726, 1974.
38. Roberts AH: Long-term prognosis of severe accidental head injury. Proc R Soc Med 69:137–140, 1976.
39. Balla J, Karnaghan J: Whiplash headache. Clin Exp Neurol Clin 23:179–182, 1987.
40. Evans RW: Some observations on whiplash injuries. Neurol Clin 10:975–997, 1992.
41. Liu YK, Chandran KB, Heath RG, Unterharnscheidt F: Subcortical EEG changes in Rhesus monkeys following experimental hyperextension-hyperflexion (whiplash). Spine 9:329–338, 1984.
42. Sturzenegger M, DiStefano G, Radanov BP, et al: Presenting symptoms and signs after whiplash injury. Neurology 44:688–693, 1994.
43. MacNab J: Acceleration extension injuries of the cervical spine. In Rothman RH, Simeone FA (eds): The Spine, 2nd ed. Philadelphia, W.B. Saunders, 1982, pp 647–660.
44. Watkinson A, Gargan MF, Bannister GC: Prognostic factors in soft tissue injuries of the cervical spine. Injury 22:307–309, 1991.
45. Grubb RL, Coxe WS: Trauma to the central nervous system. In Eliasson AL, Prensky AL, Hardin WB (eds): Neurological Pathophysiology. New York, Oxford University Press, 1978.
46. Cartlidge NEF, Shaw D: Head Injury. Philadelphia, W.B. Saunders, 1981.
47. Mathew NT: Migraine transformation and chronic daily headache. In Cady RK, Fox AW (eds): Treating the Headache Patient. New York, Marcel Dekker, 1995, pp 75–100.
48. Rapaport AM, Weeks RE, Sheftell FD, et al: Analgesic rebound headache: Theoretical and practical implications. Cephalalgia 5(Suppl 3):448–449, 1985.
49. Kudrow L: Paradoxical effects of frequent analgesic use. In Critchley M, Friedman A, Gorini S, Sicuteri F (eds): Advances in Neurology, vol. 33. New York, Raven Press, 1982, pp 335–341.
50. Vijayan N: A new post-traumatic headache syndrome. Headache 17:19–22, 1977.
51. Gutkelch AN: Post-traumatic amnesia, post-concussional symptoms and accident. Eur Neurol 19:91–102, 1980.
52. Kelly R, Smith BN: Post-traumatic syndrome: Another myth discredited. J R Soc Med 74:275–277, 1981.
53. Trash MJ, Royston C: A follow-up study of accident neurosis. Br J Psychol 146:18–25, 1985.
54. Packard RC: Post-traumatic headache: Permanency and relationship to legal settlement. Headache 32:496–500, 1992.
55. Waddell G: A new clinical model for the treatment of low-back pain. Spine 12(7):632–644, 1987.
56. Mauskop A, Alyura BT, Cracco RQ, Altura BM: Intravenous magnesium sulfate rapidly alleviates headache of various types. Headache 36:154–160, 1996.
57. Ramadan NM, Halvorson H, Vande-Linde A, et al: Low brain magnesium in migraine. Headache 29:416–419, 1989.
58. Cox RH, Shealy CN, Cady RK, et al: Significant magnesium deficiency in depression. Neurol Orthop Med Surg 17:7–9, 1996.
59. Mathew NT, Stubis E, Nigam MP: Transformation of episodic migraine into daily headache: Analysis of factors. Headache 22:66–68, 1982.
60. Mathew NT, Reuveni U, Perez F: Transformed or evaluative migraine. Headache 27:102–106, 1987.
61. Jay GW, Brunson J, Branson SJ: The effectiveness of physical therapy in the treatment of chronic daily headaches. Headache 29:156–162, 1989.
62. Cady RK, Cox R, Shealy CN, Wilkie RG: Facet rhizotomy: A 15-year experience. J Neurol Orthop Med Surg 9(2):107–108, 1988.
63. Sorgnard R, Schwartz R, Savery F, et al: Alternative or adjunctive bioelectric treatment for chronic headache pain. Western Regional Anesthesiology Symposium, 1993.

# 12

# Temporomandibular Joint Dysfunction

## CHRISTOPHER R. BROWN, DDS, MPS

The abbreviation *TMJ* is often used erroneously as a diagnostic entity. In fact, it correctly describes the temporomandibular joints, which are diarthrodial joints connecting the mandible to the skull. For delineating dysfunction of the TMjs, the abbreviation *TMD* is correct; the *D* refers to dysfunction.

TMD is a vague diagnosis. In fact, TMD does not indicate a single diagnostic entity but rather a collection of symptoms affecting or arising from the TMJs, muscles of mastication, or contiguous soft and hard tissue entities. This vagueness accounts for much confusion within the dental community as well as other disciplines that diagnose and treat facial pain. TMD is commonly used to describe anything from sore facial muscles from cheering too hard at a ball game to advanced degenerative joint disease. As a result, many patients and clinicians have found themselves in a virtual no-man's land of confusion.

It has been conservatively estimated that over 10 million people in the United States suffer from symptoms attributed to TMD. Up to 75% of nonpatient populations have at least one sign of TMJ dysfunction. Around 33% have at least one painful symptom in the face or TM joints. Although epidemiologic estimations may differ somewhat, TMD sufferers are most commonly females (female-to-male ratio of 5:1) between the ages of 15–45 years.[4] TMD costs the U.S. billions of dollars in health care and lost days of productivity.

In 1934 Costen[2] first addressed this entity by hypothesizing that lost vertical dimension in the facial structures was the main source of symptoms. As a result, the idea of opening the bite through various forms of dental reconstruction became the chief pathway to problem solving. Hence disorders of the TMJ fell into dentistry, and occlusion was conceptualized as the dominant etiologic factor. Dentistry, as a leader in TMD treatment, focused strictly on the role of occlusion and alterations of mandibular position to reduce or eliminate facial pain.

Unfortunately, the approach to treatment has often conceived of TMD as a single disease entity. The search has been for a simple answer to a complex problem that often requires multiple treatment modalities. Despite concerted efforts to discover the cure for TMD, logic dictates that the first approach, as in any disease entity, should be to formulate a working differential diagnosis. The term TMD is far too inclusive and in fact describes symptoms rather than causation. In the decades after Costen's discovery,

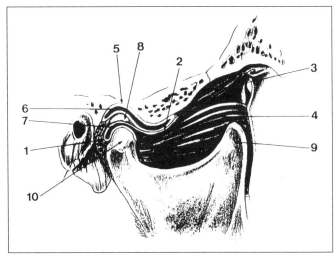

**FIGURE 1.**
Temporomandibular joint. The anatomic components: 1, retrodiscal tissues; 2, anterior capsular ligament (collagenous); 3 and 4, superior and inferior lateral pterygoid muscles; 5, articular surface; 6 and 7, superior and inferior joint space; 8, meniscus; 9, coronoid process; 10, condylar head.

scientific constructs have begun to emerge, and dentistry, with a multidisciplinary approach, has begun to find workable solutions for pain resolution.

## ANATOMY

Functionally the TMJs involve the articulation of the mandibular condyles in the temporal bones (Fig. 1). The articulating surfaces of the temporal bones consist of concave, thin bony surfaces or fossae and convex, thick bony surfaces or eminentiae. The fossae are the concavities hosting the mandibular condyles, and the eminentiae are the bony convexities anterior to the fossae. In addition, the TMJs include the articulating discs, retrodistal tissues, joint capsules, and synovium, all of which are soft tissue structures. Medially and laterally the discs insert at the medial and lateral poles of the condyles. Anteriorly, the discs are continuous with the superior belly of the lateral pterygoid muscles.

The temporomandibular capsule is a dense fibrous tissue sheet completely enclosing each joint in a 360° circle, with its insertion lines at the neck of the condyle below and at the temporal bone above. The upper and lower compartments of the TMJs have a synovial lining that appears to have a highly active immunologic ability to produce antibodies and collagenase-type materials that help to protect and ensure the continuity of the synovial fluid.

The TMJs, although considered synovial joints, have a number of attributes that distinguish them from other synovial joints in the human body:

1. The articulating surfaces of the TMJs are covered by fibrocartilage rather than hyaline.

2. The TMJs are divided into upper and lower compartments by a fibrous meniscus (disc), the purpose of which is to help facilitate both rotation and translation.

3. The TMJs are the only joints in the human body that must work in harmony with another joint—in both correct function and dysfunction. A dysfunctional joint

often creates an equal and opposite force on the opposing joint; i.e., hypomovement on the left can produce hyperfunction on the right.

4. The function of the TMJs is influenced greatly by masticatory muscles and supportive structures of the joints.

The anatomy of TMJs provides both rotational and translational movement. The TMJs are formed by the mandibular condyles as they fit into the glenoid fossae of the temporal bones. The condyle and glenoid fossae are separated by the fibrous cartilage disc (meniscus), which divides the joint into the upper and lower chambers. The articular portion of the disc, which is composed of connective tissue, is devoid of nerves or vessels. The posterior attachment of the disc, however, is richly vascularized and innervated. The disc itself is attached to the condyle both medially and laterally by collateral ligaments that permit both rotational and translational movement of the disc/condyle complex during opening and closing of the mouth. Rotational movement occurs between the condyle and the surface of the disc during early opening, whereas translation takes place in the space between the superior surface of the disc and the glenoid fossae. Synovial fluid provides lubrication to the joint and acts as a medium for transporting nutrients and waste products to and from the articular surfaces.

### Supporting Musculature

Movement of the TMJs is achieved by a series of skeletal muscles. The primary masticatory muscles include the masseter, medial pterygoid, temporalis (mouth closing), digastric muscles (mouth opening), and lateral pterygoid muscles, which are further divided into the inferior and superior belly. The lateral pterygoid muscles assist in protruding the mandible and provide stabilization for the condyle/disc complex during function.

### Innervation

The innervation of the TMJs and supporting structures is supplied primarily by the trigeminal and facial nerves. The trigeminal nerve, which provides both sensory and motor innervation, is the primary nerve that supplies the TMJs. Sensory fibers of the trigeminal nerve extend to synapses in the trigeminal spinal nucleus of the brainstem.

The trigeminal nerve is divided into three branches: ophthalmic, maxillary, and mandibular. The mandibular nerve provides sensory and/or motor branches to the medial and lateral pterygoid muscles, temporalis, masseter, and TMJs via the auriculotemporal nerve. While passing behind the TMJs, the auriculotemporal nerve emerges distal to the condyle, then traverses into the temporal area. It also supplies sensory perception to the tongue and lower teeth. The primary nerve supplies of the TMJs arise from the auriculotemporal nerve posteriorly, the masseteric nerve medially, and the posterior deep temporal nerve laterally. Although the facial nerve (cranial nerve VII) does not directly supply the TMJs, it provides motor and sensory functions to associated musculature and supporting structures, including the orbicularis oculi and anterior two-thirds of the tongue. The taste sensation of the posterior one-third of the tongue is provided by the glossopharyngeal nerve.

### Vascular Supply

The arterial supply to the TMJs originates from the superficial temporal artery (posterior to the joint), posterior auricular artery, deep auricular artery, lateral pterygoid pedicle, and masseteric artery. The three latter vessels are branches of the maxillary artery.

## CLASSIFICATION OF TEMPOROMANDIBULAR DISORDERS

Bell[3] devised one of the best classification systems for TM disorders. His system was proposed more accurately as a classification for orofacial pain rather than TMD alone and suggests correctly that TMD is a continuum of disorders rather than a single clinical entity.

I. Somatic pain
   A. Superficial somatic pain
      1. Cutaneous
      2. Mucogingival
   B. Deep somatic pain
      1. Musculoskeletal pain
         a. Muscle pain
            i. Protective splinting
            ii. Myofascial trigger point pain
            iii. Muscle spasm pain
            iv. Muscle inflammation pain
         b. Temporomandibular joint pain
            i. Disc attachment pain
            ii. Retrodistal pain
            iii. Capsular pain
            iv. Arthritic pain
         c. Osseous and periosteal pain
         d. Soft connective tissue pain
         e. Periodontal dental pain
      2. Visceral pain
         a. Pulpal dental pain
         b. Vascular pain
II. Neurogenous pain
   A. Neuropathic pain
      1. Traumatic neuroma
      2. Paroxysmal neuralgia
         a. Idiopathic neuralgia
         b. Symptomatic neuralgia
      3. Neuritic neuralgia
         a. Peripheral neuritis
         b. Herpes zoster
         c. Postherpetic neuralgia
   B. Deafferentation pain
      1. Sympathetically maintained pain syndromes
      2. Anesthesia dolorosa
      3. Phantom pain
III. Psychogenic pain
   A. Chronic facial pain
   B. Psychoneurotic pain
      1. Conversion hysteria
      2. Delusional pain

## SYMPTOMS OF TEMPOROMANDIBULAR DYSFUNCTION

The symptoms of TMD are often varied and at first may seem unrelated. An old catchphrase for TMD was "the great imposter" because of the diversity of symptoms that also may be attributed to other conditions. Any or all of the following may result from TMD:

1. TM joint noise—popping, clicking, grinding, crepitation.
2. Mandibular trismus or inability to open the mouth uniformly—can be measured by lack of opening or deviation of the mandible from midline.

3. Pain in or around the TMJs.

4. Headaches—bilateral, unilateral, occipital, or frontal; may be exacerbated by chewing or stress.

5. Neckaches.

6. Inability to fit the maxillary and mandibular teeth together—may be perceived by the patient as "not a normal bite."

7. Facial pain on chewing—located around the TMJs or perceived by the patient as a headache or earache.

8. Tinnitus.

9. Earache—bilateral or unilateral, in the absence of ear pathology.

10. Excessive ear wax—usually found in conjunction with chronic retrodistal inflammation and posterior displacement of the condyle.

11. Photosensitivity.

12. Dysphagia.

13. Palpable trigger points in the masticatory muscles.

14. Myalgia—generalized in the head and neck or focalized in the masticatory muscles.

Any tissue dominated by the three major branches or the trigeminal system or its subsets is subject to pain and dysfunction. The severity of symptoms may range from annoyance to debilitation and may fluctuate with time. It is also not unusual for patients to go through a period of quiescence. As in any nonmalignant pain entity, fluctuations of intensity and duration are to be expected.

## CAUSES OF TEMPOROMANDIBULAR DYSFUNCTION

TMD is such a broad category that it is difficult to discuss specific causes. Aside from functional disorders, the TMJs are subject to the same pathology that afflicts other synovial joints, such as various kinds of arthritis, synovitis, hyperuricemia, neoplasia, and fibrosis.[2]

Much effort seems to have been made to conceive of TMD as something magical. It is treated as if it were a totally separate entity from the rest of the body in which the laws of human physiology and physics suddenly do not apply. The bounds of reason are often ignored. Several distinct components make the TMJs somewhat unique, as previously mentioned, but overall they function much like other synovial joints. In making clinical assessments of TMJ problems, it is wise to keep in mind the function and dysfunction of other joints. This concept helps to guide the clinician toward an acceptable differential diagnosis.

### Why Do the Temporomandibular Joints Make Noise?

The TMJs pop, click, and crunch for various reasons. The most common clinical situation is displacement of the disc(s) in the anterior/medial direction with resulting distalization of the condylar head(s) within the glenoid fossae. This displacement results in the classic popping of the TMJs. Chronic displacement of the disc(s), especially in women, may lead to degeneration of the condylar head(s), distortion of the disc(s), and total dysfunction of the TMJ(s), resulting in pain. As degeneration progresses, the noises emitted by the TMJs may change to crepitation as a result of roughening of the articulating surfaces. Along with this degeneration often comes restriction of mandibular range of motion, loss of function, and increase in pain. In certain people, ischemic necrosis of the condylar heads may exacerbate the situation.

Nonpathologic anatomic variations, such as aberrations of the condylar heads, discs, capsular lining, retrodistal tissues, and articulating surfaces, also may cause the TMJs to make noise. Growths or foreign bodies within the TMJs, although rare, also must be ruled out in the presence of TM joint noise. The individual patient must be carefully assessed to determine whether the joint noises are indicative of pathology. A cursory examination can be accomplished by fingertip palpation or stethoscope. Definitive diagnosis may require the use of computed sonography, magnetic resonance imaging (MRI), and a combination of radiographs.

Several categories of pain origins account for the majority of TMD and merit special discussion because of their prevalence.

## Occlusion

The most controversial aspect of TMJ treatment is the role of occlusion. Some behavioral scientists claim there is no supporting evidence that occlusion plays any part at all in the etiology, perpetuation, or alleviation of TMD symptoms. "Lack of scientific evidence" is the battle cry. On the other side of the arena are those who claim that all symptoms can be eliminated or alleviated by restoration of the biting surfaces of the teeth. Much anecdotal evidence supports this phenomenon. Thrown into the soup are others who believe, like Costen, that restoration of the facial vertical dimension and re-alignment of the teeth and stomatognathic complex via various restorative procedures will resolve patient complaints.

The whole controversy goes back to the erroneous "one entity, one solution" way of thinking. The battle lines have been drawn, and reason has been thrown out the window.

No other joints in the body have provoked such a zealous search for a solution to pain and dysfunction. The answer is simple, in a roundabout way: there is no single answer. TMD is without a doubt multifactorial, both symptomatically and etiologically. For successful resolution, clinicians from various disciplines must work together. Many human afflictions do not fall into the strict definition demanded by the scientific community. Close scrutiny of any clinical study reveals obvious flaws compared with laboratory-controlled tests. The best that can be accomplished is a blend of academia, clinical study, and common sense. While trends can be followed and measured, epidemiologic studies must be estimated and weighed in conjunction with unique individual factors to achieve full understanding of the pain entity.

Does occlusion play a part in TMD? Of course it does, at times—but not in all cases. Occlusion may play a major factor in one patient but no role at all in another. The treating doctor, however, must have a thorough understanding of occlusion to help provide a differential diagnosis. To quote Mark Twain, "There are lies, damn lies, and statistics." Statistically and epidemiologically occlusion plays a questionable role in TMD, but this does not mean that thousands of patients whose symptoms were alleviated by treatment of occlusion were misdiagnosed and mistreated. Perhaps it means instead that subsets of pain etiologies need to be understood and analyzed for possible roles in a patient's painful lifestyle. According to an old saying, "When the only tool you own is a hammer, the whole world looks like a nail." The antithesis is also true: when clinicians refuse to look at an entity as a contributing factor, they can in truth say, "I've never seen that." Without question occlusion should be taken into consideration for a differential diagnosis. The kinematics of the stomatognathic system requires harmony of all components for normal, pain-free function. Any aspect of the system at any given time may dominate, causing dysfunction and pain. Therefore, a multidisciplinary approach usually yields the best clinical results.

## Direct Trauma

Trauma is one of the most common causes of TMD. In fact, it has been estimated that trauma accounts for the majority of TM disorders.[11]

Direct trauma to the mandible, depending on the pulse duration and force vectors, is capable of injuring the TMJs in the form of soft tissue damage or bony involvement.

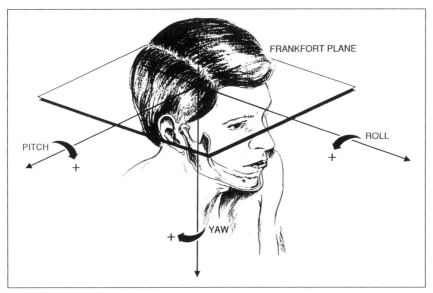

**FIGURE 2.**
Real-world forces to the head and neck are always multidirectional during trauma.

There is no such thing as a pure direct blow except under strict laboratory conditions (Fig. 2). In the real world the relevant factors in considering soft tissue damage as a result of trauma are too numerous to count. A few examples are neck position, head position, rotation of the cervical spine, movement of the head on an x/y axis, position of the mandible at the time of impact, angle of the blow, amount of soft tissue to absorb the blow, and modulus of elasticity of the individual's tissue under those particular circumstances. Even under the banner of direct trauma, all of these factors lead to other forces often thought of as indirect, such as shear, torsion, compression, and tension (Fig. 3).

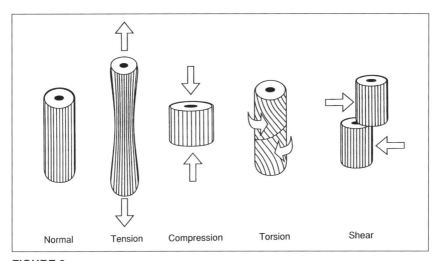

**FIGURE 3.**
Mechanisms for injury to human tissues that may occur simultaneously during both direct and indirect trauma.

Although injury categories are certainly evident, each person's physical response to trauma is unique. The term *direct* is descriptive only of the point of impact and the tissue precisely affected—not of the total injury component. Every direct injury has an indirect component as well.

Soft tissue injuries to the TMJs often result from direct blows to the mandible and are considered the result of crush-type forces. Because of the nature of the anatomy, various soft tissue components (e.g., menisci, cartilage, blood vessels) are juxtaposed between bony surfaces (e.g., condylar head, superior articulating surfaces of the bony socket, distal and medial aspects of the socket). When the condyle is forced beyond its physiologic range, especially in rapid motion, the chance of a crush-type injury exists. The result is disruption of the joint surfaces and supporting tissues on both a cellular and macro level. Hemarthrosis may result, leading not only to an acute condition but also to synovitis, which contributes to inflammation of the affected surfaces and results in long-term articular degeneration and possible degenerative joint disease.

Direct blows to the mandible or TMJs usually result in rapid onset of symptoms, but this generalization must be assessed for each patient. It is not uncommon for the victim to feel a change in occlusion, noticing soon after the trauma that the teeth do not match together normally. If the meniscus or menisci are anteriorly displaced but within the physiologic range of motion of the condylar head, the injury may be accompanied by popping or clicking of the TMJ(s) due to displacement of the menisci. Displacement may be unilateral or bilateral. If it is unilateral, the noise may be accompanied by trismus or deviation of the mandible to the side of the disc displacement—in essence, hypomobility of the affected TMJ. The opposite occurs on the contralateral side, resulting in hypermobility of the TMJs and deviation of the mandible away from the joint. If there is an influx of fluid into the joint as a result of the blow, the void left by a displaced disc may be filled by the fluid, resulting in no noticeable joint noise. Lack of joint noise often leads to misdiagnosis of TMJ injuries and to a lag time before effective treatment can be initiated.

In some cases, the force and pulse duration are such that the disc is displaced beyond the physiologic range of motion of the condylar head, resulting in disc displacement that is not "recaptured" during motion. The result is an injured TMJ that does not make noise; the mandibular range of motion is unaffected, and there may be little if any deviation of the mandible. This injury is particularly difficult to diagnose initially because of the lack of overt clinical symptoms. The clinician must be astute, and soft tissue injuries must be assumed as a result of direct blows to the mandible. A single examination may not be sufficient to develop a true diagnosis. The patient should be seen on 2-week, 6-week and up to 6-month follow-up to determine whether function is altered and whether a cellular level injury has led to an alteration in system function. In all cases of direct blows to the mandible, soft tissue crush injuries within the TMJs should be taken into consideration during the examination.

A form of direct impact to the face that is becoming more and more prevalent results from airbag inflations (Fig. 4). Almost 100% of all 1995 passenger cars have driver-side airbags, and 87% also have passenger-side systems.[18] Airbags are released from their restraints at approximately 200 mph. Although there is no question that airbags save lives, it has also been demonstrated that passengers who do not wear seat belts and passengers who sit so close to the airbags that they receive the full force of inflation may actually have a greater chance of injury in low-speed collisions.[18]

Careful review of crash test films indicates that often the dummies contacting the airbags lead with their chins. Because of the dummies' construction, forces to the TMJs have not been measured. However, dentists across the nation are reporting patients with broken teeth, facial abrasions, and disc displacements of the TMJs as a result of impact with airbags. As a rule of thumb, when a patient has been involved in a motor vehicle accident with sufficient force to inflate an airbag, a TMJ injury should be suspected.

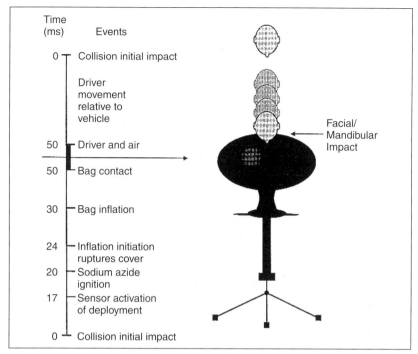

| Time (ms) | Events |
| --- | --- |
| 0 | Collision initial impact |
| | Driver movement relative to vehicle |
| 50 | Driver and air |
| 50 | Bag contact |
| 30 | Bag inflation |
| 24 | Inflation initiation ruptures cover |
| 20 | Sodium azide ignition |
| 17 | Sensor activation of deployment |
| 0 | Collision initial impact |

Facial/Mandibular Impact

**FIGURE 4.**
Airbags inflate at a rate of approximately 200 mph. Most airbags are designed to protect the 50th percentile male. Effectiveness of airbags can be compromised by such factors as the occupant's height, posture, and distance from the steering wheel. These variables can even lead to airbag-induced injuries of the head, neck, and chest.

## Indirect Trauma

Lack of understanding has made injuries due to indirect trauma an emotionally charged issue. Although there are other sources of indirect trauma, the vast majority of indirect injuries result from rear-end motor vehicle accidents (REMVAs) that lead to the clinical diagnosis of "whiplash." REMVAs account for over 25% of all MVAs and for an even greater proportion of soft tissue cervical damage.[13] In the United States, whiplash injuries often involve insurance adjusters, attorneys, and legal confrontations. Clinicians often take sides when there are really no sides to take. The clinician should determine injury and probable causation. Understanding of causation helps to understand the injuries and results in a more accurate diagnosis and improved patient healing (Fig. 5).

Because most indirect injuries to the TMJs are a result of REMVAs, certain facts about REMVAs must be taken into consideration. First of all, all REMVAs are unique; no two are alike. Crash tests are used to make specific measurements under controlled circumstances. They are at best guidelines and cannot be expected to provide all of the answers.

Low-impact and high-impact REMVAs cannot be lumped together in the same category. The dynamics and occupant kinematics are not comparable. In low-impact MVAs, factors such as seat construction, thickness of the passenger compartment fabric lining, contents of the trunk, position of the seats, and physical factors of the occupants (e.g., weight, length of neck, muscular strength, position of the neck, angles of the position of the vertebrae) are extremely important in considering the amount and type of injuries received by the victims.[13,14,16] Any or all of these factors may contribute

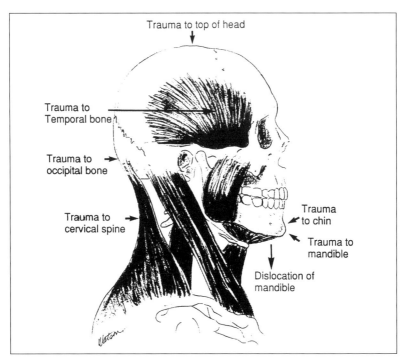

Trauma to top of head

Trauma to
Temporal bone

Trauma to
occipital bone

Trauma to
cervical spine

Trauma
to chin

Trauma to
mandible

Dislocation of
mandible

**FIGURE 5.**
Any one or all of the above injuries may result from a motor vehicle accident.

significantly to the number and degree of injuries. In high-velocity impacts, these factors tend to become less significant. The forces involved are so overwhelming and the duration pulse so short that other contributing factors are mute.

The forces in even a low-impact REMVA are often beyond human physiologic limits—and all it takes to result in tissue injury is force beyond physiologic limit. There is little relationship between the amount of dollar damage to a car and the injuries of the occupants.[5,7,10]

Human tissue injuries result from what is known as delta V (DV), the change in velocity. The DV of the automobile is not the DV of the occupants. It has been estimated that the head of an occupant in the front seat of the lead car accelerates about 2.5 times faster than the automobile.[15] Aside from direct contact, DV is what causes injuries. Many studies indicate that the maximal DV occurs to occupants within 0.1–0.2 seconds after impact (Fig. 6).[8,17] In other words, injuries to the human body have occurred within the blink of an eye. That short of an energy pulse is almost too difficult to comprehend. Yet beyond that time span, the forces have begun to dissipate and change. To understand how injuries occur in REMVAs, one must understand that an incredible amount of force is applied in an unbelievably short time. The result is often devastating tissue damage.

These principles must be understood before injuries to the TMJs as a result of REMVAs can be understood. The mechanisms of injury are not that different between direct and indirect trauma. The force vectors involved may be from different directions, but the resulting clinical injuries are strikingly similar.

In the form of a free body diagram (Fig. 7), the head, neck, and mandible are separate entities held together by various soft tissue components. In a direct blow to the mandible, for instance, there is a point of impact at which blunt trauma (or crush) may

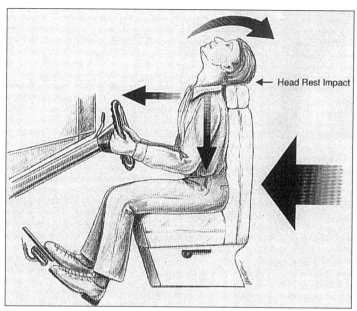

**FIGURE 6.**
The total duration of impact in rear-end motor vehicle accidents is 0.1–0.2 seconds.

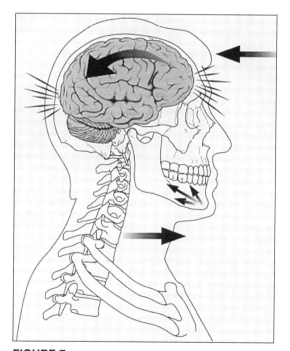

**FIGURE 7.**
Acceleration of various body parts occurs at different rates and at different moments during trauma. The result of this difference in momentum is the crushing and tearing of soft tissue at hard tissue junctions.

occur. If there is enough force, the mandible is moved along the vector line until it contacts another bony component (the skull). The transmitted force moves the skull along the same vector, which ultimately causes movement of the neck as well. Along the bony interfaces and interconnections lie various soft tissues that absorb the shock and are subjected to the type of forces already mentioned.

In an indirect injury to the TMJs from acceleration (whiplash) in a REMVA, the dynamics and chain of events change, but the results are similar. The automobile actually moves out from under the occupant. The first movement is the forward motion of the torso followed by movement of the neck—all within 0.1–0.2 seconds. There is a lag time of skull movement during this motion. Furthermore, the skull moves both translationally (for a brief period) and in an arch around the movement of the neck (rotational). Considering the components of the free body diagram (see Fig. 7), there is also a lag time of mandibular movement in comparison with the skull and cervical column. This movement is also translational and rotational by nature of the anatomy. This lag time calls on the muscles to absorb the involved forces while going from zero acceleration to movement. If the muscles did not absorb this movement, obviously the skull and mandible would fly off. The time is so short that there is often movement of the head, neck, and TMJs before the Golgi bodies have time to fire the muscle bundles for resistance, resulting in muscular damage on either a micro or macro level.[13,14] Once this absorption has been completed and the various body components are moving in relatively the same direction (but still at different vectors), the movement is interrupted when the neck and torso contact the seat and/or headrest. For a brief moment all rearward movement is stopped with multidirectional compressive forces on the "shock absorbers," which are the soft tissues. The whole process is begun again in reverse, with the skull leading the way, arching around the neck and mandible. Large compressive forces are produced on the supporting soft tissues as the body goes through the rebound stage of deceleration.

In some instances of direct trauma due to acceleration, the victim reports that his or her head hit nothing. In such cases, the following factors need to be taken into consideration.

1. There may be contact between the mandible, skull, and cervical spine. Only the soft tissue components stop bone from rubbing bone. The amount of forces involved is influenced greatly by the acceleration of the various body parts, both in unison and relatively with each other. $F = M \times A$, where F = force, M = mass, and A = acceleration.

2. The neck and skull may hit the headrest. Headrests often are not designed properly to stop cervical injuries.[9] The resulting forces in some instances may in fact be magnified. The deleterious effect (or lack thereof) of headrests is often underestimated.

3. The chin may hit the chest during the deceleration phase. Striking the chin on the chest reduces the forces on the cervical spine.[12] The law of conservation of energy dictates that the forces must go somewhere; stresses on the mandible and, therefore, the TMJs increase as a result.

Because of the shortness of the force duration, the shock, and disorientation of the occupants, the patient's account of this brief period is not always reliable.

The clinical symptoms of TMD due to indirect trauma (almost a misnomer) are similar to those of a direct blow. The only difference is the delay in onset of overt symptoms, which may occur for several reasons:

1. Acceleration-induced TMD, because of the nature of human anatomy and REMVAs, is commonly associated with cervical injuries.[19] Cervical injuries and the associated pain often take precedence over injuries to the TMJs. Cervical soft tissue injuries produce such similar symptoms that the two are often confused early in treatment.

2. There is a direct connection between the trigeminal nerves, which help to mediate noxious stimuli and motor movements of various structures of the TMJs, and the

occipital nerves originating in the cervical spine. Anatomic dissections indicate direct anastamosis of these two supposedly separate nervous components.[1,6] The result may be a change in function of the musculature of the masticatory system via the occipital nerves and the trigeminal system, leading to delayed-onset TMD without direct damage to the TMJs. A literature review by Talley et al. indicates a high correlation between cervical injuries and TMD/facial pain.[19]

3. Damage to the TMJs and their supporting structures may occur on a cellular level and may take time to cause systematic changes perceived by the patient as pain. Microdamage in the human body may lead to macrodamage, which in turn leads to dysfunction. This process may take months to occur.

4. Resulting injuries may create a repetitive strain syndrome (Fig. 8). By nature of the trauma, the occlusal surfaces of the teeth may be the only component of the masticatory system that has not been altered to some extent. As a result, the occlusion assumes the dominant role, causing a tug of war between edematous soft tissue aspects of the TM joints, dysfunctional muscles, damaged ligaments, and strained capsules. This syndrome may surface clinically as bruxism, exacerbating already compromised functional ability. The result is a syndrome not unlike the syndrome in other joints that break down first on a cellular level, leading to system breakdown as a result of repetitive strain.

5. Misdiagnosis is probably one of the leading causes of delay of treatment. People are often advised that the pain will go away. The efficacy of NSAIDs and muscle relaxers, although both are appropriate, often is not clinically verified in a given patient. Misunderstanding by the initial clinician of the signs and symptoms of TMD, which are often confusing, may delay proper treatment. The development of a good working relationship with dentists specifically trained in the diagnosis and treatment of TMD is extremely important in arriving at an accurate differential diagnosis.

## Psychogenic Origins

The exact role of emotional problems such as stress, anxiety, and depression in patients with TMD is uncertain. Diamond reports a phenomenon of "depression headache," which is a somatic characterization of depression. It has been suggested that almost any psychiatric disorder predisposes patients to tension-type headaches.[4] Too

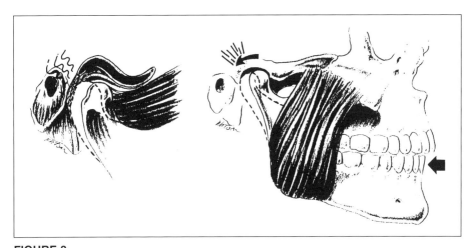

**FIGURE 8.**
Inflammation and swelling of the temporomandibular joints may result in a sudden "misfitting" of the biting surfaces (occlusion) of the upper and lower teeth, resulting in possible development of bruxism (tooth-grinding). Continuation over time may result in a painful repetitive strain syndrome.

often patients with clearly discernible signs of TMD have been diagnosed with somatization of emotional disorders, resulting in pain. The variability of pain complaints associated with frequent maladaptive behavioral and psychosocial sequelae often leads clinicians to diagnose TMD problems as purely psychogenic. Having a good working relationship with a skilled dentist can prove vital in achieving an accurate diagnosis from which to initiate treatment.

In many cases, chronic spasms of the masticatory and cervical muscles result in vague tension-type headaches. After months of pain, the patient's serotonin level is depleted, resulting in clinical depression. This is sometimes coupled with many visits to multiple doctors—all with no diagnosis, direction, or hope of recovery. Before a patient is relegated to the category of psychosomatic disorders, clinically demonstrable signs of TMD should be pursued by a dentist specifically trained in the diagnosis and management of TMD.

### Sleep Disturbances

Sleep deprivation often accompanies chronic pain. The patient's situation may become a "chicken-or-egg" dilemma. The interruption of stage IV (deep restorative) sleep is common in patients with chronic pain.[4] At times sleep disturbances are initiated by an acute episode such as trauma or surgery; when perpetuated, such disturbances result in chronic sleep deprivation.[4] One of the first lines of defense in treating TMD is to make sure that the patient is sleeping.

### TREATMENT OPTIONS

Traditionally TMD treatment is divided into two phases: phase I and phase II. Phase I includes all techniques designed for pain reduction and restoring the TMJs to a state of quiescence. Phase II corrects any discrepancies between mandibular position, teeth, and supporting structures. This is often considered the dental aspect of TMD treatment.

### Phase I

No one treatment mode, of course, helps to alleviate dysfunctional TMJs or the resulting pain. As in any problem, there are multiple ways to achieve clinical success.

As a rule of thumb, a conservative approach should be tried before advancing to more exotic methods. The best regimen is based on physical medicine. Physical modalities such as moist heat, ice massage, rest, and a soft food diet should be used as a first line of defense. A mild exercise regimen may augment healing and reduction of symptoms.

NSAIDs, muscle relaxers, and analgesics should be used as adjuncts for a limited period. Narcotics should be used with caution because of the potential for both physical and emotional attenuation. As in any chronic pain condition, tricyclic antidepressants have been found efficacious and may be used for blockage of serotonin uptake and as an adjunct for sleep.

If symptoms do not resolve rapidly, an intraoral orthotic designed to relax the musculature and reduce intercapsular inflammation should be used (Fig. 9). Pharmacologic support, as previously mentioned, may help in pain reduction.

Physical therapy modalities in conjunction with a guided rehabilitation program help to restore the patient to proper form and function. Other supportive care can be provided by speech pathologists, occupational therapists, dietitians, massage therapists, and biofeedback programs.

Surgical intervention is a final resort. Often arthrocentesis and/or arthroscopy is preferred over a full open-joint procedure. At times, because of severe degenerative joint disease, more complex surgeries or variations of joint reconstruction may be

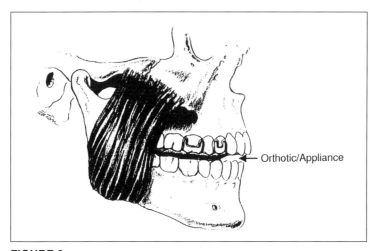

Orthotic/Appliance

**FIGURE 9.**
Appliances for treatment of temporomandibular dysfunction come in many shapes and sizes, depending on the patient's needs. Treatment goals often include decompression of swollen tissues within the temporomandibular joints, reduction of muscle spasms, orthopedic repositioning, and pain reduction.

needed. These, however, are needed rarely, and careful case selection is tantamount to ensuring success. Physical therapy rehabilitation is mandatory after any type of surgical intervention. The regimen must be carefully designed to restore the affected areas to proper physiologic function.

## Phase II

At times restoring the TMJs to proper form and function requires alterations in the dentition. Several methods can be used by themselves or in combination. These methods should not be used when the patient is in an active state of pain but rather as a finishing technique after the patient is quiescent. Most pain is a soft tissue phenomenon. Hard tissue landmarks, as indicated by radiographs, do not dictate a pain-free position for the patient. The following are common examples of phase II finishing techniques:

1. **Equilibration.** The enamel surfaces of the teeth are altered by the use of a dental handpiece to restore proper occlusal alignment with the TMJs and their supporting structures.

2. **Crown and bridge prosthetics.** Missing or broken teeth often need to be restored to provide maximal stomatognathic support during function. Various devices fall into this category, all of which aim for the same result. The required prosthesis is dictated by patient need and preference.

3. **Orthodontics.** This technique is most appropriate when patients have a gross discrepancy between the maxillary and mandibular position or the patient's teeth have had limited restorative work. Orthodontics can be quite effective when properly used and often help to correct growth disorders.

4. **Use of an appliance or orthotic on an as-needed basis.** In occasional cases, this is the most conservative and logical approach to a chronic problem—after all other physical means are exhausted. Too often, however, this technique is used when the dentist does not know how to ascertain a proper finishing technique and does not give patients other options. Long-term use of an orthotic can cause problems with the teeth and periodontium. There is also the chance of dental compensation, with the orthotic creating an acquired malocclusion.

5. **Orthognathic surgery.** This technique should be a last resort. By nature of the surgery, the clinician is using hard tissue landmarks to solve a soft tissue problem. In special cases these techniques are necessary, but such cases should be few and far between. Great care must be taken to guide the patient to as pain-free a state as possible before reconstructive surgery is attempted. Otherwise there is no target for which the surgeon can strive.

As a word of caution, too often the above techniques are used as front-line procedures for pain relief. One cannot look at radiographs, diagnostic casts of the teeth, or other hard tissue adjuncts and predict a pain-free stomatognathic position within the realm of human physiologic function. Such conclusions are often erroneous and indicate possible misunderstanding of the cause of pain. Not everyone needs perfect occlusion or aesthetically pleasing teeth to live a pain-free life. The object of TMD treatment should be resolution of the patient's pain, not restoration of the dentition to as perfect a position as possible. Many people in chronic pain have perfect occlusion, and many people with terrible occlusion and compromised stomatognathic function are pain-free. Corrective techniques are effective, however, when used properly and in the right sequence.

## The Two-Minute TMJ Examination

Screening for TMD does not have to be a long, drawn out affair. The following simple procedures will help to indicate whether there is a need for a dental consultation to rule out TMD as a contributing factor to the patient's pain complaints:
1. Maximal mouth opening
   a. Normal opening is approximately the width of three fingers without pain.
   b. Mandibular opening should be relatively straight without deviation.
2. Joint noise
   a. Popping, clicking, or grinding in one or both of the TMJs in the presence of facial pain, headaches, or neckaches is significant.
   b. Joint noise can be confirmed by patient report, manual palpation of the TMJs, or use of a stethoscope.
3. Pain on palpation of the masseter, temporalis, or intraoral muscles.
4. Otologic examination
   a. Excessive ear wax bilaterally or unilaterally in the absence of obvious pathology.
   b. Pain in the external auditory canals distal to the TMJs on insertion of the otoscope in the absence of obvious pathology.

## Multidisciplinary Pain Treatment

Just as TMD is often a manifestation of multiple precipitating factors, management requires cooperation among many health care professionals. A review of the signs and symptoms often associated with TMD brings to mind many clinical possibilities that may need to be examined to determine a proper diagnosis. No one profession can dominate the treatment of chronic pain. The artificial delineation of practice parameters, as dictated by licensure and custom, is artificial indeed when it comes to the management of pain.

The key to success in the management of chronic pain is to understand the limitations of one's own abilities and to appreciate the talents and skills of other professions. Although one profession may be the primary provider in any given situation, the various symptoms of patients with TMD probably will require team effort. Although such patients are often a challenge to treat, one of the benefits to practitioners is the opportunity to communicate with fellow professionals outside their chosen discipline. Discussion with others can produce exciting opportunities for learning and sharpening each other's diagnostic skills. Unfortunately, without these opportunities, various disciplines of the healing arts fail to communicate and misunderstand each other's abilities. The modern age of information availability and transfer is melding the once rigid walls between professions, resulting in a better, more rounded approach to management of patients with TMD and chronic pain.

## CONCLUSION

The track record of treating patients with TMD has not been good. Too many times patients wander from doctor to doctor without relief. Despite occasions when the patient's motivation is questionable, most patients simply want to get well and get on with their life. The frustration felt on the part of the practitioner who sincerely wants to help the patient often results in strained doctor–patient relationships. The key to success is knowing the symptoms associated with TMD and understanding the underlying causation. Looking outside one's profession and seeking assistance from other disciplines often leads to successful pain management.

Dentistry has come a long way since the days of "drill and fill." Opportunities abound for motivated dentists to acquire skills in the management of head and neck pain associated with TMD. Such skills are generally not taught at the undergraduate level but must be pursued in postdoctoral education. One of the most important lessons for the dentist to learn on the road to proper case management is appreciation of other professions and their role in successful treatment. Communication is the best learning tool.

The challenge of the modern managed care system with its fiscal responsibilities requires an even more concerted effort by the healing arts to form a multidisciplinary approach to pain management. Better communication among health care providers, along with development of third-party payer partnerships, will help to usher in a new era of cost-effective pain management that alleviates pain and restores hope of a better life to patients with TMD.

## REFERENCES

1. Baburr L: Occipital neuralgia alias C2–3 radiculopathy. J Neurol Orthoped Med Surg 10:133, 1989.
2. Bell W: Temporomandibular Disorders: Classification, Diagnosis, Management, 2nd ed. Chicago, Yearbook, 1982.
3. Bell W: Orofacial Pains—Classification, Diagnosis, Management. Chicago, Yearbook, 1985, pp 100–101.
4. Cady R, Fox A: Treating The Headache Patient. New York, Marcel Dekker, 1995.
5. Carroll C, et al: Objective findings for diagnosis of "whiplash." J Musculoskel Med 6:120–124, 1986.
6. Cox C, Cocks G: Occipital neuralgia. J Med Assoc State Ala Jan:25, 1979.
6a. Garcia R: TMJs evaluated in patients with cervical whiplash injury. News Journal of the American Academy of Head, Neck, Facial Pain 4(1):12–16, 1992.
7. Hursh W: Whiplash syndrome. Orthop Clin North Am Oct:791, 1988.
8. Hyde A: Crash Injuries: How and Why They Happen. Key Biscayne, Hyde Associates, 1992.
9. Insurance Institute for Highway Safety Status Report 30(8):6, 7, 1995.
10. McNab J: The Spine. Philadelphia, W.B. Saunders, 1982.
11. McNeill C, et al: Temporomandibular Disorders—Guidelines for Classification, Assessment, and Management. Chicago, Quintessence Books, 1993.
12. The Society of Automobile Engineers: Publication #670919.
13. The Society of Automobile Engineers: Publication #730975.
14. The Society of Automobile Engineers: Publication #751156.
15. The Society of Automobile Engineers: Publication #790135.
16. The Society of Automobile Engineers: Publication #930211.
17. The Society of Automobile Engineers: Publication #952724.
18. The Society of Automobile Engineers: Publication #960665.
19. Talley R, Ousley L: Cervical trauma as an etiology of TMD: Literature review. 1994 (self-published).

# 13

# Common Peripheral Nerve Injuries

FRANK J. E. FALCO, MD
FRANCIS P. LAGATTUTA, MD

Peripheral nerve injuries are commonly encountered in the evaluation of soft tissue injuries, especially in the context of overuse syndromes. Cumulative trauma in the workplace has led to an increased incidence of peripheral nerve injuries. These injuries have cost millions of dollars each year in treatment, lost wages, and lost work time. The importance of proper diagnosis and treatment cannot be overemphasized in the cost-conscious climate of health care. The practicing physician who can recognize these disorders and appropriately manage treatment is a valued asset to the health care system.

This chapter reviews the common peripheral nerve injuries involving the upper and lower extremities. The anatomy, pathophysiology, clinical presentation, diagnostic testing, and treatment options are covered for each nerve entrapment. Table 1 lists the common peripheral nerve injuries discussed in this chapter.

The peripheral nerve injuries discussed in this chapter in relationship to soft tissue injuries are otherwise known as entrapment neuropathies. Entrapment of the nerve occurs at vulnerable points along its course because of compromise within a fibrous or osseofibrous tunnel or constriction by a fibrous or muscular band. Other factors such as repetitive motion, space-occupying lesions, systemic disorders, body habitus, external pressures, and/or posturing usually contribute to the development of an entrapment neuropathy. The entrapment typically leads to focal nerve demyelination but may progress to loss of nerve axons.

## UPPER EXTREMITY NERVE INJURIES

### Suprascapular Nerve

The suprascapular nerve arises from the superior trunk of the brachial plexus with C5 and C6 nerve root fibers. The suprascapular nerve passes through the suprascapular notch before innervating the suprascapular muscle. A ligament running across the suprascapular notch produces a foramen through which the nerve passes. The nerve then courses around the spinoglenoid notch to reach and innervate the infraspinatus muscle (Fig. 1). A ligament sometimes spans from the scapular spine to the glenoid. The

243

**TABLE 1.**
Common Peripheral Nerve Injuries

| Upper extremity | Lower extremity |
|---|---|
| Axillary nerve | Lateral femoral cutaneous nerve |
| Suprascapular nerve | Femoral nerve |
| Median nerve | Femoral nerve syndrome |
|   Carpal tunnel syndrome |   Saphenous nerve syndrome |
|   Supracondylar syndrome | Obturator nerve |
|   Pronator teres syndrome | Peroneal nerve |
|   Anterior interosseous syndrome |   Cross-leg palsy |
| Ulnar nerve |   Superficial peroneal nerve entrapment |
|   Cubital tunnel syndrome | Tibial nerve |
|   Guyon's canal syndrome |   Tarsal tunnel syndrome |
| Radial nerve |   Joplin's neuroma |
|   Posterior interosseous syndrome |   Morton's neuroma |
|   Wartenberg syndrome | |

suprascapular nerve may be entrapped at either the suprascapular or spinoglenoid notch. Entrapment is frequently related to trauma but may occur spontaneously. Repetitive circling and overhead motions of the upper limb may cause trauma to the nerve. The nerve also may be stretched with shoulder adduction, as with the back swing in tennis or golf.

No pain is associated with this nerve entrapment syndrome. Weakness may be detected with resisted shoulder external rotation and abduction. Nerve conduction

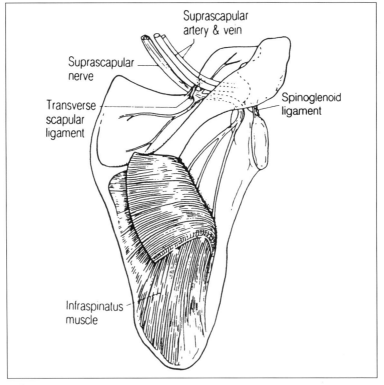

**FIGURE 1.**
Suprascapular nerve. (From Reid DC: Sports Injury Assessment and Rehabilitation. New York, Churchill Livingstone, 1992, with permission.)

slowing and denervation, as shown by needle electromyography (EMG), in the supra-spinatus and/or infraspinatus muscles with no involvement of the paraspinal or rhom-boid muscles is helpful in confirming the diagnosis.

Conservative treatment consists of rest, nonsteroidal antiinflammatory drugs (NSAIDs), local injection at the site of entrapment, and progressive rehabilitation with strengthening of the external rotators and abductors. Surgical decompression is consid-ered in patients with chronic symptoms that are unresponsive to conservative treatment. Functional electrical stimulation may clinically assist with treatment, although no liter-ature supports its effectiveness.

### Axillary Nerve

The axillary nerve arises from the posterior cord of the brachial plexus containing C5 and C6 nerve root fibers. The nerve travels through the quadrangular space formed by the scapulae, teres minor, teres major, long head of the triceps, and surgical neck of the humerus (Fig. 2). The nerve divides into anterior and posterior branches as it emerges from the quadrangular space. The posterior branch innervates the deltoid and teres minor muscles as well as provides sensation to the skin overlying the posterior deltoid. The anterior branch travels deep to the deltoid, supplying the anterior border of the deltoid and some cutaneous innervation in this region.

The axillary nerve is most frequently damaged as a result of anterior shoulder dis-location.[1] It also may be damaged by surgery. The axillary nerve may be involved with idiopathic brachial plexopathy or neuritis. Weakness of shoulder abduction may be pre-sent on examination with decreased sensation in a well-circumscribed cutaneous area overlying the lateral portion of the deltoid. Nerve conduction studies and needle EMG help to establish the diagnosis and to rule out other possible causes. Treatment consists of rest, NSAIDs, and modified activity. Prognosis is good in patients with partial as opposed to complete nerve involvement. Recovery typically takes 6–12 months with conservative treatment. Surgical decompression may be necessary if there is no im-provement with nonoperative care.

### Median Nerve

The median nerve is formed by contributions from the medial and lateral cord of the brachial plexus and contains contributions from the C5 through T1 nerve roots. The

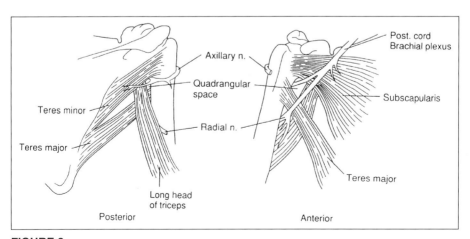

**FIGURE 2.**
Quadrangular space. (From Reid DC: Sports Injury Assessment and Rehabilitation. New York, Churchill Livingstone, 1992, with permission.)

median nerve then travels within the upper arm, where it is rarely disturbed without associated trauma. Entrapments of the median nerve typically occur within the region of the elbow, forearm, and wrist. Median nerve compression at the wrist (carpal tunnel syndrome) is the most common peripheral nerve entrapment. This disorder is discussed along with other median nerve entrapments, such as the supracondylar, pronator teres, and anterior interosseous syndromes.

### Carpal Tunnel Syndrome

Carpal tunnel syndrome (CTS), first described in 1854 by Paget, is the most common peripheral nerve entrapment.[12] CTS, also known as median thenar neuritis and partial thenar atrophy, is the result of median nerve compression by the transverse carpal ligament. The carpal tunnel is formed by the carpal bones and the transverse carpal ligament that extends across them. The median nerve passes through the tunnel along with the flexor digitorum superficialis, flexor digitorum profundus, flexor pollicis longus, and flexor carpi radialis tendons (Fig. 3).

CTS in industry has been related to forceful and repetitive activities.[9,14] The repetitive nature of work activities appears to be a greater risk factor than force for CTS.[14] The pressure within the tunnel has been shown to increase substantially with positions of flexion or extension.[3] The lowest tunnel pressure is produced in the neutral posture.[3] Increases in tunnel pressure during repetitive activity are believed to be the mechanism that leads to nontraumatic median nerve pathology.[16]

Certain disorders that may lead to carpal tunnel syndrome through compromise of the carpal tunnel space are not related to the work environment. Examples include pregnancy, gout, hypothyroidism, ganglion cysts, rheumatoid arthritis, myxedema, and amyloidosis.

Several factors increase the risk for developing CTS, which is 3–4 times more common in women than in men.[7,13] Johnson et al. demonstrated that a square wrist leads to a higher incidence of CTS;[6] the risk for developing CTS increased as the ratio of wrist thickness to wrist width reached a value of 0.7%. Other risk factors include a family history of CTS, increasing age, and occurrence within the dominant hand.

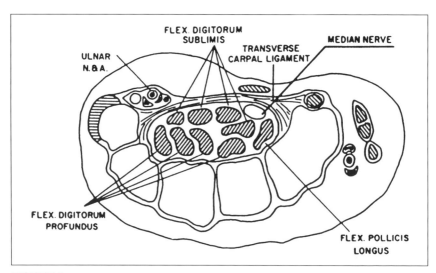

**FIGURE 3.**
Carpal tunnel. (From Primer on the Rheumatic Diseases, 9th ed. Atlanta, Arthritis Foundation, 1988, with permission.)

Certain disease processes, such as Guillain-Barré syndrome and diabetes mellitus, predispose to the development of CTS.

A patient with CTS typically complains of hand weakness or clumsiness with pain, tingling, and hypesthesia in the distribution of the median nerve. Symptoms are often bilateral and usually most pronounced in the dominant hand. Pain associated with CTS may extend proximally to the elbow and at times to the shoulder. Patients commonly describe pain that awakens them from sleep at night and is relieved with shaking the hands.

Physical examination typically reveals decreased sensation within the distribution of the median nerve to the radial three and one-half digits. The palmar aspect of the thenar eminence is spared because the palmar sensory division of the median nerve branches proximal to the tunnel. Thumb weakness and decreased two-point discrimination with flexion, abduction, and opposition movements may develop as CTS progresses. Thenar wasting typically develops in advanced cases.

Provocative testing has been used clinically to determine the presence of CTS. Tinel's sign involves gentle tapping of the median nerve at the wrist and is considered positive if symptoms are produced in the distribution of the median nerve. Phalen's test is performed by maintaining the wrist in a flexed position for 1 minute and is considered positive if numbness or paresthesias are generated in the median nerve distribution. Phalen's test has been shown to be more sensitive and specific in the evaluation of CTS than Tinel's sign.[8] Another provocative test is external wrist compression. Changes in vibration and light touch testing from wrist compression have been shown to correlate well with subjective complaints and electrodiagnostic testing.[4]

CTS is essentially diagnosed on the basis of clinical evaluation. Certain disorders that lead to CTS can be ruled out with laboratory testing and radiographs. Electrodiagnostic testing is the gold standard for the work-up in patients suspected of having CTS. In some instances, electrodiagnostic tests are normal in patients with clinical findings of CTS. In such cases, the diagnosis can be confirmed if symptoms resolve after the median nerve is anesthetized with injection of an anesthetic into the carpal tunnel.

Conservative treatment of CTS includes the use of NSAIDs, splinting, carpal tunnel injections, light duty, and sometimes complete rest. Myofascial release and tendon stretching are other treatments. Any one of these measures alone or in combination can be effective in treating early CTS. In the workplace, modification of the job site or complete ergonomic redesign is typically the most helpful approach. Failure to respond to conservative treatment or surgical intervention is often due to lack of modification in the workplace. At times, a new job assignment with less hand-intensive activities is required for return to work.

Surgery is indicated in cases of advanced CTS with objective sensory loss and/or weakness or atrophy of the abductor pollicis brevis. Postsurgical recovery time may last 6–12 weeks depending on preoperative status and extent of nerve damage. In the workplace surgery may be indicated for the patient who has failed conservative treatment, including reassignment to a job that is not hand-intensive. After surgery, the patient returns to light duty, with restrictions on hand-intensive activity, during recovery. More research is necessary before determining whether arthroscopic surgery is more effective than traditional surgical release. The employee may have difficulty in returning to the original job despite surgical intervention; they may have to return to a job with restricted hand activity. Some employees may never return to work because of continued symptoms, lack of desire, other undiagnosed disorders, or surgical complications.

## Supracondylar Syndrome

The supracondylar syndrome is a compression neuropathy of the median nerve that occurs as the nerve passes along the distal humerus just proximal to the medial epicondyle. The ligament of Struthers is found in 0.7–2.7% of individuals, extending

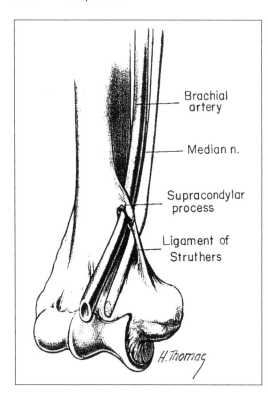

**FIGURE 4.**
Ligament of Struthers. (From Liveson JA: Peripheral Neurology: Case Studies in Electrodiagnosis, 2nd ed. Philadelphia, F.A. Davis, 1991, with permission.)

Labels in figure:
Brachial artery
Median n.
Supracondylar process
Ligament of Struthers
H.Thomas

from an anteromedial bony spur on the distal humerus to the medial epicondyle.[15] The median nerve, brachial artery, and brachial vein pass inferior to the ligament (Fig. 4). Most individuals with the supracondylar process are asymptomatic; only some individuals with the ligament of Struthers develop the supracondylar syndrome.

Patients with the supracondylar syndrome complain of localized pain above the elbow, forearm weakness, and hand numbness. Physical examination typically reveals tenderness over a palpable supracondylar spur. Neurologic findings from median nerve compromise may affect both motor and sensory nerves. Sensory deficits involve the three and one-half radial digits as well as the thenar eminence. Sensory loss in the thenar eminence is important in distinguishing a proximal entrapment of the median nerve from a distal entrapment such as carpal tunnel syndrome. Motor deficits manifest as wrist flexion and thumb weakness. Weakness with wrist flexion typifies a more proximal median nerve injury to at least the elbow level. Vascular compromise of the brachial artery may present as claudication with extension of the elbow and supination of the forearm. This same posture also may lead to a loss of the ulnar or radial pulse.

Diagnostic testing includes radiographs to identify the presence of a bony spur. Electrodiagnostic testing may reveal entrapment at the ligament of Struthers with stimulation above and below the ligament. Conservative treatment, including NSAIDs, typically is not helpful in symptomatic patients. Surgical resection of the ligament and supracondylar spur is usually indicated in the treatment of symptomatic patients.

### Pronator Teres Syndrome

Pronator teres syndrome involves entrapment of the median nerve at one of the three sites. The nerve may be entrapped by a fibrous band known as the lacertus fibrosus;

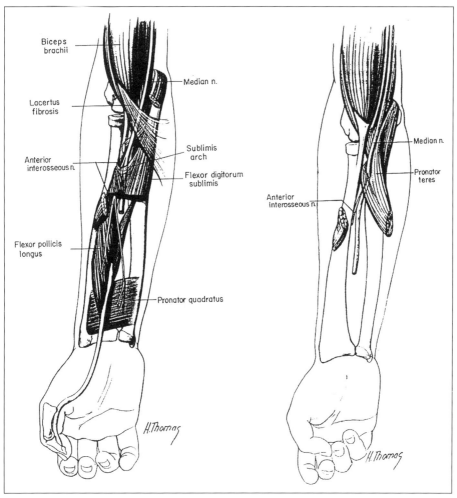

**FIGURE 5.**
Median nerve entrapment in pronator teres syndrome. (From Liveson JA: Peripheral Neurology: Case Studies in Electrodiagnosis, 2nd ed. Philadelphia, F.A. Davis, 1991, with permission.)

between the superficial and deep heads of the pronator teres; or at the arch of the flexor digitorum superficialis (Fig. 5). Compression of the median nerve at any of those locations leads to the same clinical findings.

Pronator teres syndrome is common in elderly people. The chief complaint on presentation is often pain localized to the proximal forearm region. Patients also complain of tingling and numbness involving the fingers and palm. Weakness is a less frequent complaint.

Examination often reveals tenderness with palpation of the proximal forearm. Percussion of the median nerve within the proximal forearm may produce a positive Tinel's sign. Provocative maneuvers that reproduce the pain include resisted forearm pronation with the elbow in extension and resisted finger flexion at the proximal interphalangeal joint, especially with the middle finger.

Radiographs of the humerus rule out the presence of a bone spur. Although electrodiagnostic studies may be performed to rule out other conditions such as carpal tunnel or anterior interosseous syndrome, they are not helpful in making the specific diagnosis of pronator teres syndrome.

Conservative treatment includes NSAIDs, rest, splinting, restricted job duties, and physical or occupational therapy. If there is no improvement with such treatment, surgical decompression of the nerve from the lacertus fibrosus to the pronator teres may be considered.

### Anterior Interosseous Syndrome

The median nerve divides into the main and anterior interosseous branches after it passes under the pronator teres distal to the lateral epicondyle. The main branch of the median nerve innervates the hand distally, whereas the anterior interosseous nerve innervates some of the ventral forearm musculature. The flexor pollicis longus, radial two heads of the flexor digitorum profundus, and pronator quadratus muscles are innervated by the anterior interosseous nerve. In addition to innervating these muscles, the anterior interosseous nerve provides pain fibers to the wrist.

Entrapment of the anterior interosseous nerve results from the tendinous origin of either the deep head of the pronator teres or the flexor digitorum superficialis. This condition is more common in young, muscular individuals. Pain complaints typically involve the proximal forearm and are accompanied by complaints of hand weakness, clumsiness, and loss of dexterity. Wrist pain also may be a presenting feature of anterior interosseous syndrome.

Physical examination reveals localized tenderness with palpation of the proximal forearm. A positive Tinel's sign may be present at the entrapment site. Weakness of the pronator quadratus, flexor pollicis longus, and flexor digitorum profundus can be detected clinically. Patients may have difficulty in making an "O" with the index and thumb because of weakness at the distal interphalangeal and interphalangeal joints, respectively, from involvement of the flexor pollicis longus and flexor digitorum profundus muscles (Fig. 6). Sensory abnormalities on examination are rare in this syndrome which is classically characterized by its motor effects.

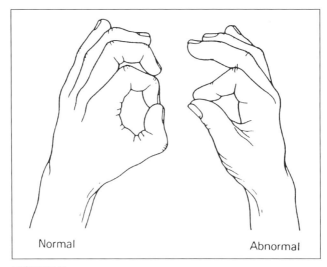

Normal                                                    Abnormal

**FIGURE 6.**
Motor deficit testing in anterior interosseous syndrome. (From Reid DC: Sports Injury Assessment and Rehabilitation. New York, Churchill Livingstone, 1992, with permission.)

Electrodiagnostic studies, which are helpful to confirm the diagnosis of anterior interosseous syndrome as well as to rule out carpal tunnel syndrome, are the only truly applicable diagnostic tool. Radiographs may be used to rule out a supracondylar spur. Treatment consists of conservative intervention such as NSAIDs, splinting, rest, or therapy. Spontaneous resolution may occur with conservative treatment. Surgical decompression of the nerve is usually indicated if there is no improvement within 3 months.

## Ulnar Nerve

The ulnar nerve is the last division off the medial cord and contains C8 and T1 nerve root fibers. It descends into the arm, entering the posterior compartment after passing through the intermuscular septum halfway down the arm. The ulnar nerve then travels posterior to the medial epicondyle between the two heads of the flexor carpi ulnaris. It innervates this muscle as well as the ulnar two heads of the flexor digitorum profundus muscle. The nerve then enters into the hand through Guyon's canal, where it divides into sensory and motor branches. The sensory branch provides sensation to the little finger and ulnar half of the ring finger. The motor branch innervates the hypothenar muscles, the two ulnar lumbricals, interossei, adductor pollicis, and deep head of the flexor pollicis brevis. The ulnar palmar and dorsal cutaneous branches travel outside Guyon's canal, arising from the ulnar nerve proximal to the wrist.

### Cubital Tunnel Syndrome

Entrapment of the ulnar nerve at the elbow is the second most common peripheral nerve entrapment of the upper extremity (Fig. 7). This entrapment, also known as cubital tunnel syndrome, is commonly encountered with overuse activities in the workplace and in patients who have suffered fractures or soft tissue injuries to the elbow region. Heavy lifting, prolonged flexion, and repetitive lifting are predisposing factors in the workplace. The cubital canal narrows with flexion, which may cause nerve compression, especially with prolonged flexion activities.

Patients with cubital tunnel syndrome present with different ulnar nerve-related complaints from hand weakness and numbness to pain along the medial elbow joint. Numbness or paresthesia occurs in the distribution of the ulnar nerve; both are exacerbated by repetitive or prolonged elbow flexion and relieved with extension. Symptoms also may result from constant pressure to the nerve as a result of leaning on the elbows. This mechanism of ulnar nerve injury is seen in patients with chronic obstructive pulmonary disease, who lean on the elbows to assist breathing. Patients may not notice hand weakness unless they are asked to perform a specific task involving grip or pinching activities.

Palpatory evaluation may reveal tenderness along the course of the ulnar nerve at the elbow. Tinel's sign may be noted with gentle percussion of the ulnar nerve over the groove of the medial epicondyle. Sensory deficits that involve the palmar and dorsal aspects of the hand as well as the ulnar one and one-half digits are consistent with cubital tunnel syndrome. If palmar and dorsal sensation from the ulnar nerve is intact, entrapment is more likely at the wrist (i.e., Guyon's canal) than at the elbow. The flexor carpi ulnaris may or may not be spared, depending on whether the entrapment occurs within the canal. Entrapments distal in the tunnel spare the branch to the flexor carpi ulnaris and do not result in wrist flexion weakness. Testing isolated distal phalangeal flexion of the little and ring fingers against resistance assesses for weakness of the ulnar-innervated portion of the flexor digitorum profundus. Interossei weakness may be evaluated by testing finger abduction and adduction.

Chronic or severe cubital tunnel syndrome leads to wasting of the interossei and hypothenar muscles, which is easily visible because of the prominence of the metacarpals. Atrophy of the lumbricals and flexor digitorum profundus may lead to clawing

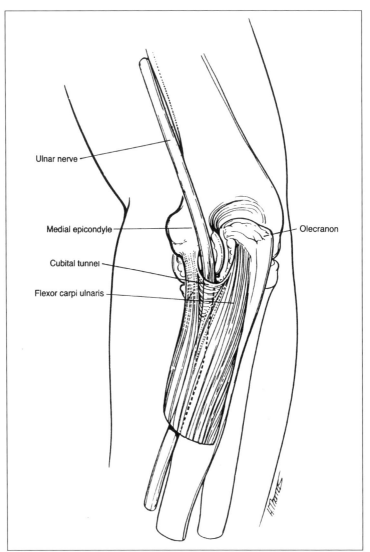

**FIGURE 7.**
Cubital tunnel. (From Liveson JA: Peripheral Neurology: Case Studies in
Electrodiagnosis, 2nd ed. Philadelphia, F.A. Davis, 1991, with permission.)

contractures of the little and ring fingers. Loss of pinch is the result of interossei and
adductor pollicis weakness. Patients cannot pinch the index finger and thumb together
without flexing the thumb at the interphalangeal joint. Unintended flexion of the interphalangeal joint of the thumb while attempting to pinch against the index finger is considered a positive Froment's sign and is due to the paralysis of the adductor pollicis
muscle.

Electrodiagnostic studies are helpful in the evaluation for cubital tunnel syndrome
in addition to the physical examination findings. Nerve conduction studies are performed proximal and distal to the elbow to assess for ulnar nerve entrapment within the
cubital tunnel. Inching techniques help to localize the entrapment more specifically.

Needle EMG evaluates motor involvement of ulnar-innervated forearm and hand muscles. Electrodiagnostic tests rule out other possible causes, such as radiculopathy, peripheral neuropathy, carpal tunnel syndrome, and Guyon's canal syndrome.

Conservative treatment for cubital tunnel syndrome includes relative rest, NSAIDs, work activity modification, splinting, and elbow pads. Surgery is indicated in patients with significant pain and/or weakness.

### Guyon's Canal Syndrome

The floor and walls of Guyon's canal are shaped by the pisiform and hamate carpals. The transverse and volar carpal ligaments that extend from the pisiform to the hook of the hamate form the roof of the canal. The ulnar nerve divides into two branches within the canal (Fig. 8). The superficial sensory branch provides sensation to the ulnar one and one-half digits. The deep motor branch innervates the hypothenar muscles, interossei, ulnar two lumbricals, adductor pollicis, and deep head of the flexor pollicis brevis. Motor branches to the hypothenar muscles arise proximally within the canal. The deep branch then continues as the deep palmar branch as it passes around the hook of the hamate, innervating the other distal muscles.

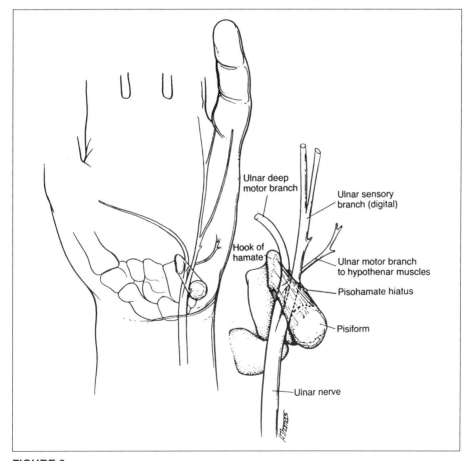

**FIGURE 8.**
Guyon's canal. (From Liveson JA: Peripheral Neurology: Case Studies in Electrodiagnosis, 2nd ed. Philadelphia, F.A. Davis, 1991, with permission.)

The most common cause for compression is repetitive trauma to the ulnar nerve at the base of the hypothenar eminence. Trauma may occur in the workplace with the holding and operation of power tools or during recreational activities such as bicycle riding. Other possible causes include ganglion cysts, fracture, abnormal muscle or fibrous bands, lipoma, ulnar artery disease, osteoarthritis, and pisiform bursitis.

Entrapment of the ulnar nerve within Guyon's canal may lead to numbness of the ulnar one and one-half digits, hypothenar weakness, and/or weakness of the other ulnar-innervated intrinsic hand muscles. The most common form of ulnar nerve compression at the wrist involves the deep palmar branch and produces intrinsic hand weakness with intact and normal sensation. The hypothenar muscles are unaffected in this setting because the entrapment occurs distal to the hook of the hamate, sparing the motor branch to these muscles. Ulnar nerve compression, on the other hand, may lead to numbness and weakness when both sensory and motor fibers are involved. Physical findings on examination depend on which fibers are involved by the entrapment.

The diagnosis is typically made from the history and physical examination. Electrodiagnostic testing helps to confirm ulnar entrapment at the wrist and to rule out other conditions such as peripheral neuropathy and cubital tunnel or carpal tunnel syndrome. Evaluation of the ulnar dorsal cutaneous nerve is helpful, because this nerve branches proximal to the wrist and therefore is spared in cases of ulnar nerve entrapment within Guyon's canal.

Conservative treatment is aimed at diminishing trauma to the ulnar nerve at the base of the hand. This goal can be accomplished by activity restriction and splinting or palmar padding in combination with NSAIDs. Surgical exploration of the canal is indicated in patients who show no improvement within several months.

## Radial Nerve

The radial nerve is an extension of the distal aspect of the posterior cord from the brachial plexus and contains C5 through C8 nerve root fibers. It provides innervation to the dorsal muscles of the arm and forearm as well as sensation to the same regions and parts of the hand. The radial nerve is least often involved in nerve entrapments of the upper extremity. It is vulnerable to traumatic injury as it courses through the spinal groove in the arm and is involved in 10–15% of humeral fractures.[11] Compression of the radial nerve may occur in the axilla, as with the use of crutches, or in the distal arm at the intermuscular septum from any type of prolonged pressure.

### Posterior Interosseous Syndrome

The radial nerve divides into sensory (superficial radial nerve) and motor (posterior interosseous nerve) branches at the level of the elbow. The posterior interosseous nerve innervates all of the muscles distal to the extensor carpi radialis longus. The extensor carpi radialis brevis and supinator are innervated by the posterior interosseous nerve before it enters the arcade of Frohse. The nerve then passes between the arcade of Froshe and the two heads of the supinator muscle as it innervates the rest of the posterior forearm muscles. Nerve compression typically occurs at the arcade of Frohse, and injury is usually the result of chronic repetitive wrist extension activities (Fig. 9).

The patient with posterior interosseous nerve syndrome complains of wrist extension weakness and inability to extend the fingers completely. Forearm pain may initially last for several days. Pain localized to the lateral elbow may occur alone or in conjunction with weakness. Physical examination may reveal decreased strength with resisted wrist extension and finger extension at the metacarpophalangeal joints. A palpable mass such as a ganglion cyst or vascular anomaly is sometimes appreciated on physical examination.

Electrodiagnostic studies sometimes reveal slowing across the arcade of Frohse and may demonstrate denervation potentials in muscles distal to the supinator.

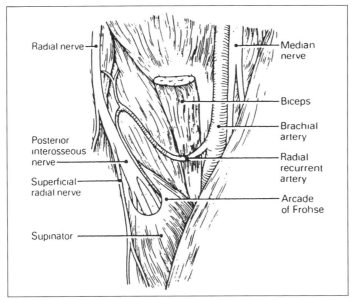

**FIGURE 9.**
Arcade of Frohse. (From Reid DC: Sports Injury Assessment and
Rehabilitation. New York, Churchill Livingstone, 1992, with permission.)

Electrodiagnostic tests are normal in cases of lateral epicondylitis and other musculoskeletal causes of lateral elbow and forearm pain.

Posterior interosseous nerve syndrome secondary to repetitive trauma often responds successfully to conservative treatment. Rest, splinting the elbow in 90° of flexion, and NSAIDs often lead to resolution of symptoms. Surgical decompression of the nerve is considered when conservative treatment fails after a trial of 2–3 months.

Posterior interosseous nerve syndrome should be considered in persistent lateral elbow pain that does not respond to typical treatment for lateral epicondylitis or other musculoskeletal conditions. Surgical decompression has been successful in alleviating lateral elbow pain due to posterior interosseous nerve syndrome.

### Wartenberg Syndrome

Compression of the superficial radial nerve in the distal forearm is known as cheiralgia paresthetica or Wartenberg syndrome. Symptoms typically include pain, numbness, and tingling in the first web space. Examination may reveal a positive Tinel's sign at the entrapment site and a false-positive Finkelstein's test. This neuropathy can result from tight watch bands, handcuffs, or casts.[5] Electrodiagnostic evaluation of the superficial radial nerve at the wrist helps to differentiate nerve injury from de Quervain's tenosynovitis. Treatment centers largely on removing the constricting object, splinting with the wrist in slight radial deviation, and NSAIDs. Surgical release may be indicated if there is no improvement with conservative treatment.

## LOWER EXTREMITY NERVE INJURIES

### Lateral Femoral Cutaneous Nerve

Entrapment of the lateral femoral cutaneous nerve is known as meralgia paresthetica. The nerve is formed by the L2 and L3 nerve roots and enters the anterior thigh

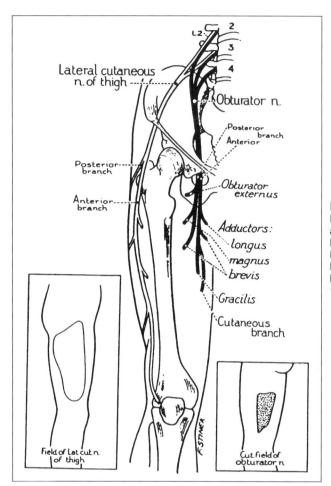

**FIGURE 10.**
Lateral femoral cutaneous and obturator nerves. (From Haymaker W, Woodhall B: Peripheral Nerve Injuries: Principles of Diagnosis. Philadelphia, W.B. Saunders, 1953, with permission.)

underneath the inguinal ligament just inferior to the anterior superior iliac spine (Fig. 10). Intrapelvic compression may result from pregnancy, obesity, abdominal tumors, uterine fibroids, and diverticulosis. Extrapelvic compression may be secondary to tight garments, belts, girdles, and trauma to the anterior superior iliac spine.

Patients with meralgia paresthetica present with complaints of burning, numbness, or tingling in the distal half of the anterolateral thigh. Symptoms may be relieved with sitting and increased with standing or hip extension. Examination reveals numbness in the anterolateral thigh. Tinel's sign may be present at the inguinal ligament. Nerve conduction studies, which are often difficult to perform in obese patients, may reveal slowing or loss in amplitude with proximal stimulation.

Conservative treatment consists of rest, NSAIDs, restriction of hip extension, and local injection. Rarely is surgical decompression performed for persistent disability.

### Femoral Nerve

The femoral nerve is composed of the L2–L4 nerve roots and innervates the sartorius, quadriceps, and pectineus muscles. The nerve provides sensation to the anterior thigh by way of the anterior femoral cutaneous nerve. The femoral nerve continues distally as the saphenous nerve, which provides sensation to the medial leg and medial foot.

## Femoral Nerve Syndrome

Although diabetic amyotrophy is the most common cause of femoral nerve neuropathy, compression may result from intrapelvic or extrapelvic causes. The majority of femoral nerve entrapments occur below the inguinal ligament. Intrapelvic compression may result from hematoma, tumor, hip osteoarthritis, hip fracture, hip arthroplasty, or surgery. Extrapelvic causes include compression from hematoma, femoral lymphadenopathy, and sustained lithotomy position.

Clinically patients present with pain in the inguinal region and dysesthesias over the anterior thigh and anterior medial leg that are exacerbated with hip extension. Symptoms are relieved with hip flexion and external rotation. Examination may reveal hip flexion weakness, knee extension weakness, decreased patellar reflex, and sensory deficits of the anterior thigh and anterior medial leg. Nerve conduction studies may reveal slowing across the inguinal ligament. Needle EMG may show denervation in the sartorius and one or more heads of the quadriceps with normal assessment of the adductor muscles.

Treatment usually consists of rest, NSAIDs, restriction of hip extension, and local injection. Surgical decompression is considered in patients with persistent complaints.

## Saphenous Nerve Syndrome

The saphenous nerve arises from the femoral nerve and travels along the medial aspect of the thigh beneath the sartorius muscle. The nerve then passes through Hunter's canal, which is formed by a connective tissue roof extending from the vastus medialis to the adductor longus, before entering the medial leg (Fig. 11). Entrapment usually occurs at the sartorius muscle or within Hunter's canal.

The most common complaint of saphenous nerve entrapment is burning pain of the medial knee and medial leg with prolonged standing and walking. The pain may occur at night and may be aggravated with knee extension. Tenderness over the distal end of Hunter's canal is present with palpation. Conservative care consists of rest, NSAIDs, restriction of knee extension, and local injection. Surgical decompression is considered in patients with chronic symptoms unresponsive to nonoperative care.

## Obturator Nerve

The obturator nerve originates from the anterior division of the lumbar plexus and contains contributions from the L2–L4 nerve roots. The obturator nerve supplies innervation to the three adductor muscles as well as the obturator externus and gracilis muscles (see Fig. 10). The nerve also provides sensation to the medial aspect of the knee and thigh. Obturator nerve entrapments, which commonly occur within the obturator canal, may develop from high retroperitoneal hemorrhage, tumor, or obturator muscle herniation. Injuries to the obturator nerve also may result from direct trauma or complications from surgery.

The patient with obturator nerve syndrome presents with pain in the groin, medial thigh, and knee as well as adductor muscle spasm. Patients also may report numbness and paresthesias along the medial aspect of the thigh and knee, which are increased with hip adduction and external rotation. Muscle testing reveals weakness of the adductor muscle group. Needle EMG may reveal denervation of the gracilis and adductor muscles with sparing of the quadriceps (which rules out a nerve root lesion).

Conservative treatment consists of rest, NSAIDs, and restriction of hip abduction and hip external rotation. Surgical decompression is sometimes necessary to alleviate symptoms fully.

## Peroneal Nerve

The common peroneal nerve receives contributions from the L4–S1 root fibers, with the main contribution coming from the L5 nerve root. The common peroneal and

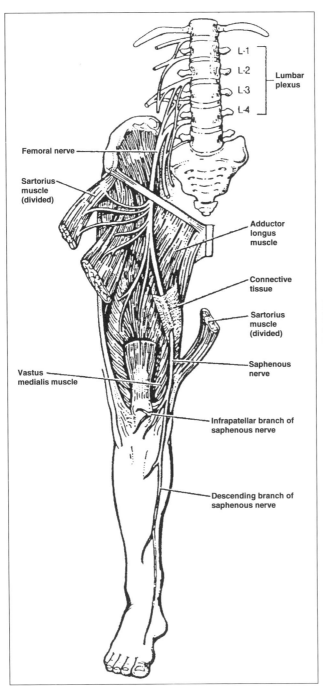

L-1
L-2
L-3
L-4

Lumbar plexus

Femoral nerve

Sartorius muscle (divided)

Adductor longus muscle

Connective tissue

Sartorius muscle (divided)

Vastus medialis muscle

Saphenous nerve

Infrapatellar branch of saphenous nerve

Descending branch of saphenous nerve

**FIGURE 11.**
Lateral femoral cutaneous and obturator nerves. (From Haymaker W, Woodhall B: Peripheral Nerve Injuries: Principles of Diagnosis. Philadelphia, W.B. Saunders, 1953, with permission.)

tibial nerves travel together as lateral and medial divisions, respectively, of the sciatic nerve. A motor branch from the peroneal division of the sciatic nerve supplies the short head of the biceps femoris muscle. The peroneal division then separates from the tibial division of the sciatic nerve in the popliteal fossa and continues as the common peroneal

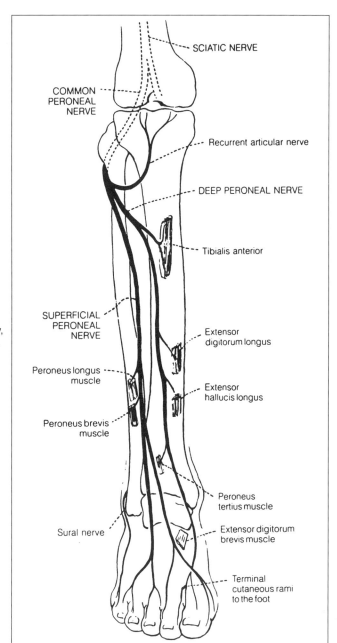

**FIGURE 12.**
Peroneal nerve. (From
deGroot J, Chusid JG:
Correlative Neuroanatomy,
2nd ed. East Norwalk, CT,
Appleton & Lange, 1988,
with permission.)

nerve. After wrapping around the fibular head, the common peroneal nerve divides into the superficial and deep peroneal nerves (Fig. 12).

The deep peroneal nerve innervates the anterior tibialis, extensor digitorum longus, extensor hallucis longus, and extensor digitorum brevis muscles. The deep peroneal nerve also provides cutaneous sensation to the web space between the first and second toes. The superficial peroneal nerve branches from the common peroneal nerve at the fibular head, passing between the fibula and peroneus muscles. The superficial peroneal nerve innervates the peroneus longus and brevis muscles. The nerve continues as a sensory nerve, dividing into the intermediate and medial dorsal cutaneous branches. These nerves provide cutaneous innervation to the distal anterolateral leg and dorsum of the foot except for the great and second toes, which are supplied by the deep peroneal nerve.

### Cross-Leg Palsy

Peroneal nerve entrapments occur most commonly at the fibular head as the nerve travels near the lateral side of the knee. The most common mechanism of injury is acute compression, traction, or laceration at the fibular head, causing a neuropraxic lesion. Also known as yoga footdrop and strawberry picker's palsy, this entrapment frequently occurs with crossed legs, bed positioning, squatting, casting, and tight boots. Predisposing factors include dieting and peripheral neuropathy. The nerve also may be entrapped as it passes through a fibroosseous tunnel between the fibular and peroneus longus muscle. Damage occasionally results from nerve infarction or tumor.

A patient with peroneal nerve entrapment complains of numbness involving the dorsal aspect of the foot. Weakness of the ankle may present as a footdrop, making it difficult to walk and climb stairs. Unopposed inversion at the foot and ankle due to weak evertors may lead to an unstable ankle, clumsy ambulation, and ankle sprains. Physical examination confirms weakness of the ankle dorsiflexors and foot evertors. Sensation is decreased along the anterolateral leg and dorsum of the foot. Tinel's sign may be present with gentle tapping at the fibular head. Nerve conduction studies may reveal slowing across the entrapment site and fibular head, and needle EMG may show denervation in muscles innervated by the superficial and/or deep peroneal nerves.

The mainstay of conservative treatment consists of NSAIDs, local injections, corrective shoes to maintain an eversion posture, and an ankle-foot orthosis for foot drop. Surgical release of the peroneal nerve may be indicated if there is no improvement with conservative care.

### Superficial Peroneal Nerve Syndrome

The superficial peroneal nerve is commonly involved in lesions of the common peroneal nerve. This nerve also may be entrapped distal to the fibular head as it exits through the fascia to become superficial or at the dorsal lateral aspect of the ankle and foot. Injuries to the superficial peroneal nerve may be secondary to forced plantarflexion or eversion.

Clinical presentation may consist of foot evertor weakness with burning dysesthesias, analgesia, and hypesthesia over the distal anterolateral leg, dorsal foot, and toes. Nerve conduction studies may reveal slowing and small action potential amplitudes. Needle EMG may reveal denervation of the peroneal brevis and longus muscles. Treatment is similar to that for common peroneal nerve entrapments.

### Posterior Tibial Nerve

The posterior tibial nerve is a continuation of the tibial division of the sciatic nerve and contains fibers from the L4–S2 nerve roots. The nerve branches off the sciatic nerve in the popliteal fossa, passing between the two heads of the gastrocnemius muscle. The gastrocnemius, soleus, plantaris, posterior tibialis, flexor digitorum longus, and flexor hallucis longus muscles, which make up the posterior leg compartment, are innervated by the posterior tibial nerve. The nerve then passes through the tarsal tunnel at the level of the ankle along with the posterior tibial vessels and tendons of the posterior tibialis, flexor digitorum longus, and flexor hallucis longus muscles (Fig. 13). The nerve then divides into the medial plantar, lateral plantar, and calcaneal nerves within the tarsal tunnel.

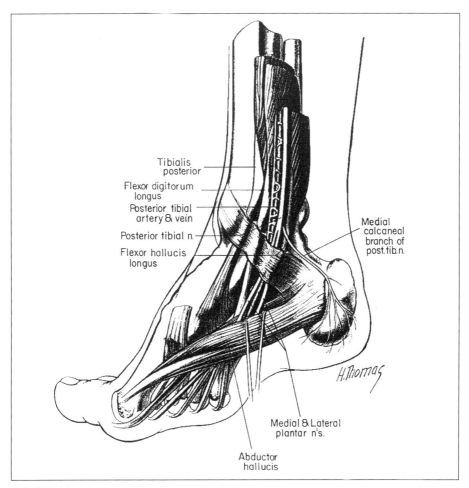

**FIGURE 13.**
Tarsal tunnel. (From Liveson JA: Peripheral Neurology: Case Studies in Electrodiagnosis, 2nd ed. Philadelphia, F.A. Davis, 1991, with permission.)

### Tarsal Tunnel Syndrome

Tarsal tunnel syndrome (TTS) is the most common posterior tibial nerve entrapment and occurs within the tarsal tunnel. This syndrome is relatively rare in comparison with carpal and cubital tunnel syndromes. Trauma, such as fracture or sprained ankle, accounts for one-third of TTS. Other potential causes include tenosynovitis, ganglion cyst, or posterior tibial vein engorgement. The medial plantar nerve is the most commonly involved of the three terminal branches.

Typical presenting symptoms include burning pain and paresthesias in the toes and sole of the foot. The symptoms are often worse at night and may awaken a person from sleep. Symptoms may be increased by activity such as ambulation and diminished with rest. Examination may reveal a positive Tinel's sign at the ankle as well as a sensory deficit in the distribution of the posterior tibial nerve. Rarely, physical examination reveals weakness of toe flexors and foot intrinsic muscles.

The medial plantar branch of the posterior tibial nerve may be compressed in the abductor tunnel distal to the tarsal tunnel. This syndrome, known as medial plantar neuropathy or jogger's foot, has been described in runners with repetitive injury to the medial plantar nerve within the tunnel. Clinically, patients experience burning and tingling over the medial two-thirds of the sole with tenderness on palpation of the medial plantar nerve at the abductor tunnel.

Nerve conduction studies confirm the diagnosis of TTS in most cases. Sensory nerve conduction studies of the medial and lateral plantar nerves are more sensitive in detecting an entrapment than evaluation of the motor nerves.[10] Mixed nerve techniques also may be used, although normal motor fibers may obscure abnormal sensory conduction findings. Electrodiagnostic testing should include the medial and lateral plantar nerves, because one or both nerves may be involved in TTS. Needle EMG studies may show fibrillations and positive sharp waves in involved intrinsic muscles of the feet. A high false-positive rate of denervation potentials may be seen in normal individuals secondary to foot trauma.[2] Therefore, an abnormal EMG in the symptomatic foot should be compared with the asymptomatic side to determine the significance of the findings. A diagnostic anesthetic injection into the tarsal tunnel helps to confirm the diagnosis when electrodiagnostic tests are unrevealing in a clinically evident case of TTS.

Initial treatment of TTS consists of rest, ice, elevation, and NSAIDs. Supportive footwear may be used in patients who do not respond to early care. The footwear or orthotics attempt to correct abnormal foot mechanics with a medial heel wedge or a long medial arch support to decrease pronation. Tarsal tunnel injections with an anesthetic and corticosteroid in combination with other forms of conservative treatment may be helpful in expediting the resolution of symptoms. Resistant cases may require surgical decompression.

### Joplin's Neuroma

The medial plantar digital nerve is a terminal sensory branch of the medial plantar nerve that supplies sensation to the medial side of the hallux. The nerve is superficial and susceptible to injury from trauma to the great toe or chronic compression, as with a tight shoe. Clinically there is usually pain along the medial portion of the great toe. Physical examination may reveal pain with palpation of the medial plantar digital nerve just proximal to the interphalangeal joint and loss of sensation along the medial edge of the great toe.

### Morton's Neuroma

Morton's neuroma is due to entrapment of the interdigital nerve within the third and fourth interspace (Fig. 14). The neuroma is believed to result from repeated trauma to the interdigital nerve, as with barefoot running, high heel shoes, repetitive stooping, and shortened heel cords. Morton's neuroma is more common in women than in men and typically occurs between the ages of 40 and 60 years.

The patient typically complains of pain that is localized on the plantar aspect of the foot between the two metatarsal heads, radiates to the toes, and occasionally radiates proximally. The pain usually occurs with weight-bearing activity such as walking and abates with rest. The pain rarely progresses to night pain. Occasionally the patient complains of tingling, burning, or dysesthesias between the third and fourth toes. Tenderness to palpation may be present along with exacerbation of symptoms on passive toe extension. Sensory impairment typically involves the affected interdigital web and toes.

Nerve conduction studies sometimes reveal conduction slowing along the interdigital nerve with a decrease in action potential amplitude; typically, however, they are difficult to perform and not effective in evaluation for interdigital neuroma. Conservative treatment consists of NSAIDs, metatarsal pads, orthotics with medial longitudinal arch support, metatarsal bar to increase toe plantarflexion, and local injection. Surgical excision of the neuroma is considered after all conservative efforts have been exhausted.

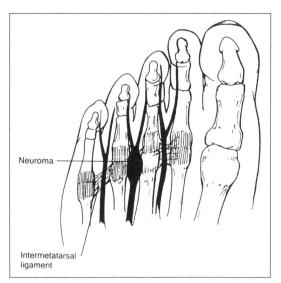

**FIGURE 14.**
Morton's neuroma. (From Mann RA:
Entrapment neuropathies of the foot.
In DeLee JC, Drez D (eds): Orthopaedic
Sports Medicine: Principles and
Practice. Philadelphia, W.B. Saunders,
1994, with permission.)

## CONCLUSION

Peripheral nerve injuries commonly develop from overuse or repetitive nerve trauma at vulnerable points along the anatomic course of the nerve. The injury usually occurs within a fibrous or osseofibrous tunnel, from constriction by a fibrous or muscular band, or at a bony prominence. The physician needs a keen awareness of the clinical presentation of the entrapment syndromes to make a correct diagnosis. Electrodiagnostic evaluations play an important role in confirming the diagnosis of certain entrapment syndromes. Treatment consists of rest, ice, NSAIDs, restriction of extremity motion, work activity modification, orthotic devices, and local injections. Surgical intervention is considered in patients with persistent disabling symptoms that do not respond to conservative treatment or with significant neurologic deficits.

## REFERENCES

1. Blom S, Dahlback LO: Nerve injuries in dislocations of the shoulder joint and fractures of the neck of humerus. Acta Chir Scand 136:461–466, 1970.
2. Falck B, Alaranta H: Fibrillation potentials, positive sharp waves and fasciculations in the intrinsic muscles of the foot in healthy subjects. J Neurol Neurosurg Psychiatry 46:681–683, 1983.
3. Gelberman RH, Hergenroeder PT, Hargens AR, et al: The carpal tunnel syndrome: A study of carpal canal pressures. J Bone Joint Surg 63A:380–383, 1981.
4. Gelberman RH, Szabo RM, Williamson RV, et al: Sensibility testing in peripheral nerve compression syndromes: An experimental study in humans. J Bone Joint Surg 65A:632–638, 1983.
5. Gerstner DL, Omer GE: Peripheral entrapment neuropathies in the upper extremity. Part 2: Recognizing and treating ulnar and radial nerve syndromes. J Musculoskel Med 5:37–49, 1988.
6. Johnson EW, Gatens T, Poindexter D, et al: Wrist dimensions: Correlation with median sensory latencies. Arch Phys Med Rehabil 64:556–557, 1983.
7. Kopell HP, Goodgold J: Clinical and electrodiagnostic features of carpal tunnel syndrome. Arch Phys Med Rehabil 67:290–292, 1986.
8. Kuschner SH, Ebramzadeh E, Johnson D, et al: Tinel's sign and Phalen's test in carpal tunnel syndrome. Orthopedics 15:1297–1302, 1992.
9. Occupational disease surveillance: Carpal tunnel syndrome. Centers for Disease Control. JAMA 262:88, 1989.
10. Oh SJ, Sarala PK, Kuba T, et al: Tarsal tunnel syndrome: Electrophysiological study. Ann Neurol 5:327–330, 1979.
11. Packer JW, Foster RR, Garcia A, et al: The humeral fracture with radial nerve palsy: Is exploration warranted? Clin Orthop 88:34–38, 1972.

12. Paget J: Lectures on Surgical Pathology. Philadelphia, Lindsay & Blakiston, 1854.
13. Phalen GS: Reflections on 21 years' experience with the carpal tunnel syndrome. JAMA 212:1365–1367, 1970.
14. Silverstein B: The prevalence of upper extremity cumulative trauma disorders in industry. Doctoral dissertation, University of Michigan, Ann Arbor, MI, 1985.
15. Suranyi L: Median nerve compression by Struthers ligament. J Neurol Neurosurg Psychiatry 46:1047–1049, 1983.
16. Szabo RM, Chidgey LK: Stress carpal tunnel pressures in patients with carpal tunnel syndrome and normal patients. J Hand Surg 14A:624–627, 1989.

# 14

# Selective Spinal Injections: A Clinical Overview

## ROBERT E. WINDSOR, MD
## KRYSTAL W. CHAMBERS, MD

Selective spinal injection is a relatively new phrase that implies discrete, well-controlled injection technique directed at specific target organs in and around the spine. The term has been used with increasing frequency as the use of fluoroscopy to aid needle placement has become more popular. Fluoroscopic direction of needle placement increases the accuracy and efficacy of several types of selective spinal injections. Indeed, many types of spinal injections cannot be reasonably performed without the use of fluoroscopy.

## EPIDURAL CORTISONE INJECTIONS

The first epidural injections were into the lumbar region. Lumbar epidural injections as a treatment of low back pain (LBP) and sciatica were first introduced in 1901 when several investigators injected cocaine epidurally.[13,49] This practice was short-lived, and epidural injections largely fell from the clinical armamentarium until 1925 when Viner injected 20 cc of 1% procaine and Ringer's solution, normal saline, or petrolatum, using the sacral route for sciatica.[71] He reasoned that a counterirritant may stimulate resolution. In 1930, Evans reported his experience with injecting up to 120 cc of procaine and saline into the sacral epidural space.[23] He claimed a 60% cure rate. Robechhi and Capra reported the first experience with epidural injection of cortisone for the treatment of LBP and sciatica via a sacral route.[56] Since that time, epidural injections have gained in popularity.

As with most areas of medicine, clinical use of epidural injections for the treatment of LBP and sciatica has preceded well-controlled clinical trials to evaluate efficacy. This has led to controversy and a poorly formed body of literature. Investigators have reported their experience with varying volumes of fluid (ranging from 2–120 cc),[14,65] various routes of injection (sacral hiatus, paramedian, midline, transforaminal, and indwelling catheter for prolonged blockade),[11,17,22,28,70,72] various injectants (normal saline, xylocaine, bupivicaine, methylprednisolone, betamethasone, triamcinolone, morphine sulphate),[7,11,16,17,18,32,56] and various techniques for localizing the epidural space (hanging drop, loss of resistance, contrast injection).[2,17,22,57,73] Inconsistencies in indications and protocols have been striking.[11,16,20,55]

This section does not discuss in detail the controversies surrounding the use of epidural injections. It focuses on what is currently considered to be mainstream use of epidural procedures as well as certain biases held by the author. Where bias is a factor, it is pointed out. The term *lumbar epidural cortisone injection*, when used generically, refers to all techniques of epidural injections.

Lumbar epidural cortisone injections are indicated for the treatment of acute and relapsing lumbar radiculopathy and central canal and foraminal stenosis.[11,16,20,55] They are also indicated for other conditions that occasionally cause one or more of these syndromes, such as spondylolisthesis, scoliosis, and compression fractures. A blind technique (which does not use fluoroscopic visualization) yields improper needle positioning even in experienced hands in up to 40% of injections via the caudal route and 30% of injections via the translaminar route.[21,22,44,53,73,74] In other words, without fluoroscopic visualization even experienced hands place the needle in a position that does not allow the injectant to bathe the target organ adequately in up to 40% of cases. This does not necessarily mean that all inadequate needle placements are outside the epidural space. They may be epidural, but because of local anatomic variation (e.g., median raphe, perineural fibrosis, large herniated disc, spondylosis)[22,53] the medication does not flow where the injectionist intends. Relying on "appropriate" regional anesthesia after instillation of local anesthetic as part of the injectant also may be misleading because of the large dermatomal overlap.[29] Fluoroscopic visualization and contrast injection demonstrate fluid flow patterns that would not be noted with a blind technique. For these reasons the author and others believe that fluoroscopic visualization of needle positioning and contrast flow is critical to optimize outcome.

A translaminar epidural may be performed by either a midline or paramedian approach. With a midline approach, the patient is typically seated in a forward-flexed posture or curled in a fetal position with the affected limb downward. The lumbar region is palpated by the injectionist for an interspinous space at the intended level. After appropriate sterile preparation and local anesthesia, an epidural needle (typically a Touhy or Hustead needle) is inserted. As the needle is advanced, the injectionist intermittently checks for loss of resistance, that is, the disappearance of resistance to digital pressure on the plunger of a glass or plastic syringe filled with air or an air-fluid mixture.[2] Loss of resistance generally indicates that the epidural space has been reached. At this point, contrast may be injected to confirm placement of the needle and to watch its flow pattern. If the needle is properly positioned, the injection of contrast demonstrates a typical cloudlike pattern known as an epidurogram. The epidurogram ceases to spread immediately upon halting the injection of contrast. The injectionist then watches the flow of the contrast to confirm that it reached its intended target. Other possibilities for the contrast pattern are an outline of fascial structures (if the needle is too shallow) or a myelographic pattern. The same approach generally can be performed in the prone position, although sometimes this position is difficult because of hypertrophic spinous processes and reduction in the size of the interspinous space. In the prone position the lumbar spine assumes a slightly extended posture and thus a narrowed interspinous space becomes even narrower. This problem can be somewhat ameliorated by placing a pillow under the stomach of the patient.

The cloudlike pattern of an epidurogram (Figs. 1 and 2) is easily differentiated from a fascial injection or a subarachnoid injection. A fascial injection is dense and spreads in a linear pattern from the point of injection in a caudal and lateral direction. As in an epidurogram, the spread of contrast stops with cessation of injection. A subarachnoid injection typically diffuses rapidly and continues to spread beyond the time the injection has stopped. In addition, a subarachnoid injection is homogeneous and may pulsate rhythmically with the beat of the heart.

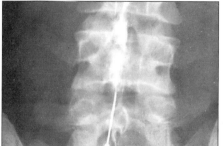

**FIGURE 1.**
Paramedian lumbar epidurogram.

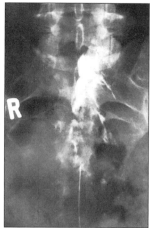

**FIGURE 2.**
Caudal epidurogram.

A paramedian approach is preferred by the author and many other injectionists who use fluoroscopic guidance. This technique is generally performed with the patient in the prone position. The epidural needle is placed down to the lamina inferior to the intended interlaminar space of entry. The needle is then "walked off" the lamina into the interlaminar space. At this point, the needle is advanced using loss of resistance as a guide. The needle should be inserted on the pathologic side. Spread of contrast often is confined to the side of entrance, even if the needle tip is in a midline position. If bilateral spread is desired and the injection is confined to the ipsilateral side, the needle may simply be pulled out of the epidural space by 1–2 cm and redirected to cross the midline. This maneuver can be easily accomplished without pulling the needle all the way out or even into subcutaneous tissue.

Transforaminal epidural injections are generally performed for two reasons: (1) medication did not flow in the desired direction because of local anatomic variation or abnormality or previous surgery at the level of pathology or (2) the injectionist wishes to place the medication within the epidural space more precisely than may be done with the above techniques. In addition, if the volume of injectant is limited to ½–1 cc of local anesthetic, it may be used for diagnostic purposes. If the patient's extremity pain dramatically reduces within 30 seconds, it may be reasonably assumed that the anesthetized nerve root mediates the pain. The assumption is buttressed when a previous root block performed in the same manner at a distant level failed to reduce pain.

The technique is performed by directing a 22- or 25-gauge, 3½- or 6-inch spinal needle into the foramen, using a slightly posterolateral and caudal-to-cephalad approach. The skin entrance site should allow a 30–45° angle in the sagittal plane, a 15–30° angle in the axial plane, and a 30–45° angle in the coronal plane. From this point of entrance the needle is placed downward to the base of the transverse process and then "walked off" (a process described below) inferiorly and into the foramen. The tip of the needle must be placed at the 6 o'clock position with reference to the pedicle in the superior aspect of the foramen. In this position the chances of injuring the nerve root or injecting into the epidural sleeve are minimized. In patients with a hypertrophic facet joint, a 30° bend placed approximately 1 cm from the end of the needle with the convex side of the bend on the same side as the bevel may facilitate proper placement. This technique can be used advantageously by rotating the needle as it is advanced to influence the direction in which the needle travels. By having greater maneuverability, the injectionist may enter the skin more medially than otherwise would be possible. This advantage helps to prevent injury to abdominal organs in larger people. In addition, it also helps in skiving around structures such as the iliac crest, hypertrophic facet joints, or large transverse processes.

A double-needle technique is useful, however, for directing a needle around a fusion mass or maneuvering through tight spaces, as occasionally seen at the lumbosacral region with high iliac crests, large L5 transverse processes, or hypertrophic facet joints. This technique is described in more detail below.

The sacral hiatus has been used as a portal to the spine for many reasons. Initially it was used to inject large volumes of local anesthetic or normal saline and cortisone to treat LBP.[9,14,26] More recently it has been used to pass catheters selectively into the anterior epidural space and to inject specific regions. In addition, selective catheter placement has been used to disrupt and inject structures such as perineural adhesions and perineural cysts.[58]

The procedure is performed with the patient in the prone position, a pillow under the pelvis, the hips internally rotated, and the gluteal musculature relaxed.[8] The skin is cleaned from a posterior to anterior direction only; this technique avoids spreading bacteria from the perianal region to the region of the sacral hiatus. The sacral cornua, which generally lie immediately adjacent to the hiatus, are palpated by the injectionist, and the soft tissues and sacral periosteum immediately caudal to this region are infiltrated with a small amount of local anesthetic. A 22- or 25-gauge, $3\frac{1}{2}$-inch spinal needle is then inserted into the skin downward to the periosteum at a 30–45° angle in the horizontal plane with the bevel down. The needle is then "walked up" into the sacral hiatus. When it reaches the hiatus, it should be approximately in the horizontal position. The needle tip should not be advanced beyond the posterior superior iliac crests to prevent inadvertent penetration of the thecal sac. The needle position should be viewed in the sagittal and coronal planes under fluoroscopic visualization to confirm placement; then contrast should be injected. Typically, 1–2 cc of contrast flows to the superior endplate of S1. If the needle is not in the sagittal plane, the injected contrast occasionally stays on one side of a median raphe.[22] If the pathology is on the contralateral side, the needle should be repositioned.

Medications and volumes have been a topic of debate in the past. Clinicians have used as little as 2 and as much as 120 cc volume of fluid for injection via a sacral route,[14,65] and the first report of epidural injection used cocaine.[13,49] This debate has largely resolved over time, and most injectionists use a total volume of 6–12 cc via a translaminar approach, 2–6 cc via a transforaminal approach, and 10–12 volume via a sacral route. With fluoroscopic visualization, the question of a set volume becomes almost moot, because the goal is to make certain that the target organ is adequately bathed. The closer to the target that the needle can be safely placed, the lower the volume necessary to achieve the desired purpose.

The injectant generally includes a dilute solution of local anesthetic and cortisone. Many injectionists use a combination of 1% xylocaine and saline with the cortisone, although many others (including the author) use a combination of xylocaine, bupivicaine, and cortisone. Most injectionists currently use 80–160 mg of methylprednisolone or 12–18 mg of betamethasone, although others use triamcinolone. In the author's experience, methylprednisolone has a longer onset of action and slightly longer half life than either betamethasone or triamcinolone; however, the betamethasone and triamcinolone appear to have a shorter onset of clinical activity (24–48 hours) than methylprednisolone. There is no strong evidence that one preparation works better than another. Other medications, such as narcotics, hyaluronidase, and sympathetically active agents (e.g., clonidine) are occasionally injected epidurally in selected clinical conditions.

## ZYGAPOPHYSEAL (FACET) JOINT PROCEDURES

Bogduk has provided an excellent description of the zygapophyseal (facet) joint.[6] The zygapophyseal joints are the diarthrodial joints that lie on either side of the posterior spinal column. They are formed by the approximation of the superior articular process of the lower vertebra and the inferior articular process of the upper vertebra. They are covered by a fibrous capsule on the dorsal, superior, and inferior surfaces and by the ligamentum flavum on the anterior surface. The capsule is lined by a typical synovial membrane, which helps to protect and nourish the joint. A cartilaginous meniscoid structure lying at the periphery of the joint also helps to protect and stabilize it. Capsular redundancy at the superior and inferior extents of the joint is known as the superior and inferior capsular recess, respectively. Fat lies within these recesses. Both recesses are incompetent at their apex. The joint is innervated by the medial branch of the posterior primary ramus of the level of the joint and the level immediately above the joint. Selby et al. report an ascending branch arising from the segment beneath the joint, but Bogduk and others have been unable to confirm this finding.[64] In addition, Ray reports a large, ascending branch, arising from the posterior ramus of S1, that gives significant, if not primary, innervation to the L5–S1 facet joint.[51]

Goldthwait first suggested the facet joint as a source of pain in 1911.[27] The facet joint was thought to be the primary cause of LBP until 1934 when Mixter and Barr reported that the lumbar disc could herniate and compress nerve roots.[43] At that point, medical attention was turned to therapy directed at the disc.[39]

Since that time, a number of investigators have demonstrated that the facet joint can be a source of pain and may refer pain into the lower extremities.[3,32,34,41,45] Schwarzer et al. demonstrated that the facet joints may be the primary cause of LBP in up to 39% of cases.[60] Various attempts have been made to map out individual referral zones for the lumbar spine, but the overlap is so large that such attempts are essentially useless for helping to isolate the painful joint.

The injection of cortisone and local anesthetic into a facet joint was a popular procedure through most of the 1970s and 1980s. It remains popular in certain regions of the United States.[3–5,39,45,56] Good to excellent results with facet joint cortisone injections have been reported in 18–63% of cases.[12,18,19,35,37,38,40,45,47] A study by Barnsley et al. indicated that this procedure does not work well for whiplash injuries.[1] The procedure has recently come under intense scrutiny and is now highly controversial. After performing analyses of the literature dealing with facet joint cortisone injections, multiple investigators have found no evidence that they are effective for treatment of LBP of facet joint etiology.[30,33,52,54] Schwarzer et al. reported that no clinical findings accurately predict the presence of facet joint pain.[60] They further assert that the only accurate means of determining whether a patient has LBP of facet joint etiology is to perform double diagnostic intraarticular facet joint injections or facet joint nerve blocks. Because the majority of LBP appears to be of disc etiology[61] and consistent clinical indicators of facet joint pain appear to be lacking, it is quite possible that selection criteria used in the past for patient enrollment in facet joint injection studies have been inadequate.

Like most other joints in the body, the facet joint is a diarthrodial joint and can become inflamed. As a result, intraarticular cortisone injections can be a powerful component in the overall treatment of an inflamed facet joint. The conundrum is to determine accurately who has facet joint pain and who does not, let alone differentiating inflammatory pain from mechanical pain.

Several methods are available for performing a lumbar facet joint injection. The most popular method in the United States is a straight, posterolateral approach.[18,19] The patient is placed prone on a procedure table, and the x-ray beam is directed obliquely through the lumbar region until the joint line of the facet joint to be injected is visualized. Using a 22- or 26-gauge, $1/2$-inch needle, a posterolateral trajectory is used to place the needle tip within the facet joint capsule. If an en pointe approach is used (in which the needle trajectory is parallel with the fluoroscopic beam so that it appears as a dot) and if the injectionist attempts to place the needle within the middle of the facet joint with respect to its superior-to-inferior extent, it is usually difficult to achieve an intraarticular position because of the overhanging lateral curve of the superior articular process. This lateral curve is not seen on fluoroscopic visualization because of the relatively small amount of bone mass that composes the overhang. However, with this technique the needle is usually easily placed within the superior or inferior recess of the facet joint capsule by directing the needle to the superior or inferior extent of the joint line, respectively.

The author's preferred technique is a slight modification of the above. The positioning of the patient and direction of the x-ray beam are the same, but the skin is penetrated by the needle in a more medial position on the back. The needle is then directed to the posterior aspect of the lamina and "walked off" laterally into the facet joint. By using this slight modification and taking a slightly more sagittal approach, the needle usually may be placed within the facet joint with little trouble.

Another technique is commonly used in European countries. The patient is placed in a prone position, and the fluoroscopic beam is directed in an anterior-to-posterior direction. The facet joint is visualized, and the needle is directed to the inferior aspect of the joint. The needle is then advanced in a cephalad direction until it comes to rest in a mass of soft tissue. At this point, the needle is generally within the inferior recess.

Once the injectionist considers the needle to be intraarticular or at least intracapsular, a $\frac{1}{2}$-cc volume of contrast is injected. The contrast should migrate rapidly to the superior recesses, joint line, and inferior recess in that order. In the author's experience, unless contrast is injected, the needle will be placed in an extraarticular and extracapsular position at least one-half of the time, with a higher frequency in older patients. Therefore, the author strongly recommends the use of contrast injection to confirm placement. In addition, when contrast is injected, architectural abnormalities, such as synovial cysts, abnormal communication with the epidural space, or ruptured capsules, can be detected.

A normal potential space posterior to the ligamentum flavum may communicate with a facet joint capsule. When contrast is injected into a facet joint that communicates with this potential space, extravasation of contrast is seen. The contrast appears to flow into the epidural space, but in fact it flows into the potential space. Communications between the facet joint capsule and epidural space are traumatic or degenerative in nature and should be considered abnormal. Determining whether the contrast has spread into the epidural space vs. the potential space requires the use of postinjection cross-sectional computed tomographic scanning. In addition, one facet joint may communicate with another facet joint on the same or opposite side via the potential space. This space is much more common in the cervical spine.

Facet joint denervation is another method of treating LBP of facet joint etiology.[4,10,51,59,63,66,67,69] Several methods are in use, including injection of phenol or absolute alcohol, cryotherapy, and radiofrequency. Radiofrequency facet joint denervation is the procedure used by the author and is described below[3–5,10] (Fig. 3).

The target organ is the medial branch of the posterior primary ramus.[3–5,50] This branch separates from the main trunk of the posterior primary ramus as it passes through the foramen. It hugs the bone as it passes under the accessory mammillary ligament and then innervates the joint. At the point that the branch passes beneath the ligament, it is most vulnerable to destruction. This region is consistently marked by the junction of the superior articular process and the transverse process at its superior extent.

The author typically uses a 10-cm, 22-gauge probe with a 5-mm exposed tip. The naked end is placed along the bony surface of the transverse process at the above described region so that as much of the naked tip is adjacent to the branch as possible. A 30-second stimulation at 50 and 2 HZ at 1 V is performed. If radicular stimulation

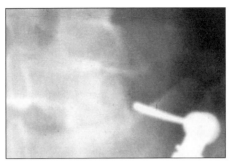

**FIGURE 3.**
Radiofrequency facet nerve ablation. The radiofrequency probe is in position for ablation of the
medial branch of the dorsal ramus of L5.

occurs, the probe is repositioned. If there is no radicular stimulation, a 60-second lesion is performed with the probe temperature maintained between 75 and 80° C. This procedure should be performed at the same level as the denervated joint and the level above because of the two-level innervation of the lumbar facet joint. An ascending branch has been described by some, but most researchers believe that the lumbar facet joints are supplied by only two levels. If there is an ascending branch, its reported location would make it difficult to destroy consistently without risking other structures.[64]

Good-to-excellent results of this procedure have been touted to be between 75 and 80% for patients with facet joint pain at 6 months and 55–65% at 1 year.[10,42,48,66,67] Recognized complications include infection; hematoma formation; nerve root injury; cutaneous anesthesia, hypesthesia, or dysesthesia; and cutaneous burn.

## SACROILIAC JOINT INJECTIONS

The sacroiliac (SI) joint is a complicated structure of which little is known. The SI joint is discussed in other parts of this volume and will not be reviewed here. This section focuses on clinical issues surrounding SI joint injection.

Currently a great deal of controversy surrounds the SI joint.[21,24,25,36,62,68] Some clinicians believe that no clinical examination techniques accurately define SI joint pathology, whereas others believe that clinical examination is useful. Clearly, this degree of disagreement allows ample room to debate any and every step of a treatment algorithm.

The injection technique begins with the patient in the prone position on a fluoroscopy table (Fig. 4). Under fluoroscopic imaging the inferior recess usually appears as an upside-down Y. From this angle it is difficult to determine how to enter the joint. To determine the angle of entry more accurately, the tube is slowly rotated to the side opposite the joint to be injected under direct visualization. If the tube is stationary, the patient's contralateral hip must be elevated. During this process, the limbs of the upside-down Y will slowly come together until they are indistinguishable. When this occurs, rotation should stop and the inferior recess should be quite clear. The inferior recess should be placed in the center of the fluoroscopic field to decrease parallax, and a metallic marker, such as the tip of a spinal needle, should be placed on the skin at a point 1–2 cm inferior to the inferior recess and parallel to the x-ray beam.

At this point, the skin and subcutaneous tissues should be anesthetized with 1% lidocaine. A 22- or 25-gauge, 3½-inch spinal needle should be inserted down to the sacrum, immediately medial to the inferior recess and approximately 1–2 cm proximal to its distal extent. The next step is to "walk" the needle laterally until it slips easily into the inferior

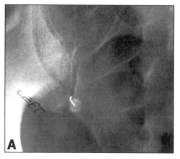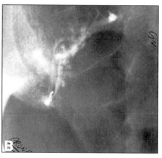

**FIGURE 4.**
Sacroiliac joint injection. *A,* A 22-gauge, 3½-inch spinal needle has been placed in the inferior recess of the left SI joint. *B,* An arthrogram after contrast injection.

recess; care must be taken not to push the needle all the way through the recess. Once the needle appears to be properly positioned, a fraction of a cubic centimeter of nonionic contrast is injected to confirm the intraarticular position of the needle. If injection cannot occur because of high resistance, the bevel is rotated until the needle tip is probably embedded in articular cartilage. If the needle is properly positioned, the contrast migrates in a cephalad direction along the joint line. If the needle is malpositioned, the injected contrast outlines a fascial plane. If too much contrast is injected at this point, the recess may be obscured, making further injection attempts difficult. If the needle is extraarticular, repositioning should be attempted at the same level of the joint. If the needle cannot be properly placed at this point because it cannot gain purchase on an articular surface, the sacrum may be posteriorly positioned to the ilium. In this case, the needle is extracted; it should reenter the skin slightly lateral to the original injection point and be placed downward to the ilium in a position similar to that described above but lateral to the inferior recess. If this maneuver does not work, entry should be attempted at the redundant portion of the capsule that actually extends immediately inferior to the joint.

Once the intraarticular location of the needle tip has been confirmed by a partial arthrogram, further injection is necessary to achieve the desired purpose. If the injection is for diagnostic purposes, one should continue to inject an additional 1–2 cc of contrast under direct visualization until the joint is full or extravasation is demonstrated. The injectionist should record and grade pain complaints in intensity, quality, and distribution. If pain is created upon injection, infiltration of the joint with 1 or 2% lidocaine is attempted. An SI joint that produces the same quality and distribution or at least the same intensity of pain as the patient's chief complaint may be significant, especially if the pain is decreased by at least 50% within 30 seconds of injection of lidocaine.[62] This concept is based on the provocative analgesia model and has yet to be proven. Serial spot films, including at least one lateral view, may be clinically useful.

If the purpose of the injection is to inject cortisone, a spot film should be taken after the initial partial arthrogram, and the remaining portion of the joint should be filled with a solution containing local anesthetic and a cortisone preparation.

## SELECTIVE SPINAL INJECTION NEEDLE TECHNIQUES

### En Pointe

The first and simplest technique is referred to as an en pointe or pinpoint technique. The target organ is placed in the center of the fluoroscopic field to reduce parallax. The patient or the tube is rotated so that the target organ is properly oriented and the plane of entry can be easily visualized. The injectionist then places the needle over the target organ as seen on the fluoroscopic monitor. The needle is directed into the target organ along the needle's long axis so that the needle is seen as a pinpoint. Care must be taken to prevent skiving.

## Skiving

Skiving refers to the change of a needle's course as it passes through tissues (Fig. 5). It may be a help or a hindrance. If an en pointe technique is used, it is generally a nuisance, but if its action is planned or modulated, it can be an aid. Skiving occurs most prominently at soft tissue density inferfaces, as when going through a fascial plane. The needle's path changes in a direction opposite the bevel. To augment this action, the

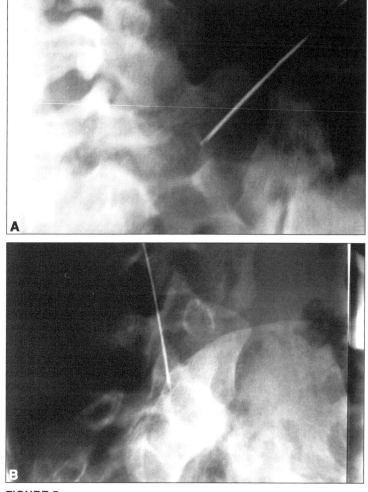

**FIGURE 5.**
*A,* Double-needle approach to the right S1 superior articular process (SAP) (A-P view). *B,* The double-needle system has been placed down to the right S1 SAP (oblique view). There is a rudimentary S1–S2 segment present.

*(Continued on following page.)*

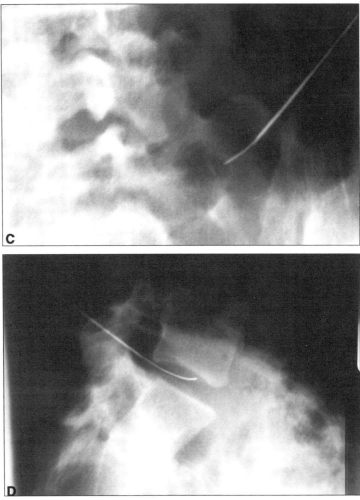

**FIGURE 5** *(Continued).*
*C,* The double-needle system has been retracted and the 22-gauge, 6-inch
curved spinal needle has been advanced to begin the initial approach to the
L5–S1 intervertebral disc (A-P view). *D,* Intradiscal placement of the 22-gauge,
6-inch curved spinal needle using a double-needle technique (lateral view).
*(Continued on following page.)*

needle can be bent before insertion 30–45° away from the bevel, approximately 1–2 cm
proximal to its distal extent. This maneuver increases the amplitude of direction change
when the needle goes through tissue changes. The amplitude of direction change is also
increased by using a smaller gauge needle. Skiving is helpful when the injectionist
needs to go around structures or through tight crevices, as in a lumbar selective root
block around a hypertrophic facet joint and into a stenotic foramen.

## Parallax
Parallax occurs in fluoroscopic imaging when a structure appears to be at a different position relative to another structure than it actually is because of improper positioning in the fluoroscopic field. For example, if a metallic marker is placed over the

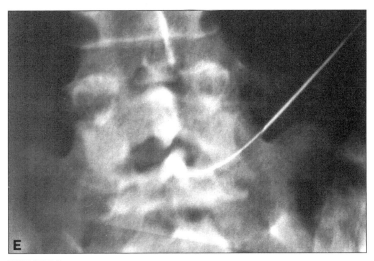

**FIGURE 5** *(Continued)*.
*E,* Intradiscal placement of a 22-gauge, 6-inch curved spinal needle using a double-needle technique (A-P view). There is a rudimentary S1–S2 segment present.

T12 spinous process in the center of the fluoroscopic field and the field is subsequently moved inferiorly so that the marker is at the top of the field, the marker no longer appears to be over the T12 spinous process. It appears to be over the T8 or T9 spinous process, depending on the size of the patient.

Parallax can be inconvenient at best and dangerous at worst. If the injectionist does not have an excellent knowledge of how one structure relates to another in a three-dimensional construct, the needle may pass through the wrong structures, such as blood vessels or nerves. Although parallax is almost always avoidable by repositioning the tube or patient, its effects can be minimized if the injectionist has a good sense of triangulation.

## Triangulation

An injectionist uses triangulation when the starting position is anywhere but the en pointe position described above (Fig. 6). The injectionist must estimate the angle of trajectory of the needle to contact the target organ in a three-dimensional structure as represented on a two-dimensional screen. To do so, the injectionist must have a good idea of how deep the target organ is beneath the skin. This skill simplifies and expedites many procedures in which an en pointe technique is not practical.

## Double-needle Technique

A double-needle technique (Fig. 7) is used to decrease the incidence of infection during procedures such as discography and to aid difficult needle placement as in nerve root blocks or thoracic discography. To use this technique, the author gently curves a 22-gauge, 6-inch spinal needle 180°, starting at the base of the needle. The needle is curved in a direction opposite the bevel. The needle is then placed through the lumen of an 18-gauge, 3½-inch spinal needle so that the 6-inch spinal needle curves in the same direction as the bevel of the 18-gauge spinal needle. An additional bend may be placed on the distal end of the 22-gauge needle, as described in the section on skiving, to expedite needle placement at the site of the target organ.

A double-needle technique is most commonly used during L5–S1 discography. The technique used by the author is a posterolateral, cephalad-to-caudad approach. The

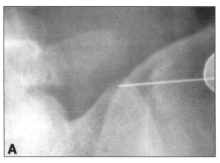

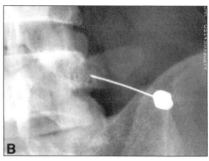

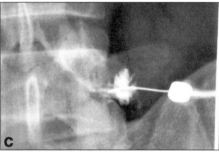

**FIGURE 6.**
Triangulation in a left L5 selective nerve root block. *A,* A 22-gauge, 1½-inch spinal needle is inserted lateral and inferior to the left L5 transverse process. *B,* The spinal needle is advanced to the base of the L5 transverse process to determine depth and angle of injection. *C,* The needle has been directed into the superior left L5–S1 foramen. Contrast material has been injected and a "perisheathogram" is demonstrated.

22-gauge, 6-inch/18-gauge, 3½-inch spinal needle system is placed downward on the lateral aspect of the S1 superior articular process so that the bevel of the 18-gauge needle is medially placed. The system is then retracted 2–3 cm, and the 22-gauge needle is unsheathed. The 22-gauge needle is then rotated 180° and advanced to the anterior aspect of the S1 superior articular process at the lower third of the disc space. The 22-gauge needle is then rotated 180° back to its original position so that with further advancement it will pass posterior and inferior to the L5 nerve root and into the L5–S1 disc.

## Walking the Needle

The term *walking* (Fig. 8) is commonly used by injectionists. It refers to placing a needle tip downward on a bony surface and gently, repetitively retracting the needle. With a combination of torquing the needle and moving the needle-holding hand in a direction opposite the desired direction, the needle tip is bounced or "walked" along the

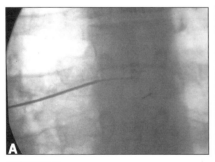

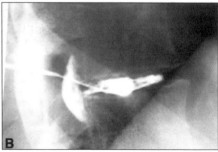

**FIGURE 7.**
Double-needle technique. *A,* A 22-gauge, 6-inch curved/18-gauge, 3½-inch spinal needle system is used to enter a thoracic disc. *B,* Lateral view of a thoracic discogram using the double-needle technique.

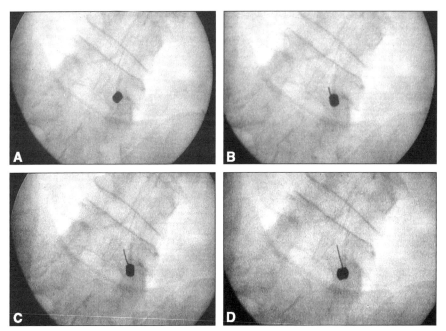

**FIGURE 8.**
Walking technique. *A*, A 22-gauge 3½-inch spinal needle has been placed on the L5 lamina in an en pointe fashion. *B–D*, The spinal needle is gently retracted, torqued, and advanced along the surface of the bone until the target is reached.

bony surface into the intended target organ. This technique is often used for injecting a facet joint or performing a selective nerve root injection.

## CONCLUSION

The study of selective spinal injection is a developing science. The proper use of fluoroscopic imaging helps to make relatively safe many types of injections that were formerly considered dangerous. Furthermore, the use of fluoroscopic imaging has made many types of injections precise and well controlled. Thus, many injections that were thought to require repetition, such as epidural cortisone injection, may need to be performed only once. It has been well demonstrated that blind (nonfluoroscopic) epidural cortisone injections may be poorly placed up to 45% of the time.[73,74] In addition, the intelligent use of selective spinal injections is paramount to optimal outcome in a cost-effective manner.

The increasing use of fluoroscopic imaging during selective spinal injections has expedited the development of many "new" needle techniques. Only a few are outlined in this chapter. Beginning injectionists are cautioned not to use these needle techniques or to perform procedures with which they are unfamiliar without proper training.

## REFERENCES

1. Barnsley L, Lord S, Wallis B, Bogduk N: Lack of effect of intraarticular corticosteroids for chronic pain in the cervical zygapophyseal joints. N Engl J Med 330:1047–1050, 1994.
2. Barry P, Kendall P: Corticosteroid infiltration of the epidural space. Ann Phys Med 6:267–273, 1962.
3. Bogduk N: Lumbar dorsal ramus syndrome. Med J Aust 2:537–541, 1980.

4. Bogduk N, Long D: Percutaneous lumbar medial branch neurotomy. Spine 5:193–200, 1980.
5. Bogduk N, Macintosh J, Marshland A: Technical limitations to the efficacy of radiofrequency neurotomy for spinal pain. Neurosurgery 20:529–534, 1987.
6. Bogduk N, Twomey L: Clinical Anatomy of the Lumbar Spine, 2nd ed. Melbourne, Churchill Livingstone, 1991.
7. Breivik H, Hesia PE, Molnar I, Lind B: Treatment of chronic low back pain and sciatica: Comparison of caudal epidural injections of bupivacaine and methylprednisolone with bupivacaine followed by saline. Adv Pain Res Ther 1:927–932, 1976.
8. Brown DL: Atlas of Regional Anesthesia. Philadelphia, W.B. Saunders, 1992, pp 293–301.
9. Brown J: Pressure caudal anesthesia and back manipulation. Northwest Med 59:905–909, 1960.
10. Burton CV: Percutaneous radiofrequency facet denervation. Appl Neurophysiol 39:80–86, 1976/77.
11. Bush K, Hillier S: Controlled studies of caudal epidural injections of triamcinolone plus procaine for the management of intractable sciatica. Spine 16:572–575, 1991.
12. Carrera G: Lumbar facet joint injection in low back pain and sciatica. Neuroradiology 137:661–664, 1980.
13. Cathelin F: Mode d'action de la cocaine injecte dans l'espace epidural par le procede du canal sacre. C R Soc Biol 53:478, 1901.
14. Clark CJ, Whitwell J: Intraocular hemorrhage after epidural injection. BMJ 2:581–586, 1961.
15. Coomes E: A comparison between epidural anesthesia and bed rest in sciatica. BMJ 1:20–24, 1961.
16. Cuckler J, Bernini PA, Weisel SW, et al: The use of epidural steroids in the treatment of lumbar radicular pain. A prospective, randomized, double blind study. J Bone Joint Surg 67:63–66, 1985.
17. Dallas T, Lin R, Wu WH, Wolskee P: Epidural morphine and methylprednisolone for low back pain. Anesthesiology 67:408– 411, 1987.
18. Destouet J, Murphy W: Lumbar facet block: Indications and technique. Orthop Rev 14:57–65, 1985.
19. Destouet J, Gilula LA, Murphy WA, Monsees B: Lumbar facet joint injection: Indication, technique, clinical correlation, and preliminary results. Radiology 145:321–325, 1982.
20. Dilke T, Burry HC, Grahame R: Extradural cortisone injection in the management of lumbar nerve root compression. BMJ 2:635–637, 1973.
21. Dreyfuss P, Dreyer S: Lumbar Zygapophyseal (Facet) Joint Injections. In Contemporary Concepts in Spine Care. North American Spine Society, 1994.
22. El-Khoury G, Ehara S, Weinstein JN, et al: Epidural steroid injection: A procedure ideally performed under fluoroscopic control. Radiology 168:554–557, 1988.
23. Evans W: Intrasacral epidural injection in the treatment of sciatica. Lancet ii:1225–1229, 1930.
24. Fortin J, Aprill CN, Ponthieux B, Pier J: Sacroiliac joint: Pain referral maps upon applying a new injection/arthrography technique. Part I: Asymptomatic volunteers. Spine 19:1475–1482, 1994.
25. Fortin J, Dwyer AP, West S, Pier J: Sacroiliac joint: Pain referral maps upon applying a new injection/arthrography technique. Part II: Clinical evaluation. Spine 19:1483–1489, 1994.
26. Goebert H, Jallo ST, Gardner WS: Sciatica: Treatment with injections of procaine and hydrocortisone acetate. Results in 113 patients. Anesth Analg 27:130–134, 1960.
27. Goldthwait JE: The lumbosacral articulation: An explanation of many cases of lumbago, sciatica and paraplegia. Boston Med Surg J 164:365–372, 1911.
28. Gordon J: Caudal extradural injections in the treatment of low back pain. Anesthesia 35:515–516, 1980.
29. Haymaker W, Woodhall B: Peripheral Nerve Injuries: Principles of Diagnosis, 2nd ed. Philadelphia, W.B. Saunders, 1967.
30. Helbig T, Lee C: The lumbar facet syndrome. Spine 13:61–64, 1988.
31. Helliwell M, Robertson JC, Ellis RM: Outpatient treatment of low back pain and sciatica by a single extradural corticosteroid injection. Brit J Clin Pract 228–231, 1985.
32. Hirsch D, Inglemark B, Miller M: The anatomical basis for low back pain. Acta Orthop Scand 33:1–17, 1963.
33. Jackson R, Jacobs RR, Montessano PX: Facet joint injection in low-back pain. Spine 13:966–971, 1988.
34. Kellergren JH: Observations on referred pain arising from muscle. Clin Sci Mol Med 3:175–190, 1938.
35. Lau LSW, Littlejohn GO, Miller MH: Clinical evaluation of intra-articular injections for lumbar facet joint pain. Med J Aust 143:563–565, 1985.
36. Laslett M, Williams M: The reliability of selected pain provocation tests for sacroiliac joint pathology. Spine 19:1243–1249, 1994.
37. Lewinnek GE, Warfield CA: Facet joint degeneration as a cause of low back pain. Clin Orthop 213:216–222, 1986.
38. Lilius G, Laasonen EM, Myllynen P, et al: Lumbar facet joint syndrome: A randomized clinical trial. J Bone Joint Surg 71B:681–684, 1989.
39. Lippett AB: The facet joint and its role in spine pain. Spine 9:746–750, 1984.
40. Lynch MC, Taylor JF: Facet joint injection for low back pain. J Bone Joint Surg 68B:138–141, 1986.
41. McCall IW, Park WM, O'Brien JP: Induced pain referral from posterior lumbar elements in normal subjects. Spine 4:441–446, 1979.

42. McCulluch JA, Organ LW: Percutaneous radiofrequency lumbar rhyzolysis. Can Med Assoc J 116:30–311, 1977.
43. Mixter WJ, Barr JS: Rupture of intervertebral disc with involvement of the spinal cord. N Engl J Med 211:210–215, 1934.
44. Mehta M, Salmon N: Extradural block. Confirmation of the injection site by x-ray monitoring. Anaesthesia 40:1009–1012, 1985.
45. Mooney V, Robertson J: Facet joint syndrome. Clin Orthop 115:149–156, 1976.
46. Moran R, O'Connell D, Walsh MG: The diagnostic value of facet joint injections. Spine 12:1407–1410, 1986.
47. Murtagh FR: Computed tomography and fluoroscopy guided anaesthesia and steroid injection in facet syndrome. Spine 13:686–689, 1988.
48. Oudenhoven RC: Articular rhizotomy. Surg Neurol 2:275–278, 1974.
49. Pasquier M, Leri D: Injectio intra-et extradurales de cocaine a dose minime dans le traitement de la sciatique. Bull Gen Ther 142:196, 1901.
50. Pedersen HE, Blunck CFJ, Gardener EJ: The anatomy of posterior rami and meningeal branches of the spinal nerves (sinu-vertebral nerves): With an experimental study of their function. J Bone Joint Surg 38A:377–391, 1956.
51. Ray CD: Percutaneous Radiofrequency Facet Nerve Blocks: Treatment of the Mechanical Low Back Syndrome [monograph]. Burlington, MA, Radionics, 1982.
52. Raymond J, Dumas J: Intra-articular facet block: Diagnostic test or therapeutic procedure? Radiology 151:333–336, 1984.
53. Renfrew D, Moore TE, Kathol MH, et al: Correct placement of epidural steroid injections: Fluoroscopic guidance and contrast administration. AJNR 12:1003–1007, 1991.
54. Revel ME, Listrat VM, Chevalier XJ, et al: Facet joint block for low back pain: Identifying predictors of a good response. Arch Phys Med Rehabil 73:824–828, 1992.
55. Ridley M, Kingsley GH, Gibson T, Grahame R: Outpatient lumbar epidural steroid injections in the management of sciatica. Br J Rheum 27:295–299, 1988.
56. Robechhi A, Capra R: Prime esperienze cliniche in campo eumatologico. Minerva Med 98:1259–1263, 1952.
57. Rowlingson JC, Kirschenbaum L: Epidural analgesic techniques in the management of cervical pain. Anesth Analg 65:938–942, 1986.
58. Salinger D: Epidural endoscopy to treat post surgical perineural adhesions. Presented at the North American Spine Society 11th Annual Conference, Vanouver, BC, Canada, October, 1996.
59. Schuster G: The use of cryoanalgesia in the painful facet syndrome. J Neurol Orthop Surg 3:271–274, 1982.
60. Schwarzer AC, Aprill CN, Derby R, et al: The clinical features of patients with pain originating from the lumbar zygapophysial joints. Spine 19:1132–1137, 1994.
61. Schwarzer AC, Aprill CN, Derby R, et al: The relative contributions of the disc and zygapophysial joint in chronic low back pain. Spine 19:801–806, 1994.
62. Schwarzer AC, Aprill CN, Bogduk N: The sacroiliac joint in chronic low back pain. Spine 20:31–37, 1995.
63. Si!vers RH: Lumbar percutaneous facet rhizotomy. Spine 15:36–40, 1990.
64. Selby DK, Paris SV: Anatomy of the facet joints and its correlation with low back pain. Contemp Orthop 312:1097–1103, 1981.
65. Snoek W, Weber H, Jorgensen B: Double blind evaluation of methylprednisolone for herniated lumbar discs. Acta Orthop Scand 48:635–641, 1977.
66. Shealy CN: Percutaneous radiofrequency denervation of spinal facets and treatment for chronic back pain and sciatica. J Neurosurg 43:448–451, 1975.
67. Shealy CN: Facet denervation in the management of back and sciatic pain. Clin Orthop 115:157–164, 1976.
68. Slipman C: Accuracy of provocative sacroiliac joint maneuvers. Arch Phys Med Rehabil [submitted for publication].
69. Sluyter M: Percutaneous Thermal Lesions in the Treatment of Back and Neck Pain. Burlington, MA, Radionics, 1981.
70. Stanley D, McLaren MI, Euinton HA, Getty CJM: A prospective study of nerve root infiltration in the diagnosis of sciatica: A comparison with radiculography, computed tomography, and operative findings. Spine 15:540–543, 1990.
71. Viner N: Intractable sciatica: The sacral epidural injection—an effective method of giving relief. Can Med Assoc J 15:630, 1925.
72. Warr A, Wilkinson JA, Burn JMB, Langdon L: Chronic lumbosciatic syndrome treated by epidural injection and manipulation. Practicioner 209:53–59, 1972.
73. White AH, Derby R, Wynne G: Epidural injections for the diagnosis and treatment of low back pain. Spine 5:78–86, 1980.
74. White A, Derby R, Wynne G: Injection techniques for the diagnosis and treatment of low back pain. Orthop Clin North Am 553–567, 1983.

# 15

# Imaging of the Lumbar Spine

## STEPHEN A. ANDRADE, MD

Imaging of the lumbar spine has advanced significantly since the time when only radiographs and myelography were available. Today the most commonly used imaging techniques include computed tomography (CT) scanning, magnetic resonance imaging (MRI), discography, and CT-discography. In many centers the use of myelography is steadily declining.[15] Physicians from a wide variety of medical specialties now treat pain arising from the lumbar spine. Nonradiologist, nonsurgeon physicians must develop some measure of familiarity with the use of CT, MRI, discography, and myelography. They must learn which imaging study provides the best information about the suspected diagnosis. In the current medical economic climate the cost of an imaging study should be considered, but the quality of medical care should not be compromised. Physicians must learn the cost:benefit ratio of each study ordered.

This chapter, written for the nonradiologist, nonsurgeon physician, reviews and compares the indications and limitations of magnetic resonance imaging, discography, CT scanning, and myelography of the lumbar spine.

## MAGNETIC RESONANCE IMAGING

MRI is considered to be the premier modality for imaging the lumbar spine. It is superior to CT scanning for visualizing spinal neoplasms, infections, and hematomas as well as inflammatory processes affecting the disc, vertebral bodies, or paravertebral soft tissue.[26,27] Contained disc herniations can be distinguished from extruded disc herniations with MRI.[13] MRI is more effective in demonstrating sequestered disc fragments than CT scanning and myelography.[24] Some authors believe that MRI is superior to CT, myelography, and discography because it directly acquires images in any desired plane, does not require ionizing radiation, and evaluates each level of the lumbar spine, including the distal spinal cord.

Patients with certain biomedical implants, such as pacemakers, spinal cord stimulators, cerebral aneurysm clips, or cochlear implants cannot undergo an MRI study.[16] In addition, patients with orbital metallic foreign bodies cannot be scanned safely. Claustrophobia should not be considered a contraindication to MRI because administration of sedative agents usually overcomes the problem. At times general anesthesia under the direction of an anesthesiologist is necessary.

A sagittal MR image of the lumbar spine provides a general overview of multiple motion segments. On a T2-weighted image the cerebrospinal fluid (CSF) appears as a

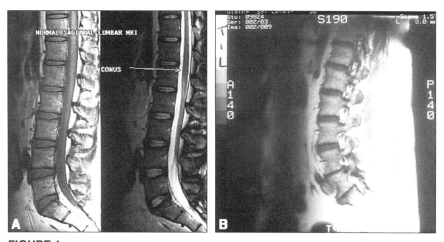

**FIGURE 1.**
*A,* On T2-weighted sagittal MR image, the cerebrospinal fluid appears as a bright signal intensity (white) on the right. The T1, on the left, and T2 sagittal MR exam covers multilumbar levels and the distal spinal cord. *B,* The sagittal MR image allows visualization of the neuroforamina.

bright signal. The spinal cord is visualized and the nerve roots and vessels can be seen within the neuroforamen (Fig. 1). An axial MR image through a disc provides a view of the relationship of the disc to the nerve roots and thecal sac (Fig. 2).

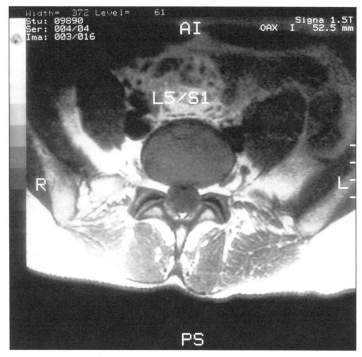

**FIGURE 2.**
Axial MR image of the L5–S1 disc.

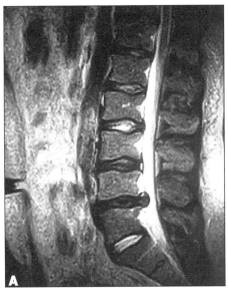
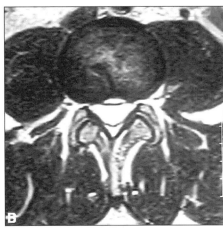

**FIGURE 3.**
*A,* The high-intensity zone in the posterior anulus is seen as a white area surrounded by a darker intensity on the T2-weighted fast-spin echo sagittal MRI examination of L3–L4 disc. *B,* The axial view of the high-intensity zone. Note the white area of the posterior disc.

The MRI provides information not only about the anatomic relationships within the lumbar spine but also about the physiologic state of the soft tissue. Once a disc begins to mature, the water content within the disc decreases. On a T2-weighted image this change is seen as a low-intensity signal (dark).[22] Anular disruptions, which can be detected with high-quality MRI, result, and anular tears begin to form.

Aprill and Bogduk[2] used provocative discography to study the so-called high-intensity zone (HIZ) seen in the posterior anulus of a disc on fast-spin echo T2-weighted MRI (Fig. 3). CT-discography was used to evaluate the internal morphology of these discs.

They found an 89% correlation between pain production and presence of an HIZ. CT-discography revealed that discs with a high-intensity zone showed evidence of grade 4 anular disruption (Fig. 4). Schellhas et al.[34] recently confirmed the work of Aprill and Bogduk.

MRI is more accurate in diagnosing disc herniation than CT and CT-myelography. In the same study nerve root compression was sometimes demonstrated with myelography and CT-myelography when it was not visualized with MRI.[38] In general, however, a soft tissue cause for nerve root compression is better seen with MRI.

Recurrent or persistent sciatica after disc surgery can be a perplexing problem. The cause of pain may be a recurrent disc herniation. Therefore, it is crucial to distinguish between recurrent disc herniation and postoperative scar tissue on the imaging study. Gadolinium-enhanced MRI is highly accurate in this particular setting.[18,31] On T1-weighted, gadolinium-enhanced MRI (Fig. 5) scar tissue appears as an area of high signal intensity (white).

MRI allows visualization of hypertrophic bony changes, such as osteoarthritic spurring associated with zygapophyseal joint degeneration. According to Modic,[27] however, "the distinction between hypertrophy of the ligamentum flavum and overgrowth is difficult to distinguish because of similar signal intensities." Therefore, some authors believe that CT scanning is the study of choice for viewing osseous changes that result

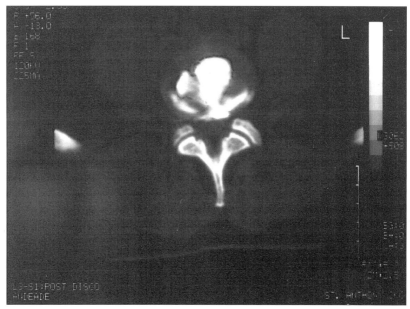

**FIGURE 4.**
CT-discography image of a grade 4 anular disc disruption.

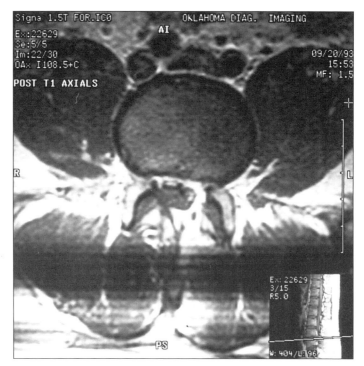

**FIGURE 5.**
Gadolinium-enhanced, T1-weighted axial MR image. Note white (high-intensity) area in the left posterior paracentral region. This area is scar tissue.

in spinal stenosis.[15,27] Other causes of spinal stenosis, such as intra- or extradural tumors and synovial cysts, are more accurately assessed with MRI.[19,25,37]

MRI of the lumbar spine is exquisitely sensitive, as Boden's prospective MRI study of asymptomatic patients emphasizes.[4] Critics are concerned that the high degree of sensitivity of MRI may lead to unnecessary surgery. It must be remembered that MRI depicts only the anatomy of the lumbar spine; it does not have the capability to document the presence or absence of pain. Therefore, provocative or analgesic spinal injection techniques such as discography, transforaminal selective epidural nerve root blocks, or zygapophyseal joint injections are frequently necessary to confirm or eliminate the sites of anatomic abnormality shown on MRI as sources of pain.

In the current climate of cost-consciousness and managed care, guidelines for the appropriate use of lumbar MRI have been offered. According to the recommendations of the North American Spine Society (NASS), MRI is not needed until 7 weeks after the onset of symptoms in patients with persistent pain. However, NASS also recommends that "in situations of major acute injury or symptoms of infection, neoplasia or progressive neural dysfunction, MRI may be appropriate to the initial workup."[16]

## LUMBAR DISCOGRAPHY

Lindbolm is credited with the introduction of lumbar discography.[23] Holt's work in the late 1960s cast lumbar discography as an unreliable test with a false-positive rate of 35%.[17] In 1988 Simmons and Aprill[36] reviewed Holt's work and concluded that he based his lumbar discography data on outdated techniques. In 1990 Walsh performed a prospective study of lumbar discography that included asymptomatic and symptomatic individuals. He concluded that the false-positive rate of "properly" performed lumbar discography approaches zero.[39] Although lumbar discography is still controversial,[28,32,33] it has been endorsed by the North American Spine Society.[14]

Lumbar discography is a provocative diagnostic test designed to determine whether a suspected disc level is a source of pain. A needle is placed in the centrum of the disc, and nonionic water-soluble contrast media is injected into the disc (Fig. 6). The injection results in a measurable increase in intradiscal pressure. Derby has related pain generation to the pressure produced during disc injection. According to his data, discs that are the source of pain become painful at lower pressure thresholds.[8,9] The presence of nociceptors within the periphery of the anulus of the disc has been described previously.[5] Roberts et al., using immunohistologic techniques, confirmed that mechanoreceptors are located in the peripheral anulus and anterior longitudinal ligament.[30] Type III mechanoreceptors have nociceptive functions and may become sensitized by an inflammatory process. Aprill and Bogduk have suggested that the high-intensity zone seen with T2-weighted fast-spin echo MRI is actually "nuclear material trapped between the lamellae of the anulus fibrosus, which has become inflamed, and this accounts for the brighter signal."[2]

The data of Derby, Aprill and Bogduk, and Roberts help to explain why a painful disc produces pain on discographic testing and a nonpainful disc does not. The presence of anular tears in degenerative discs has been documented with discography (Fig. 7). Through these tears nuclear material migrates toward the outer anulus of the disc. The nuclear material stimulates an antibody–antigen reaction that leads to the release of inflammatory products. The inflammatory process sensitizes the type III mechanoreceptors.[30] The pressure threshold at which these receptors "fire" is reduced; consequently, when the disc is tested with discography, pain is produced at a measurably lower pressure.

Discographically normal nucleogram patterns (Fig. 8) result from the collection of injected nonionic contrast medium within the nucleus of the disc. The contrast medium

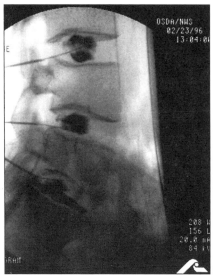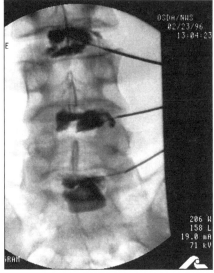

**FIGURE 6.**
Anteroposterior and lateral views of lumbar discography. Contrast medium was injected into the nucleus of the disc, producing a nucleogram.

does not communicate with the outer anulus. Therefore, there is no evidence of anular fissures through which nuclear material can communicate with the outer anulus. Hence the type III mechanoreceptors are not sensitized, and typically this type of disc is found to be nonpainful at discography.

Recommended standards for lumbar discography technique and interpretation of data collected during the study have been published.[1,6,7,14] Whenever possible, the discographic study should include a nonpainful control level. The nonpainful control level validates the patient's complaint of pain at other disc levels.

Comparison studies between CT-discography and myelography[20,21,35] have found that CT-discography is more accurate than myelography in demonstrating disc pathology. A comparison of lumbar discography with MRI may be inappropriate. Both are radiologic imaging techniques, but unlike MRI, lumbar discography is a pain-provocative test. It has been suggested that CT-discography demonstrates anular tears better than MRI.[29] Lumbar discography should be considered as an adjuvant to MRI; that is, discography is best used to confirm or eliminate the possible sites of pain generation suggested by MR imaging.

Lumbar discography has been used in a wide variety of clinical settings, such as evaluation of persistent pain after lumbar fusion, far lateral disc herniations, painful disc levels in scoliotic patients, and recurrent disc herniations. Specific indications for the use of lumbar discography have been set forth by the North American Spine Society.[14] Lumbar discography is recommended for patients with persistent low back or leg pain that has failed to improve with nonoperative or operative treatment when other noninvasive imaging studies have not explained definitively the origin of persistent symptoms.

Potential complications of lumbar discography include infection, neural injury, hemorrhage, dural puncture, and paralysis. In the hands of experienced discographers, such complications are rare. With a double-needle technique the incidence of discitis associated with lumbar discography is 0.7%;[10] in another study, the incidence was 0.1–0.2%.[14]

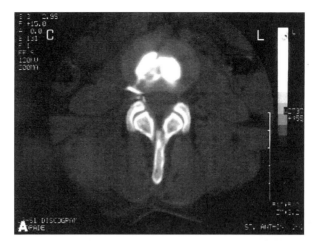

**FIGURE 7.**
*A*, Example of radial anular fissure on CT discography. *B*, Lateral view of lumbar discography. Note contrast medium spreading posteriorly from central nucleus through anular fissure on the L4–L5 disc.

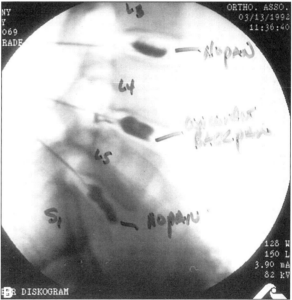

## COMPUTED TOMOGRAPHY OF THE LUMBAR SPINE

Reconstruction of rotating x-ray fan-beam projections into two-dimensional images is the basis of CT image creation.[3] The soft tissue imaging capabilities of CT allow visualization of intervertebral discs, ligaments, muscle, and vessels.

CT imaging is superior to MRI for the viewing of cortical bone detail, although MR is far superior to CT for evaluation of bone marrow space. Lateral stenosis can be demonstrated with unique clarity when three-dimensional reformatting of CT images is used.[15] Because of its lower cost CT scanning is the first-choice imaging study for the lumbar spine at certain centers.[15] Supporters of MRI counter that, although CT is less expensive, it yields less information and requires the use of ionizing radiation. Furthermore, visualization of intradural structures with CT requires intrathecal injection of contrast media.

An appropriate CT scan of a lumbar motion segment should include the area from the inferior aspect of the pedicle above to the superior aspect of the pedicle below. This approach allows visualization of the inferior aspect of the cranial vertebral body, disc,

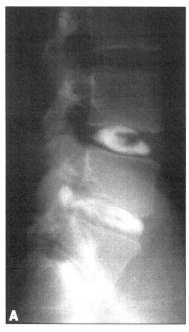

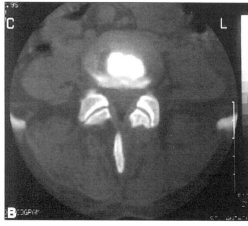

**FIGURE 8.**
A, Lateral view of lumbar discography. Note L3–L4 disc, an example of a normal nucleogram. Contrast is localized in the nucleus. B, CT-discography examination of a normal nucleogram.

zygapophyseal joints, neuroforamen, neural canal, and superior aspect of the caudal vertebral body.[11] The use of soft tissue and bone windows facilitates visualization of these structures.

Caution must be taken in visualizing the L5–S1 disc level. The posterior aspect of the L5–S1 disc on CT scanning is convex in the axial view and may be misconstrued as a disc bulge or herniation. This effect, which is due to the lumbosacral angulation in relationship to the CT imaging angle at the L5–S1 disc level, may be overcome by using reformatted sagittal images.[15]

CT scanning is more accurate than myelography for evaluating disc herniations, according to Heitoff.[15] Herniations are effectively demonstrated with CT, but contained vs. noncontained herniations are better distinguished with MRI. Anular tears are not visualized with CT, although degenerative changes such as loss of disc height, the intradiscal vacuum effect (Fig. 9), and calcification in the disc can be demonstrated well with CT. Considering the clinical importance of anular tears, as suggested by Aprill and Bogduk, MRI is favored over CT scan if the suspected low back pain arises from the disc and is not secondary to nerve root compression.

One particular strength of CT is the ability to visualize osseous disease. Pars interarticularis defects and hypertrophic bony overgrowth of the zygapophyseal joints are well demonstrated with CT.[11,15]

## LUMBAR MYELOGRAPHY

Myelography is an invasive procedure that requires the intrathecal injection of radiographic contrast media and ionizing radiation to create an image (Fig. 10). Potential complications include postmyelographic spinal headaches, arachnoiditis, allergic reactions, and, on rare occasions, infection such as meningitis or epidural abscess.

The use of small-gauge spinal needles (26- or 25-g) reduces the incidence of spinal headaches after dural puncture. Spinal headaches are treated conservatively with

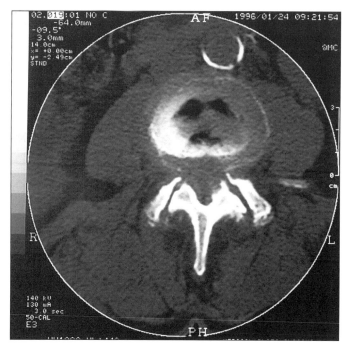

**FIGURE 9.**
Axial CT examination of a degenerated lumbar disc. Note dark area in central disc, the so-called vacuum disc. Bony hypertrophy of the zygapophyseal joints is also visualized.

bedrest, oral analgesics, and an increase in oral fluid intake. A trial of intravenous fluids containing caffeine sodium benzoate has been reported in the anesthesiology literature. When the spinal headache is intractable, treatment with lumbar epidural autologous "blood" patches may be highly effective.

Iophendylate (Pantopaque) contrast medium, which was used in the past for myelography, has been associated with arachnoiditis. However, since the introduction of nonionic water-soluble contrast media, the incidence of myelography-associated arachnoiditis has decreased. Some authors contend that CT-myelography is the best method to diagnose arachnoiditis, but MRI serves reasonably well.

Nonfilling of a nerve root sheath, as seen with myelography, indicates the presence of a compressive lesion within the neuroforamen. The nature of the lesion is not defined with myelography alone. CT or MR imaging is needed to define the nature of the compressing lesion (Fig. 11). Sagittal MR images provide a direct view into the neuroforamen; thus, lesions occupying this region can be visualized. Axial CT and MR images provide additional information about the patency of the neuroforamen. CT and MRI are noninvasive procedures, whereas myelography is invasive.

Critics of myelography suggest that CT and MRI should replace myelography as an imaging study of the lumbar spine because the effectiveness of CT and MRI in demonstrating disc herniations is well established.[15,21,38]

## SUMMARY

Nonradiologist, nonsurgeon physicians who treat patients with back pain and leg pain should strive to improve their knowledge of the various imaging tools. The indi-

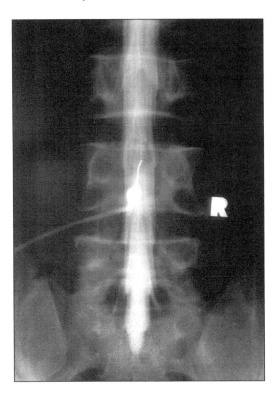

**FIGURE 10.**
Anteroposterior view of lumbar myelography.

cations for their use should be clear so that the most appropriate imaging study can be ordered.

MRI provides a detailed anatomic overview of extradural and intradural structures of the lumbar spine, including information about the physiologic state of the intervertebral disc and demonstration of anular tears. Gadolinium-enhanced MRI can be used to distinguish between postoperative scar and recurrent disc herniation. Inflammatory processes, infections and spinal neoplastic lesions are well demonstrated with MRI. MRI is noninvasive and does not require ionizing radiation for image creation. It is contraindicated in certain patients with biomedical implants.

CT imaging is an effective method for studying the lumbar spine. It provides detailed anatomic images of selected areas within the lumbar spine. Osseous changes associated with degeneration and trauma are also effectively demonstrated with CT. CT is inferior to MR in displaying information in the sagittal and coronal planes and in visualizing earlier stages of disc degeneration and intradural pathology. Although it is a noninvasive technique, CT requires the use of ionizing radiation.

Lumbar discography is a provocative diagnostic imaging study of the intervertebral disc. CT, MRI, myelography, and CT-myelography provide information only about anatomic changes and cannot determine whether they generate pain. However, the high-intensity zone seen on T2-weighted fast-spin echo MRI may be a visual image of a painful lesion. The combination of CT and discography provides a detailed view of internal disc pathology. Lumbar discography is an invasive procedure and requires the use of ionizing radiation. Complications associated with lumbar discography are rare.

Myelography is an invasive procedure requiring the use of ionizing radiation. It effectively demonstrates compressive lesions. Although the nature of the lesion cannot be distinguished with myelography alone, the combination of CT imaging and myelography

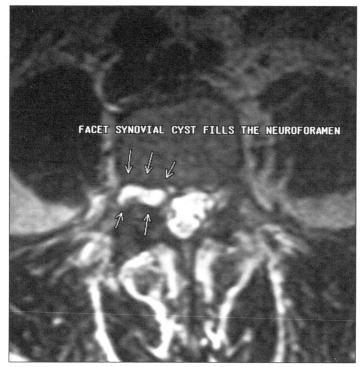

**FIGURE 11.**
Axial MR examination of lumbar zygapophyseal cyst filling the right neuroforamen.

provides an effective method for studying intradural pathology. Myelography is relatively insensitive to central disc protrusions compared with CT or MRI.

Complaints of low back pain and leg pain are common. Fortunately, most symptoms are self-limiting and of short duration. Therefore, CT, MRI, myelography, and discography are not needed in most patients. When a patient fails to improve with appropriate conservative treatment measures, however, the use of these imaging studies becomes paramount for directing subsequent care.

**Acknowledgment.**    The author gratefully acknowledges the assistance of Michael Pollack, M.D., Radiologist and Medical Director, Oklahoma Diagnostic Imaging, Oklahoma City, Oklahoma, in the preparation of this chapter.

## REFERENCES

1. Andrade SA: A response to Dr. Bogduk's "Proposed discography standards." Int Spinal Inject Soc Newslett 2(2):123–124, 1994.
2. Aprill CN, Bogduk N: High intensity zone: A diagnostic sign of painful lumbar disc on magnetic resonance imaging. Br J Radiol 65:361–369, 1992.
3. Barnes GT, Lakshminarayanan AV: Computed tomography: Physical principles and image quality considerations. In Sagel S, Lee J, Stanley R (eds): Computed Body Tomography with MRI Correlation, 2nd ed. New York, Raven Press, 1989, pp 1–21.
4. Boden SD: Abnormal magnetic resonance scans of the lumbar spine in asymptomatic subjects: A prospective investigation. J Bone Joint Surg 72A:403–408, 1990.
5. Bogduk N: Clinical Anatomy of the Lumbar Spine, 3rd ed. New York, Churchill-Livingstone, 1990.
6. Bogduk N: Proposed discography standards. Int Spinal Inject Soc Newslett 2(1):10–13, 1994.

7. Derby R: A second proposal for discography standards. Int Spinal Inject Soc Newslett 2(2):108–122, 1994.

8. Derby R: Pain provocation in normal nucleograms during discography. Prevalence and relationship to intradiscal pressure. Int Spinal Inject Soc Newslett 2(6):16–27, 1993.

9. Derby R: Lumbar discometry. Int Spinal Inject Soc Newslett 1(5):10–19, 1993.

10. Fraser RD: Discitis after discography. J Bone Joint Surg 69B:31–35, 1987.

11. Gado M, Sartor K, Hodges F: Spine. In Lee J, Sagel S, Stanley R (eds): Computed Body Tomography with MRI Correlation, 2nd ed. New York, Raven Press, 1989, pp 991–1062.

12. Gresham JL: Evaluation of the lumbar spine by discography and its use in selection of proper treatment of the herniated disk syndrome. Clin Orthop 67:29–41, 1969.

13. Grenier N: Normal and disrupted lumbar longitudinal ligaments: Correlative MR and anatomic study. Radiology 171:197–205, 1989.

14. Guyer RD: Contemporary Concepts in Spine Care—Lumbar discography. Position statement for the North American Spine Society Diagnostic and Therapeutic Committee. Spine 20:2048–2059, 1995.

15. Heitoff K: The Lumbar Spine. Philadelphia, W.B. Saunders, 1990.

16. Herzog R: Contemporary concepts in spine care—Magnetic resonance imaging: Use in patients with low back or radicular pain. Spine 20:1834–1838, 1995.

17. Holt EP Jr: The question of lumbar discography. J Bone Joint Surg 50A:720–726, 1968.

18. Hueftle MG: Lumbar spine: Post-operative magnetic resonance imaging with Gd-DTPA. Radiology 167:817–824, 1988.

19. Jackson DE Jr: Intraspinal synovial cysts: MR imaging. Radiology 170:527–530, 1989.

20. Jackson RP: Foraminal and extraforaminal lumbar disc herniation: Diagnosis and treatment. Spine 12:577–585, 1987.

21. Jackson RP: The neuroradiographic diagnosis of lumbar herniated nucleus pulposus. I: A comparison of computed tomography (CT), myelography, discography, and CT-discography. Spine 14:1356–1361, 1989.

22. Kricun R, Kricun M: MRI and CT of the Spine—Case Study Approach. New York, Raven Press, 1994.

23. Lindbolm K: Diagnostic puncture of intervertebral disks in sciatica. Acta Orthop Scand 17:213–239, 1948.

24. Masaryk TJ: High-resolution MR imaging of sequestered lumbar intervertebral disks. AJR 150:1155–1162, 1988.

25. Maupin WB: Synovial cysts presenting as neuroforaminal lesions: MR and CT appearance. AJR 153:1231–1232, 1989.

26. Modic MT: Vertebral osteomyelitis: Assessment using MR. Radiology 157:157–166, 1985.

27. Modic MT: The spine. In Higgins CB, Hriack H (eds): Magnetic Resonance Imaging of the Body. New York, Raven Press, 1987, pp 511–524.

28. Nachemson A: Lumbar discography—Where are we today? Spine 4:555–567, 1989.

29. Osti OL: MRI and discography of anular tears and intervertebral disc degeneration. A prospective clinical comparison. J Bone Joint Surg 74B:431–435, 1992.

30. Roberts S: Mechanoreceptors in intervertebral discs, morphology, distribution and neuropeptides. Spine 20:2645–2651, 1995.

31. Ross JS: MR imaging of the post-operative lumbar spine: Assessment with gadopentetate dimeglumine. AJR 155:867–872, 1990.

32. Shapiro R: Response to lumbar discography: An outdated procedure. J Neurosurg 64:686, 1986.

33. Shapiro R: Current status of lumbar discography. Radiology 159:815, 1986.

34. Schellhas K: Lumbar disc high-intensity zone: Correlation of magnetic resonance imaging and discography. Spine 21:79–86, 1996.

35. Simmons EH: An evaluation of discography in the localization of symptomatic levels in discogenic disease of the spine. Clin Orthop 108:57–69, 1975.

36. Simmons JW, Aprill CN: A reassessment of Holt's data on "the question of lumbar discography." Clin Orthop 237:120–124, 1988.

37. Sze G: Malignant extradural tumors: MR imaging with gadolinium-DTPA. Radiology 167:217–223, 1988.

38. Takahashi M: Comparison of magnetic resonance imaging with myelography and CT-myelography in the diagnosis of lumbar disc herniation. Neuro Imag Clin North Am 3:487–516, 1993.

39. Walsh TR: Lumbar discography in normal subjects: A controlled prospective study. J Bone Joint Surg 72A:1081–1088, 1990.

# 16

# Electrodiagnostic Testing

FRANK J. E. FALCO, MD
GARY GOLDBERG, MD

Electrodiagnostic testing can be used to supplement the history and physical examination of a patient suspected of having a neuromuscular condition. Nerve conduction studies, electromyography (EMG), and somatosensory-evoked potentials allow an objective physiologic evaluation of the peripheral and central nervous systems. These different electrodiagnostic techniques are used to localize and characterize pathophysiologic processes within the nervous system. Electrodiagnostic testing is commonly used in the evaluation of peripheral neuropathy, compression neuropathy, radiculopathy, myelopathy, and myopathy.

This chapter focuses on the role of electrodiagnostics in the assessment of soft tissue injuries. The fundamentals of electrodiagnostic testing, equipment, indications, contraindications, and limitations are also discussed, along with the use of intraoperative electrodiagnostic monitoring.

## INSTRUMENTATION

The equipment used to perform electrodiagnostic evaluations includes the electrodes, amplifiers, display device, and speaker. Most modern electrodiagnostic equipment incorporates the use of computers for storage, analysis, and display of signals.

Surface electrodes are usually round or square and made of steel, platinum, silver, nickel, or lead. The typical electrodes are approximately 1 cm$^2$ in size. The electrodes are used in recording action potentials of peripheral nerve conductions, muscle, and somatosensory-evoked potentials. A ground electrode made of the same type of material but larger is used to reduce electrical artifact and to serve as a common reference site for the differential amplifier to which the recording electrodes are connected.

Intramuscular needle electrodes are used during the EMG evaluation and are sometimes used for recording nerve action potentials to improve recording quality in patients with obesity or edema, in whom the electrical resistance of the skin and subcutaneous tissues may be exceedingly high. Subdermal needle electrodes also may be used instead of surface electrodes during somatosensory-evoked potential studies to overcome skin impedance. There are several different types of EMG needle electrodes. The monopolar needle is made of stainless steel with a diameter of approximately 1 mm. Teflon is used along the length of the needle for insulation with the exception of the bared distal tip. The needle is used in conjunction with a surface (reference) electrode and measures voltage differences between the electrode tip and the surface. The coaxial concentric needle is a hollow stainless steel cannula with an insulated wire within the bore of the needle. The wire is typically one-tenth of a millimeter in diameter and is usually made of nichrome, silver, or platinum. A separate surface electrode to serve as a reference is not needed when the coaxial needle is used. The exposed shaft serves as the reference for the exposed tip of the wire (recording electrode) in measuring electrical activity. The third type of EMG needle is the bipolar concentric needle, which, like the coaxial, is a stainless steel cannula but contains two insulated wires with bare tips at the recording surface. Voltage differences are measured between the two wires, with the cannula serving as the ground electrode. The other two types of EMG needle electrodes require the use of a separate electrode to serve as the ground. The concentric needles record smaller amplitudes than the monopolar needle because the recording electrodes are close together. The concentric needles consequently reduce unwanted electrical noise and record from a more confined region of the muscle.

Action potentials recorded during the electrodiagnostic evaluation range from microvolts to millivolts. Filters and amplifiers are used to produce visible action potentials that can be displayed on the cathode ray tube. A series of amplifiers is used to magnify the recorded signal, and filters reduce undesired electrical noise (artifact) that obscure the electrical potential.

Two types of percutaneous stimulators are used to elicit nerve action potentials. The constant voltage stimulator maintains a constant voltage regardless of the skin resistance. The constant current stimulator uses constant amperage with variation in the voltage. Either type of stimulator may be used for percutaneous nerve stimulation. Transcutaneous magnetic stimulation is under investigation as a painless alternative to percutaneous electrical stimulation.

Action potentials displayed on a cathode ray tube are analyzed to extract various parameters that differentiate normal and abnormal electrophysiology. Portions of the action potential have been arbitrarily described as negative when above the isoelectric baseline and positive when below the baseline. An audio amplifier and loud speaker are used during the EMG evaluation to permit interpretation of the various sounds associated with the electrical activity of resting muscle and with motor unit potentials recorded during active recruitment.


## PERIPHERAL NERVES

### Anatomy and Physiology

The motor axons found in peripheral nerves project from anterior horn cells (motor neurons) in the anterior gray matter of the spinal cord. The motor neurons are located within the spinal cord, whereas the sensory neurons are located outside the spinal cord within the dorsal root ganglion (DRG). The DRG is found just distal to the spinal nerve within the primary dorsal ramus inside the intervertebral foramen. Motor fibers carry motor impulses from the spinal cord to the peripheral muscles, whereas the sensory fibers relay information about sensation from the periphery to the spinal cord.

The three components that make up the peripheral nerve are the endoneurium, perineurium, and epineurium (Fig. 1). The endoneurium is the connective tissue that surrounds each individual axon. The perineurium supports each fascicle, which is a separate bundle of axons within the nerve. The epineurium wraps around a group of fascicles.

Nerve fibers are either myelinated or unmyelinated, which has a significant effect on the nerve conduction velocity. Schwann cells provide the myelin covering to the axon, which provides physiologic insulation for electrical conduction. Myelin does not

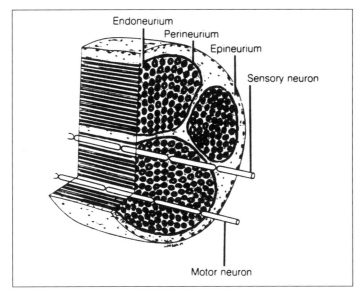

**FIGURE 1.**
Peripheral nerve components. (From deGroot J, Chusid JG: Spinal nerves and plexuses. In deGroot J, Chusid JG (eds): Correlative Neuroanatomy, 2nd ed. East Norwalk, CT, Appleton & Lange, 1988, with permission.)

completely cover the entire length of the axon. Nodes of Ranvier are short unmyelinated segments located along the nerve axon. The nodes are equidistant from one another, similar to the spacing of the Schwann cells. Action potentials travel along the myelinated nerve axon by "jumping" from one node to the next as opposed to continuous propagation in the unmyelinated nerve (Fig. 2). This process, termed saltatory conduction, results in significantly faster conduction velocities compared with unmyelinated nerve fibers.

The myelinated type A and unmyelinated type C fibers are the two fiber types found in mammalian peripheral nerves. There are several subtypes of fibers within these two general classifications (Table 1). The Aα fibers are found in motor nerves and sensory nerves that convey proprioception information. Temperature and touch sensa-

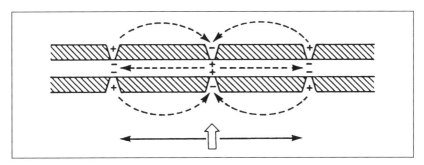

**FIGURE 2.**
Saltatory conduction. Open arrow = stimulus. Broken arrow = local current. Solid arrow = propagating impulses in both directions. (From Kimura J: Anatomy and physiology of the peripheral nerve. In Kimura J (ed): Electrodiagnosis in Diseases of Nerve and Muscle: Principles and Practice, 2nd ed. Philadelphia, F.A. Davis, 1989, with permission.)

**TABLE 1.**
Nerve Fiber Types

| Fiber Type | Function | Fiber Diameter (μm) | Conduction Velocity (m/s) | Spike Duration (ms) | Absolute Refractory Period (ms) |
|---|---|---|---|---|---|
| A α | Proprioception; somatic motor | 12–20 | 70–120 | 0.4–0.5 | 0.4–1 |
| β | Touch, pressure | 5–12 | 30–70 | 0.4–0.5 | 0.4–1 |
| γ | Motor to muscle spindles | 3–6 | 15–30 | 0.4–0.5 | 0.4–1 |
| δ | Pain, temperature, touch | 2–5 | 12–30 | 0.4–0.5 | 0.4–1 |
| B | Preganglionic autonomic | <3 | 3–15 | 1.2 | 1.2 |
| C dorsal root | Pain, reflex responses | 0.4–1.2 | 0.5–2 | 2 | 2 |
| sympathetic | Postganglionic sympathetics | 0.3–1.3 | 0.7–2.3 | 2 | 2 |

From Ganong WF: Review of Medical Physiology, 13th ed. East Norwalk, CT, Appleton & Lange, 1987, with permission.

tion are carried by Aδ fibers, whereas pain is transmitted by Aδ and C fibers. The Aα fibers have the largest diameters and fastest conduction velocities. Nerve conduction studies evaluate only the myelinated Aα motor and sensory fibers because they have lower thresholds for electrical stimulation than other fiber types.

There are two phases during the generation of an action potential, the subthreshold and threshold phases. An action potential is produced with a depolarization of approximately 15–20 mV above the resting membrane potential from a subthreshold to threshold level.[7] No action potential is generated in the subthreshold range. An action potential is generated once the threshold membrane potential is reached and is an all-or-none response (Fig. 3). The depolarization results from a change in the permeability of the membrane to sodium ions, which causes a rapid change in the resting membrane potential from negative to positive. Shortly thereafter, an increase in potassium ion

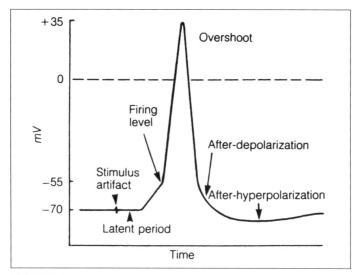

**FIGURE 3.**
Nerve action potential. (From deGroot J, Chusid JG: Signaling in the nervous system. In deGroot J, Chusid JG (eds): Correlative Neuroanatomy, 2nd ed. East Norwalk, CT, Appleton & Lange, 1988, with permission.)

influx and a decrease in sodium ion permeability lead to repolarization of the membrane potential to the resting level. Immediately after the action potential, there is a period of hyperpolarization known as the refractory period, during which the nerve is resistant to further stimulation before slowly returning to the resting membrane potential.

Nerve conduction studies are performed by creating a nerve action potential through external electrical stimulation with a percutaneous stimulator. The stimulator has a cathode and an anode. The cathode is negatively charged and attracts positively charged ions (cations), whereas the positive anode attracts negatively charged ions (anions). This change in electrical charge by the cathode and anode depolarizes the nerve locally. Unlike physiologic nerve impulses, which travel in one direction, electrically induced depolarization generates impulses that propagate in both directions along the nerve (see Fig. 2).

## Nerve Conduction Studies

Stimulation and recording of action potentials along the nerve in the direction in which physiologic conduction normally takes place is termed orthodromic. Nerve conduction studies in the direction opposite to normal physiologic conduction are termed antidromic. Most motor conduction studies are orthodromic with stimulation of the nerve proximal to the recording electrode, which records a compound muscle action potential (CMAP) when placed over a distal muscle. Sensory nerve studies are commonly performed antidromically with stimulation proximal to the recording electrodes, which have been placed over a distal sensory cutaneous nerve to record a sensory nerve action potential (SNAP).

Several nerve conduction parameters that are measured during testing reflect the electrophysiologic properties of the nerve. The *latency* is a measurement of the conduction time in milliseconds from nerve stimulation to the recording of the action potential. The *distal motor latency* is the time from stimulation of the distal motor nerve to the recording of the CMAP, which includes the time for the action potential to travel along the nerve as well as the time to cross the myoneural junction and to generate the CMAP. The distal motor latency is typically recorded to the point of the initial negative deflection of the CMAP. The *distal sensory latency* is the time from stimulation of the distal sensory nerve to the recording of the SNAP. Some practitioners measure to the onset of the SNAP, whereas others use the peak of the SNAP to determine the distal latency. The distal sensory latency is a measurement of nerve conduction time without the physiologic time delays involved in generating a CMAP, as is the case with the distal motor latency.

Nerve conduction velocity (NCV) is the measurement of the speed at which an action potential propagates along the nerve, expressed in meters per second. The conduction velocity is determined by stimulating the nerve distally and proximally. A proximal latency is determined in the same manner as described above for distal latencies with the exception that the point of nerve stimulation is more proximal. The distance between the two sites of stimulation is measured along the length of the nerve in centimeters. This distance reflects the length of nerve across which the action potential has propagated. The NCV is determined by dividing the distance between the stimulation sites by the difference between the distal and proximal latencies. The NCV is a direct measure of nerve velocity for sensory as well as motor nerves. Any distal delays in the muscle are "subtracted" when using the difference between the proximal and distal latencies; therefore, this difference reflects only the conduction time along the measured nerve segment. Because the distal sensory latency is a direct measurement of nerve conduction time, a sensory NCV also can be determined by dividing the distance between the stimulation site and recording electrode by the distal sensory latency.

The amplitude of the action potential in general reflects the number of functioning axons within the peripheral nerve. This may not always be the case for CMAP amplitudes. Certain disorders, such as disuse muscle atrophy, myopathic processes, or neuromuscular junction disorders, may result in small CMAPs without affecting the number of nerve axons. Motor action potential amplitudes are usually measured from the base to the negative peak of the action potential, whereas the SNAP may be measured in either the same manner or from the negative peak to the positive peak of the action potential. The latter is more easily applied to sensory action potential amplitude measurements since SNAPs are more consistently biphasic than CMAPs.

The duration of the action potential is another parameter measured during nerve conduction studies. The action potential duration is the length of time in milliseconds spanned by the complete action potential—a measure of the width of the potential.

The action potential is a reflection of the differences in the axons found in the peripheral nerve. A$\alpha$ fibers within the nerve have different inherent conduction velocities. The fastest conducting fibers deliver an impulse faster than slower conducting fibers over the course of the nerve. This difference is more pronounced with proximal stimulation. The evoked potential from distal stimulation has a greater amplitude and a shorter duration than the evoked potential from proximal stimulation. This normal variation in the evoked potential is termed temporal dispersion. Despite changes in the amplitude and duration with temporal dispersion, the area beneath the action potential remains the same.

Several factors that affect nerve conduction should be taken into consideration in performing electrodiagnostic studies. Temperature has a direct affect on NCV and distal latencies. There is a decrease in NCV of approximately 2.4 meters per second and an increase in distal latency of about 0.3 milliseconds with each drop of 1°C in nerve temperature.[2,8,9,18] The nerve action potential amplitude and duration are inversely affected by temperature changes. The amplitude and duration increase with decreasing nerve temperature. To guard against false abnormal conduction results from cool limbs, skin temperatures should be measured and extremities should be warmed if found to be cool. Limbs are typically warmed with hot packs, warm running tap water, or electric heating pads if the skin temperature is less than 30–32°C.[2]

Age also has an effect on NCV and latencies. Because of the lack of complete myelination, conduction velocity is significantly less in newborns and infants than in adults. Conduction velocity does not approach adult values until 3–5 years of age.[1] Typically NCVs decrease and distal latencies increase with advancing age, generally beginning after the age of 60 years.[16,22,23,29] More recent studies suggest that this may not be the case in healthy elderly people and that changes in conduction may be secondary to subclinical disease and are not necessarily related to advancing age.[13,15]

Gender and height also have an effect on nerve conduction studies. Height or limb length has more of an effect on nerve conduction than gender. Gender appears to be merely a reflection of changes in height, especially with lower extremity nerve conduction studies.[5,14,15] In general, NCV decreases and distal latency increases as height or limb length increases. Recent literature suggests that gender has an effect on upper extremity nerve conduction parameters.[13,19]

The most common nerves evaluated by conduction studies are the median, ulnar, and radial nerves in the upper extremity and the peroneal, tibial, and sural nerves in the lower extremity. The two similar techniques typically used to evaluate these six nerves differ only in the method of determining the distal stimulation site. One technique identifies an anatomic region from which to stimulate the nerves distally, whereas the other technique uses standard measured distances proximal to the recording electrodes to locate the distal stimulation site. The authors prefer using the measured distance techniques, which are described below for the six nerves.

The motor fibers are evaluated orthodromically by stimulating the nerve 8 cm proximal to the surface recording electrode, which is placed over the motor point of the muscle (Figs. 4 and 5). The sensory nerves are studied antidromically by stimulating the nerve 14 cm proximal to the recording electrode. Ring electrodes are typically placed over the fingers to record sensory action potentials generated from the median and ulnar nerves (see Fig. 4). Sural nerve action potentials are recorded with a surface electrode (see Fig. 5). Radial SNAPs are recorded either with ring electrodes over the thumb or surface electrodes placed over the superficial radial nerve with stimulation 10 cm proximal to the recording ring or surface electrode (see Fig. 4).

Nerve conduction studies of peripheral nerves in asymptomatic individuals have been developed and published in the literature. Some of these data are presented in Table 2 for the median, ulnar, radial, peroneal, tibial, and sural nerves. This normative information can help to determine whether the results from conduction studies are normal. Adherence to temperature control, measurements for stimulation, and other conduction parameters helps to reduce false-positive abnormalities.

### Late Nerve Conduction Responses

Standard conduction studies are used to investigate distal peripheral nerve segments typically restricted to the forearm or leg. Two specialized conduction techniques permit the evaluation of the proximal segments of the peripheral nerve. These studies are known as late responses because of the relatively long time delay from stimulation to generation of action potentials compared with conventional nerve conduction studies.

The F-wave response is a late response that assesses conduction along the motor axon from the anterior horn cell to the muscle. This response is assessed by distal stimulation

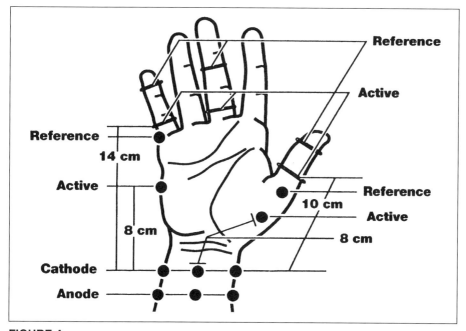

**FIGURE 4.**
Electrode placement and stimulation sites for nerve conduction studies of upper extremity peripheral nerves. (From Falco FJE, Hennessey WJ, Braddom RL, Goldberg G: Standardized nerve conduction studies in the upper limb of the healthy elderly. Am J Phys Med Rehabil 71:263–271, 1992, with permission.)

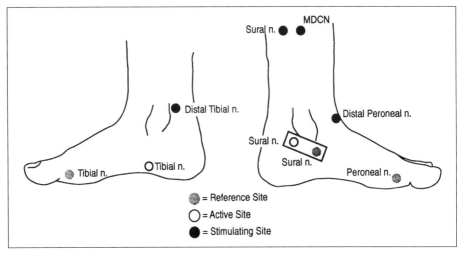

**FIGURE 5.**
Electrode placement and stimulation sites for nerve conduction studies of lower extremity peripheral nerves. (From Falco FJE, Hennessey WJ, Goldberg G, Braddom RL: Standardized nerve conduction studies in the lower limb of the healthy elderly. Am J Phys Med Rehabil 73:168–174, 1994, with permission.)

of a mixed peripheral nerve typically at the wrist, foot, or knee. Because F-wave latencies are much longer than distal motor latencies and significantly smaller than CMAP amplitudes, adjustments are made in the equipment to capture the response on the oscilloscope. The cathode is placed proximal to the anode over the peripheral nerve. An impulse is generated in both directions of the peripheral nerve after maximal stimulation. One impulse travels distally to the muscle, generating a CMAP known as the M (muscle) or direct response. The other impulse travels proximally along the nerve and antidromically activates the motor neurons within the spinal cord. The resulting impulse then propagates orthodromically along the nerve to the muscle, producing a late response known as the F-wave (Fig. 6). The F-wave allows evaluation of the proximal portion of the peripheral nerve, which is helpful in detecting proximal pathology such as early Guillain-Barré syndrome and radiculopathy. The F-wave latency normally increases

**TABLE 2.**
Standard Nerve Conduction Parameters

|  | Nerve | Distal Latency* | Velocity |
|---|---|---|---|
| Motor nerves | Median | 3.7 ± 0.3 msec | 56.7 ± 3.8 m/sec |
|  | Ulnar | 3.2 ± 0.5 msec | 61.8 ± 5.0 m/sec |
|  | Peroneal | 4.5 ± 0.8 msec | 49.9 ± 5.9 m/sec |
|  | Tibial | 3.4 ± 0.5 msec | 54.9 ± 7.6 m/sec |
| Sensory nerves | Median | 3.2 ± 0.2 msec | 56.9 ± 4.0 m/sec |
|  | Ulnar | 3.2 ± 0.25 msec | 57.0 ± 5.0 m/sec |
|  | Radial | 2.3 ± 0.4 msec | — |
|  | Sural | 3.5 ± 0.25 msec | — |

* Motor distal latencies are measured to the onset of the action potential; sensory distal latencies are measured to the peak of the action potential.
From DeLisa JA, MacKenzie K, Baran EM: Manual of Nerve Conduction Velocity and Somatosensory Evoked Potentials, 2nd ed. New York, Raven Press, 1987, with permission.

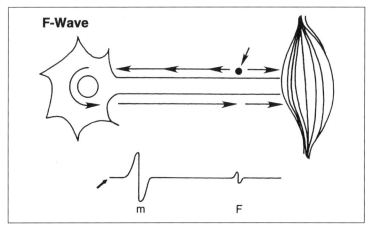

**FIGURE 6.**
F-wave. m = m response, F = F-wave. (From Weber RJ: Motor and sensory conduction and entrapment syndromes. In Johnson EJ (ed): Practical Electromyography, 2nd ed. Baltimore, Williams & Wilkins, 1988, with permission.)

with more distal stimulation along the nerve. The F-wave usually can be elicited from any skeletal muscle in adults.

The H-reflex is the electrodiagnostic equivalent to the monosynaptic reflex arc. Therefore, this conduction study evaluates proximal motor and sensory segments in addition to the spinal cord relay. Although the H-reflex can be elicited in any skeletal muscle of an infant, it can be produced only with stimulation of the tibial nerve and to a lesser degree the median nerve in adults.[10,11,20] The H-reflex latency is affected by temperature, height, and age.

The H-reflex is typically recorded from the soleus muscle with tibial nerve stimulation and the flexor carpi radialis muscle with median nerve stimulation. The cathode is placed proximal to the anode along the nerve. The percutaneous stimulator is adjusted in an attempt to stimulate only the large sensory nerve fibers with submaximal

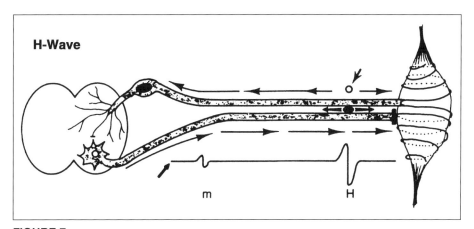

**FIGURE 7.**
H reflex. m = m response, H = H reflex. (From Weber RJ: Motor and sensory conduction and entrapment syndromes. In Johnson EJ (ed): Practical Electromyography, 2nd ed. Baltimore, Williams & Wilkins, 1988, with permission.)

stimulation. The IA afferent sensory fibers are activated, sending an orthodromic sensory impulse towards the spinal cord. The impulse is then relayed via the spinal cord to the anterior horn cells, which are activated and send a motor action potential orthodromically to the distal muscle, producing the H-reflex response (Fig. 7). A direct or M response may precede the H-reflex, depending on whether there was activation of motor fibers during stimulation. The H-reflex can still be obtained in the presence of motor fiber activation, but the H-reflex may be abolished if too many motor fibers are activated during stimulation. One popular explanation is that antidromically produced motor impulses from the stimulation collide with the orthodromically generated motor impulses from the IA fibers, preventing the production of the H-reflex.[24] The H-reflex disappears and is replaced by the F-wave with an increase from submaximal to maximal stimulation.

## SOMATOSENSORY PATHWAY

### Anatomy and Physiology

Light touch, pressure, vibration, and position sensations are transmitted from the periphery to the sensory cortex by the somatosensory pathway (Fig. 8). The sensory fibers that convey this information from the surroundings enter the ipsilateral dorsolateral fasiculus of the spinal cord. These fibers continue in a cephalad direction to the cervicomedullary junction within the dorsal columns and synapse with either the cuneate or gracile nucleus. Axons from these nuclei decussate to the contralateral side of the medulla oblongata, forming the medial lemniscus. These fibers travel rostrally and terminate at either the ventral posterolateral (VPL) or ventral posteromedial (VPM) nuclei. Axons from the VPL and VPM project to the somatosensory cortex.

### Somatosensory-evoked Potentials

Somatosensory-evoked potentials (SSEPs) are performed by stimulating a peripheral nerve and recording the evoked potential over the scalp. Although peripheral nerves can be stimulated percutaneously anywhere along their pathway, typically they are stimulated distally with the cathode oriented proximal to the anode. The large myelinated IA fibers are activated with the lowest threshold for stimulation. The nerve impulses are conducted orthodromically along the somatosensory pathway, terminating at the sensory cortex. The scalp responses are dominated by inputs conducted along the dorsal column pathway, which are the first to arrive at the cortical level. Scalp electrodes are placed over the primary somatosensory cortex using standardized locations from the 10–20 international system (Fig. 9).[21] This system defines electrode placement as either 10% or 20% of the sagittal distance from the nasion to the inion or of the coronal distance between the right and left preauricular areas. Signals are obtained by averaging techniques from electrodes placed along the somatosensory pathway and on the scalp overlying relevant regions of primary somatosensory cortex.

Electrodiagnostic evaluation of the somatosensory pathway from SSEPs allows assessment of proximal portions of sensory nerves as well as the spinal cord, brainstem, midbrain, and cortex. SSEPs are useful in the evaluation of proximal peripheral neuropathies such as Guillain-Barré syndrome. Sometimes SSEPs are used to evaluate proximal peripheral nerve entrapments, such as the lateral femoral cutaneous nerve, that would be more difficult to evaluate with traditional nerve conduction techniques. Plexopathy, myelopathy, multiple sclerosis, traumatic brain injury, and spinal stenosis with myelopathy or multiple radiculopathy are other conditions in which SSEPs can provide useful information. SSEPs are commonly used during scoliosis surgery to monitor the physiologic condition of the spinal cord during distraction of the spine.

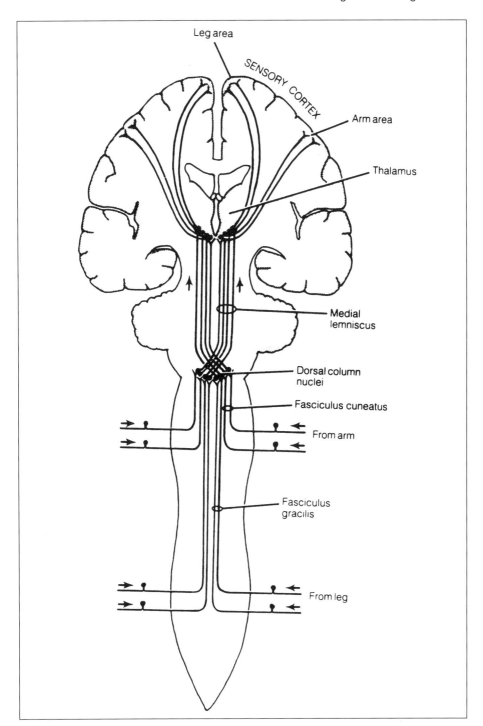

**FIGURE 8.**
Somatosensory pathways. (From deGroot J, Chusid JG: The spinal cord. In deGroot J, Chusid JG (eds): Correlative Neuroanatomy, 2nd ed. East Norwalk, CT, Appleton & Lange, 1988, with permission.)

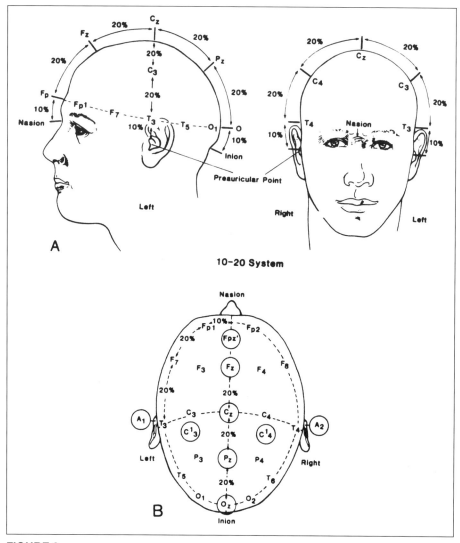

**FIGURE 9.**
International 10-20 system for electrode placement. *A,* Sagittal and coronal views, *B,* Scalp view. (From Jasper H: The ten-twenty electrode system of the international federation. Report of a committee on clinical examination in EEG. Electroencephalogr Clin Neurophysiol 10:371–375, 1958, with permission.)

## MOTOR UNIT

### Anatomy and Physiology

The motor unit is composed of an anterior horn cell, axon, and muscle fibers innervated by the motor axon (Fig. 10). The number of muscle fibers innervated by the motor axon is called the "size" of the motor unit. The size of the motor unit varies according to the function of the muscle. Large muscles that require power have motor units with hundreds to over a thousand muscle fibers. Muscles that perform precision movements, such as the extraoccular muscles, have as low as one fiber per motor unit.

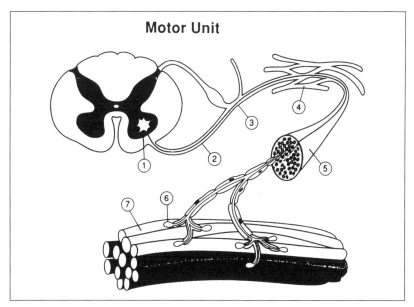

## Motor Unit

**FIGURE 10.**
Motor unit. 1 = anterior horn cell, 2 = nerve root, 3 = spinal nerve, 4 = plexus, 5 = peripheral nerve, 6 = neuromuscular junction, 7 = muscle fiber. (From Dumitru D (ed): Electrodiagnostic Medicine. Philadelphia, Hanley & Belfus, 1995, with permission.)

There are two general types of muscle fibers (Table 3). The fibers are characterized according to their twitch speed. Slow-twitch fibers are designated as type I; they have a slow-twitch speed and high concentration of oxidative enzymes and are resistant

**TABLE 3.**
Muscle Fiber Types

| | | | |
|---|---|---|---|
| Commonly used designations | | | |
| Fiber types | Type I | Type II A | Type II B |
| Twitch and fatigue characteristics | Slow (S) | Fast resistant (FR) | Fast fatigue (FF) |
| Twitch and enzymatic properties | Slow oxidative (SO) | Fast oxidative-glycolytic (FOG) | Fast glycolytic (FG) |
| Properties of muscle fibers | | | |
| Resistance to fatigue | High | High | Low |
| Oxidative enzymes | High | High | Low |
| Phosphorylase (glycolytic) | Low | High | High |
| Adenosine triphosphate | Low | High | High |
| Twitch speed | Low | High | High |
| Twitch tension | Low | High | High |
| Characteristics of motor units | | | |
| Size of cell body | Small | Large | Large |
| Size of motor unit | Small | Large | Large |
| Diameter of axons | Small | Large | Large |
| Conduction velocity | Low | High | High |
| Threshold for recruitment | Low | High | High |
| Firing frequency | Low | High | High |
| Frequency of miniature end-plate potentials | Low | High | High |

From Kimura J: Anatomy and physiology of the skeletal muscle. In Kimura J (ed): Electrodiagnosis in Diseases of Nerve and Muscle: Principles and Practice, 2nd ed. Philadelphia, F.A. Davis, 1989, with permission.

to fatigue. Fast-twitch fibers are designated as type II with several different subcategories. In general, type II fibers have a fast-twitch speed, high concentration of glycolytic enzymes, and a low resistance to fatigue with the exception of type IIA fibers. Each motor unit is composed entirely of either type I or type II fibers. The fiber types are never mixed within a single motor unit, although the muscle itself has varying degrees of each fiber type.

## Electromyography

Needle EMG provides a direct look at the motor unit by measuring the motor unit action potential (MUAP). The MUAP is generated by the simultaneous production of an action potential in the muscle fibers of a single motor unit. As described earlier, several different types of specialized needle electrodes can be inserted into the muscle to measure these potentials. These units are visualized on the oscilloscope during active muscle contraction. The normal MUAP is usually biphasic or triphasic and is therefore a compound muscle fiber action potential. There are several measurable parameters which differentiate normal from abnormal motor units. The amplitude, duration, and number of phases are typically measured during the EMG (Fig. 11). These parameters depend on factors such as age, temperature, anatomic muscle, and contraction strength.

Needle EMG can conveniently be broken down into four steps. The first step involves inserting the EMG needle into the selected muscle while the muscle is at rest. This maneuver evaluates the insertional activity of the muscle, which is characterized as small discharges of electrical activity when the needle passes through normal muscle. The needle is advanced, withdrawn, and readvanced into different directions

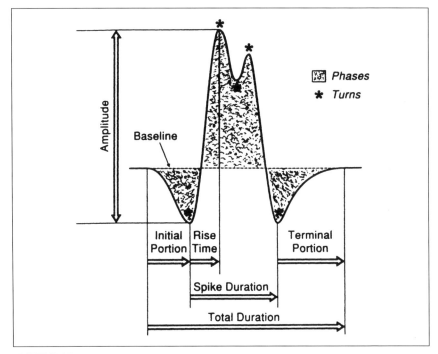

**FIGURE 11.**
Motor unit action potential. (From Dumitru D: Needle electromyography. In Dumitru D (ed): Electrodiagnostic Medicine. Philadelphia, Hanley & Belfus, 1995, with permission.)

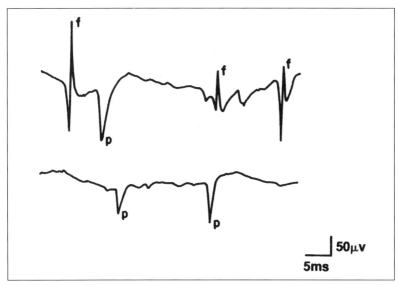

**FIGURE 12.**
Positive sharp waves and fibrillation potentials. f = fibrillation potential, p = positive
sharp wave. (From Dumitru D: Needle electromyography. In Dumitru D (ed): Electrodiagnostic Medicine. Philadelphia, Hanley & Belfus, 1995, with permission.)

within the muscle to evaluate as much of the muscle as possible. An increase or
decrease in insertional activity is considered abnormal but should be correlated with the
rest of the EMG evaluation. The second step involves observing for any muscle activity
with both the needle and muscle at rest. Normal muscle is silent at rest. The presence
of electrical activity in an otherwise motionless muscle is generally abnormal, with the
exception of an electrode located close to an area containing neuromuscular junctions
near the motor point of the muscle. Step three is assessment of the MUAPs during voluntary muscle contraction in terms of amplitude, duration, and number of phases. The
last step is an analysis of the MUAP recruitment in relation to the firing rate or the
number of recruited units. Recruitment can be abnormally slow or fast. Recruited units
are described either as normal or reduced to varying degrees.

Spontaneous activity is characterized by involuntary discharges with the muscle at
rest (step 2 of the EMG evaluation). Normally, muscle fibers should discharge only as
part of a motor unit discharge. Spontaneous discharge of muscle fibers is an indication
of either abnormality of the innervation of the muscle fiber or abnormality intrinsic to
the muscle fiber itself. Spontaneous activity is more commonly present with neurogenic lesions, although they are also present in primary muscle disorders. A spontaneous discharge of a muscle fiber is called a fibrillation and gives rise to a characteristic
electrical signal called a *fibrillation potential.* Fibrillation potentials are biphasic or
triphasic waveforms of short duration and small amplitudes. They have an initial positive deflection and are spikelike in appearance. Positive sharp waves are similar to fibrillation potentials in that they have an initial positive deflection but differ in that they
have a longer duration and sawtooth appearance (Fig. 12). Positive sharp waves and
fibrillation potentials appear in muscle 1–3 weeks after denervation.[4,30]

Fasciculations, myokymic potentials, and complex repetitive discharges are other
forms of spontaneous electrical activity that may be encountered during an EMG study.
In contrast to a fibrillation and positive sharp wave, which occur at the muscle fiber
level, a *fasciculation* is the spontaneous discharge of a motor unit and is associated with

lower motor neuron disorders, such as poliomyelitis, amyotrophic lateral sclerosis, and spinal muscular atrophy. Fasciculations also may be seen in chronic peripheral nerve or nerve root entrapments resulting in motor fiber irritation. *Myokymia* represents spontaneous repetitive discharges of a motor unit and is observed in multiple sclerosis, radiation plexopathy, hyperventilation-induced hypocalcemia, and Guillain-Barré syndrome. *Complex repetitive discharges* (CRDs) result from the formation of closed electrical circuits within the muscle that fire repetitively at high rates for short periods that begin and stop abruptly. The CRDs can be seen with chronic polyneuropathies, radiculopathy, polymyositis, Duchenne muscular dystrophy, and spinal muscular atrophy.

MUAP disturbances detected by needle EMG result from one of two possible types of lesions. A neurogenic lesion involves the lower motor neuron, whereas a myogenic lesion involves the muscle. A chronic neurogenic lesion is characterized by MUAPs with long durations and increased amplitudes. The increased amplitude and duration are due to the creation of larger units through the incorporation of denervated muscle fibers into surviving motor units by means of collateral sprouting of motor axons. These types of potentials are seen in chronic poliomyelitis, radiculopathy, peripheral nerve entrapment, chronic neuropathy, and amyotrophic lateral sclerosis. MUAPs representative of myogenic lesions are smaller in amplitude and duration. These changes in the MUAP result from muscle fiber degeneration or dysfunction within the territory of the motor unit. The number of functioning muscle fibers in the motor unit decreases. Myogenic MUAPs are seen in primary myopathies, polymyositis, and myasthenia gravis. Evaluation of the MUAP amplitude and duration helps to distinguish primary disorders of the lower motor neuron from disorders of the muscle.

Motor unit potentials in normal muscle are biphasic or triphasic, although up to one-third may be polyphasic.[6] A polyphasic motor unit is a potential with five or more phases. An increase in the number of polyphasic MUAPs is due to an increase in temporal dispersion, which in turn is due to the asynchrony of muscle fibers discharging within the motor units of surviving axons of a neurogenic lesion. Muscle fibers are incorporated into existing motor units by axonal sprouting. The axons that reach the denervated fibers are small and thinly myelinated. These immature axons transmit impulses more slowly to the newly embraced fibers, resulting in temporal dispersion of the activation of muscle fibers in the motor unit and a polyphasic MUAP results. An increase in the number of polyphasic MUAPs is an indication of ongoing reinnervation. The temporal dispersion eventually resolves as the axons mature and the polyphasic effects reverse. This resolution is a manifestation of maturation of the motor axon sprouts, which results in greater synchrony of activation of the muscle fibers in the expanded motor unit.

MUAP recruitment during voluntary contraction is helpful in the differentiation of lower motor neuron disorders from myopathies. The number of available motor units that can be recruited is decreased in disorders involving the lower motor neuron. As a result, the remaining motor units have to fire at a faster rate to provide the same contractile force. Therefore, recruitment in the presence of a neurogenic lesion displays on the oscilloscope fewer motor units that fire at a more rapid rate. In myogenic lesions, the available number of motor units is unchanged, but the force generated by each unit is decreased. Consequently, more motor units have to fire to produce the necessary contractile force. Therefore, recruitment of motor units is greater and more rapid than expected in myopathic disorders when the patient attempts to generate muscular force. Activated motor units rapidly increase their firing rate to a maximal level.

Muscle weakness that is modified by the performance of exercise may be due to neuromuscular junction pathology. Junctional transmission pathophysiology can be detected by electrodiagnostic methods. Myasthenia gravis, a neuromuscular junction disorder affecting the number of acetylcholine receptors on the postsynaptic membrane surface, is characterized by weakness, especially of facial and jaw muscles, that increases with muscle use. Lambert-Eaton myasthenic syndrome (LEMS) is a presynaptic neuromuscular junction disorder manifested by an improvement in strength immediately after a period of exercise. LEMS appears to be an abnormality of the voltage-activated calcium channels in the membrane of the presynaptic terminal.

Both conditions have specific physiologic effects that permit diagnosis through the use of a repetitive nerve stimulation technique as well as by examining the effect of muscle exercise on neuromuscular transmission. This is accomplished by looking at the CMAP amplitude produced by nerve stimulation before and after the performance of a sustained isometric muscle contraction for 1 minute. In myasthenia gravis, the effect of exercise is initially to correct a decrement in the CMAP amplitude associated with repetitive nerve stimulation at approximately 3 stimuli per second. One minute after exercise, during the period of posttetanic exhaustion, the decrement is exaggerated beyond that initially seen before exercise. In LEMS, the effect of exercise is to increase the CMAP amplitude significantly with repetitive nerve stimulation performed immediately after exercise. Electrodiagnostic studies can be extremely helpful in establishing a specific diagnosis in these rare conditions associated with general muscular weakness modified by exercise.

## SOFT TISSUE NEUROMUSCULAR DISORDERS

### Compression Mononeuropathy

Nerve conduction studies are helpful in determining the presence of a peripheral nerve entrapment syndrome, sometimes referred to as a compression mononeuropathy. These disorders typically result from local compression of the peripheral nerve and are often associated with repetitive trauma and/or nerve stretch. One of the best-recognized entrapment syndromes commonly related to repetitive trauma is carpal tunnel syndrome, which involves compression of the median nerve at the wrist. It is the most common entrapment syndrome among industrial workers as well as in the general population.

A compression neuropathy results from sustained injury to a nerve either from chronic repetitive injury or continuous compression. It may be the result of a cumulative trauma disorder or mechanical compression from arthritis or trauma. The compressive effects to the nerve have been classified according to the degree of structural changes. The physical effects from the compression lead to physiologic changes in the nerve that can be assessed with nerve conduction studies.

Neurapraxia, axonotmesis, and neurotmesis are the three categories used to describe nerve injury. Neurapraxia results from local demyelination of some of the axons within the nerve due to mechanical compression. This condition leads to a decrease in the number of impulses that can pass the obstruction, i.e., conduction block, and may result in weakness or sensory abnormalities such as paresthesia or anesthesia in the distribution of the nerve. Focal nerve conduction slowing across the region of myelin disruption is also typically seen. Nerve conduction studies document the conduction block from neurapraxia by stimulating the nerve proximal and distal to the entrapment (Fig. 13). With stimulation proximal to the conduction block, the resulting action potential typically has a delayed distal latency, which may be abnormally slowed because of local demyelination of some of the axons. In addition, the action potential amplitude produced with proximal stimulation is smaller than that generated distally because of the conduction block involving some of the axons affected by the entrapment.

In axonotmesis and neurotmesis, the degree of nerve damage is significant enough to result in axonal death and resorption. The difference between these two

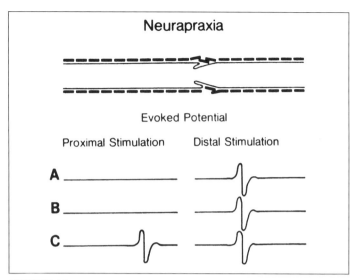

**FIGURE 13.**
Neurapraxia. A = total conduction block immediately after injury, B = total conduction block one week after injury, C = resolution of neurapraxia several weeks after injury. (From Weber RJ: Motor and sensory conduction and entrapment syndromes. In Johnson EJ (ed): Practical Electromyography, 2nd ed. Baltimore, Williams & Wilkins, 1988, with permission.)

conditions is the extent to which supporting structures of the axon are affected by the injury. Axonotmesis typically results from an acute or chronic nerve compression that affects the axon and myelin sheath but does not harm the supporting tissues. Neurotmesis, on the other hand, is the complete separation of the nerve, such as a laceration injury, which disrupts all of the supporting structures in addition to the axon and myelin sheath. This process has a profound effect on nerve regeneration after the injury. Nerve regeneration after an axonotmetic lesion is more likely because of the intact supporting structures, including the nerve sheath. In contrast, nerve regeneration is often incomplete and disorganized after a neurotmetic insult, which may lead to misdirected reinnervation resulting in neuroma formation or synkinesis.

The degeneration of the distal axonal segment and myelin sheath that occurs with axonotmesis or neurotmesis is known as Wallerian degeneration. Loss of conduction across the level of injury occurs immediately after the axon is disrupted by either axonotmesis or neurotmesis. Axonal stimulation proximal to the injury site does not produce a distal action potential because the impulse is not conducted across the disrupted axon (Fig. 14). Distal axon excitability may remain intact for 4–5 days after the injury until the completion of Wallerian degeneration.[17] During this interval, it is difficult to distinguish a neurapraxic lesion with complete conduction block due to focal demyelination from axonotmesis or neurotmesis with nerve conduction studies. When Wallerian degeneration is complete, with development of secondary changes in the denervated muscle fibers, fibrillations and positive sharp waves are then seen in the affected muscles. This process may take 2–3 weeks, depending on the length of the affected axons. Needle EMG is not helpful in differentiating neurapraxia from axonotmesis in the acute period because of this delay.

Nerve conduction studies are helpful in determining the presence or absence of peripheral nerve entrapment. A compression neuropathy is usually characterized by a neurapraxic or mixed neurapraxic/axonotmetic lesion, depending on the extent of the

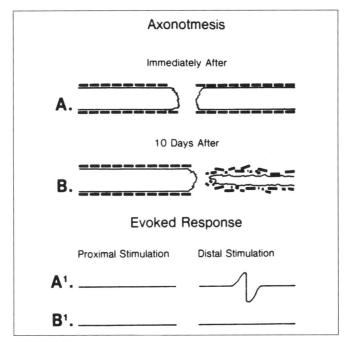

**FIGURE 14.**
Axonotmesis. A = immediately after injury, B = 10 days after injury, A¹ = evoked response immediately after injury with proximal and distal stimulation, B¹ = evoked response 10 days after injury with proximal and distal stimulation. (From Weber RJ: Motor and sensory conduction and entrapment syndromes. In Johnson EJ (ed): Practical Electromyography, 2nd ed. Baltimore, Williams & Wilkins, 1988, with permission.)

injury. Nerve entrapments rarely lead to a complete axonotmetic lesion. Sensory and/or motor fibers can be affected by different degrees by an entrapment syndrome, as assessed with the combination of motor and sensory nerve conduction studies.

Distal nerve compression neuropathies, such as carpal tunnel syndrome (median nerve entrapment at the wrist), reveal specific findings on nerve conduction studies. The distal latency is abnormally prolonged because the site of stimulation is proximal to the site of compression. Segmental nerve conduction velocity across the level of involvement is decreased because of local demyelination of the compressed nerve segment. As described earlier, the action potential amplitude may be increased with stimulation distal to the site of entrapment, indicating that distal axons beyond the point of demyelination continue to conduct in a relatively normal manner.

More proximal peripheral nerve entrapments, such as cubital tunnel syndrome or tardy ulnar palsy (entrapments of the ulnar nerve at the elbow), display similar findings from nerve conduction studies when there is focal demyelination of the nerve at the level of injury. Although the distal latency is normal because the site of stimulation is distal to the entrapment, the conduction time is abnormally prolonged and the conduction velocity of the involved nerve segment is decreased. The same changes in the action potential amplitude are seen with stimulation distal and proximal to the site of entrapment.

One common conduction technique used to increase sensitivity in detecting an entrapment neuropathy is comparison of the distal latency of the presumed entrapped nerve with another peripheral nerve. Abnormalities are detected by a statistically significant prolongation in conduction time of the affected nerve relative to the unaffected nerve. This technique is helpful in detecting nerve entrapments of milder degrees; it is routinely used to study a patient suspected of having carpal tunnel syndrome when traditional conduction studies are normal. Distal latencies of the median nerve can be compared with the ulnar or radial nerve to detect a relative slowing of median nerve conduction across the carpal tunnel.

EMG helps to determine whether a compression neuropathy has led to loss of motor axons through Wallerian degeneration. Entrapments are typically either neurapraxic or a mixed neurapraxic and axonotmetic lesion. If an entrapment syndrome is purely neurapraxic, the prognosis for full restoration of nerve function is better than in the presence of significant denervation. The greater the degree of denervation, the less likely that conservative treatment will be successful in managing the entrapment.

Electrodiagnostic evaluations are indicated in patients suspected of having nerve compression injuries that have not responded to conservative treatment. Electrodiagnostics not only establishes the diagnosis but also rules out other conditions, such as radiculopathy or peripheral neuropathy. Electrodiagnostic studies also help to determine prognosis and whether surgery is indicated to preserve nerve function.

## Radiculopathy

Radiculopathy leads to nerve root dysfunction, which results in specific signs and symptoms within the distribution of the affected nerve root. The injury typically occurs proximal to the peripheral sensory nerve cell, the dorsal root ganglion (DRG). One (monoradiculopathy) or multiple (polyradiculopathy) nerve roots may be involved, depending on the extent of the disorder. Sensory and/or motor fibers are involved, resulting in clinical findings that often follow precise dermatomal and/or myotomal patterns. Radiculopathies may be caused by soft tissue disorders such as disc herniation, ligamentous constriction, or tumor. They may result from bony encroachment of the nerve roots, such as foraminal or lateral recess stenosis. Radiculopathies are also thought to result from inflammatory components that are released from degenerated intervertebral discs and lead to chemically mediated nerve root injury or from inflammation in response to herniated disc material.

The electrodiagnostic evaluation can be invaluable in the assessment of a patient suspected of having a radiculopathy. Electrodiagnostic studies not only determine the specific nerve root level involved, but also exclude other neurologic conditions, such as peripheral neuropathy or compression neuropathy.

Sensory nerve conduction studies are usually unaffected in the presence of a radiculopathy because the site of injury is often proximal to the DRG. Abnormal findings during sensory nerve studies indicate an injury distal to the nerve root. Conduction studies of motor nerves may reveal a drop in CMAP amplitude due to Wallerian degeneration if there is an axonotmetic injury to the nerve root. On rare occasions a drop in nerve root conduction velocity may be associated with a severe loss of axons. Neurapraxic nerve root injuries have no effect on peripheral motor conduction parameters.

Late responses assist in the evaluation of suspected radiculopathies because they allow evaluation of the proximal portion of the nerve, including the root. Unfortunately, F-wave studies are rarely abnormal in the presence of radiculopathy for a number of reasons. F-waves evaluate motor fibers along the entire length of the nerve, and abnormality at the root level may be masked by the rest of the nerve. Because F-waves are recorded in muscles with more than one nerve root, slowing along the affected root may be obscured by the other normal conducting root levels. Another drawback with F-wave studies is that an abnormality may be due to injury anywhere along the motor nerve and not necessarily at the root level.

H reflex studies are more helpful than F-waves in evaluating radiculopathies, because both motor and sensory fibers at the root level are assessed. In the early stages of a radiculopathy, the H reflex may be the only identifiable electrodiagnostic abnormality, because EMG changes take 2–3 weeks to develop. Although the H reflex is sometimes helpful in the evaluation of radiculopathy, it has several drawbacks. The H reflex is elicitable in adults only from the soleus muscle on a consistent basis. Therefore, only the S1 nerve root can be evaluated by this technique. Abnormal H reflex results do not necessarily reflect an abnormality at the root level; the abnormality may be anywhere along the motor or sensory nerves that make up the reflex arc. Because an unelicitable H reflex from a previous S1 radiculopathy typically is permanent, later H reflex testing is not helpful.

Needle EMG gives the most information about a radiculopathy. A study is consistent for radiculopathy if two or more muscles within the distribution of a nerve root supplied by different peripheral nerves are abnormal and muscles receiving innervation from adjacent nerve roots are unaffected. Needle EMG findings can objectively determine the acuteness or chronicity of the radiculopathy, the degree of denervation, and prognosis for recovery. Although it takes 2–3 weeks before denervation findings from Wallerian degeneration are manifested by needle EMG, a decrease in recruitment of motor units can be detected on volition early in the radiculopathy. This finding may be present in neurapraxic as well as axonotmetic root dysfunction.

Although very helpful, the needle EMG evaluation has several shortcomings. Radiculopathies more commonly affect sensory nerve root fibers only; the EMG is normal in the presence of sensory radiculopathies. Needle EMG is normal early in the development of a radiculopathy affecting motor fibers because of the absence of denervation potentials and in radiculopathies secondary to neurapraxic injuries. The EMG study can determine the presence of a radiculopathy but not the underlying cause.

SSEPs complement nerve conduction studies and needle EMG especially in the evaluation of a sensory radiculopathy. The SSEP study allows evaluation of sensory fibers at the nerve root level. No other standard conduction technique can evaluate the proximal sensory nerve with the exception of the H reflex study. The SSEPs typically are more sensitive in detecting polyradiculopathies than abnormalities involving a single root level because the peripheral nerves are made up of multiple nerve roots that may obscure the presence of a monoradiculopathy. Cutaneous nerve stimulation can be used instead of mixed nerve stimulation to try to restrict conduction to a single nerve root level. Direct stimulation of the skin in the middle of a dermatome also has been advocated as a way to evaluate single root levels. A normal study may result, regardless of the peripheral stimulation method, because the long somatosensory pathway may diminish any abnormalities over the relatively short root segment.

Electrodiagnostic studies are indicated in a patient suspected of having a radiculopathy when there has been no clinical improvement or when symptoms have progressed. Electrodiagnostic testing is also helpful in the patient with vague symptoms involving an extremity to rule out radiculopathy and other conditions such as peripheral neuropathy or compression mononeuropathy. Although imaging studies can document anatomic abnormalities, such as a herniated disc or spinal stenosis, electrodiagnostic studies can detect the presence of associated nerve root dysfunction and determine the clinical significance of anatomic abnormalities. Needle EMG can determine the specific level or levels involved in radiculopathy and thus may assist in surgical planning when imaging studies are equivocal.

## Peripheral Neuropathy

The fact that many disorders can produce peripheral neuropathies presents a diagnostic dilemma to the clinician (Table 4). Making the proper diagnosis can be difficult despite a thorough history, physical examination, and diagnostic testing. Physicians frequently refer patients for electrodiagnostic testing to confirm or rule out the presence

**TABLE 4.**
Disorders Associated with Peripheral Neuropathies

| Axonal | Demyelinating |
|---|---|
| Critical illness | Guillain-Barré syndrome |
| HIV infection | HIV infection |
| Collagen vascular diseases | Hepatitis B |
| Amyloidosis | Epstein-Barr virus |
| Cryoglobulinemia | Cytomegalovirus |
| Sarcoidosis | Toxoplasmosis |
| Lyme disease | Lyme disease |
| Antibiotics | Systemic lupus erythematosus |
| Chemotherapeutic agents | Diphtheria |
| Heavy metals | Chronic inflammatory polyneuropathy |
| Vitamin deficiencies | Waldenström's macroglobulinemia |
| Malabsorption | Osteosclerotic myeloma |
| Diabetes | Diabetes |
| Chronic renal failure | Amiodarone toxicity |
| Hypothyroidism | Hypothyroidism |
| Hyperlipidemia | Monoclonal gammopathy |
| Hepatic failure | Leukoencephalopathies |
| Chronic obstructive pulmonary disease | Buckthorn berry intoxication |
| Hereditary motor-sensory neuropathy (types II, V) | Hereditary motor-sensory neuropathy (types I, II, IV) |
| Porphyria | Lymphoma |

of a peripheral neuropathy. Electrodiagnostic testing is helpful in determining the existence of a peripheral neuropathy and may assist in the diagnosis. Peripheral neuropathies can be characterized as either a primary demyelinating process or a condition associated with loss of axons. Although nerve conduction studies rarely lead to a specific diagnosis, they can identify whether the peripheral neuropathy is demyelinating or axonal (see Table 4). This information, when integrated with the clinical presentation of the neuropathy, often leads to a correct diagnosis or to the appropriate selection of further diagnostic studies.

Peripheral neuropathies that lead to the loss of myelin primarily affect nerve conduction (Fig. 15). Although peripheral neuropathies tend to involve all segments of the nerve, the distal nerve segments in the extremities are usually most affected. Therefore, ordinary nerve conduction studies can uncover demyelinating effects in distal nerve segments by revealing decreased nerve conduction velocity, prolongation of distal latencies, and increased temporal dispersion. In certain instances, such as Guillain-Barré syndrome or diabetes mellitus, peripheral neuropathies affect nerve roots or proximal portions of peripheral nerves. The proximal nerve segments can be evaluated with F-wave, H reflex, and SSEP testing.

Neuropathies that affect primarily the axon as opposed to the myelin have the most substantial effect on action potential amplitude (see Fig. 15). The amplitude is directly dependent on the axonal diameter and number of axons. The recorded nerve or muscle action potential amplitude will decrease with a reduction in axonal diameter or in the number of normally conducting axons. Therefore, peripheral axonal neuropathies routinely result in a drop in amplitude. Because the myelin is not affected by axonal neuropathies, the nerve conduction velocity is typically preserved as long as

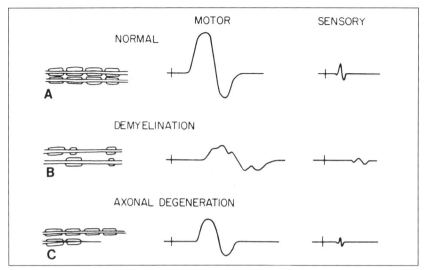

**FIGURE 15.**
Peripheral neuropathy. A = evoked potentials in normal axons, B = evoked potentials in axons undergoing segmental demyelination, C = evoked potentials in axons undergoing axonal degeneration. (From Kraft GH: Peripheral neuropathies. In Johnson EJ (ed): Practical Electromyography, 2nd ed. Baltimore, Williams & Wilkins, 1988, with permission.)

some axons still function normally. Conversely, the nerve conduction velocity may be slowed in the presence of a severe axonal neuropathy with extensive loss of myelinated fibers.

EMG also plays an important role in the evaluation of peripheral neuropathy and helps to distinguish a demyelinating process from an axonal disorder. Sampling muscles at rest in the presence of a purely demyelinating neuropathy does not reveal an increase in insertional activity or abnormal spontaneous activity. In contrast, needle EMG reveals positive sharp wave and fibrillation potentials in the distal muscles affected by an axonal neuropathy. Demyelinating neuropathies affect the myelin along different segments of the axons within the nerve. As a consequence, impulses traveling along the different axons do not reach the muscle at the same time. This may lead to voluntary MUAPs with an increase in duration and possibly a decrease in amplitude. Voluntary MUAPs in an axonal neuropathy are typically polyphasic and have an increase in duration. Over time, the MUAPs display an increase in amplitude as reinnervation and reorganization of the motor unit occur.

Nerve conduction studies and EMG can distinguish between demyelinating and axonal peripheral neuropathies. They also may be used to assess any differential effect on sensory fibers compared with motor fibers and thus help the treating physician to eliminate specific disease processes that may be responsible for the neuropathy. This information, along with the clinical presentation of the neuropathy and appropriate additional diagnostic testing, can further narrow down the potential causes of the neuropathy. Although peripheral neuropathies can be classified as either primarily demyelinating or axonal, secondary axonal degeneration or demyelination, respectively, may be associated with the primary process. Some peripheral neuropathies present as a combination of a demyelinating and axonal process, producing a mixed picture.

Electrodiagnostic evaluations are indicated as part of any complete work-up of a patient suspected of having a peripheral neuropathy. Although electrodiagnostic testing can determine the presence of a peripheral neuropathy, it cannot establish specific diagnoses. Nevertheless, electrodiagnostic tests play an integral role and help the clinician by establishing the presence of the peripheral neuropathy and ruling out other potential disorders, such as radiculopathy, compression neuropathies, and myopathy.

## Myopathy

Primary muscle disorders that lead to generalized clinical weakness are best detected by needle EMG. A thorough review of myopathic disorders is beyond the scope of this chapter.

Certain findings on the needle electromyogram are characteristic of a myopathic process. Initially, the MUAP has a short duration and a low amplitude, which reflect the loss of muscle fibers with the distribution of the motor unit. Late in the myopathic progress, the duration of the MUAP increases as it becomes polyphasic with the incorporation of late components. The motor units are less capable of developing force with voluntary contraction because of the loss of muscle fibers. Therefore, more motor units have to be activated to produce a specific degree of strength with contraction. This phenomenon is displayed during EMG as an increase in the recruitment frequency of motor units with minimal contraction. Very late in their course, myopathic processes are associated with a significant amount of fiber degeneration, and the muscle is replaced by fibrous tissue. In this late stage, insertion activity decreases because of the loss of muscle tissue, and the dysfunctional muscle shows little if any electrical activity.

In the work-up of myopathy, care must be taken in coordinating certain tests with EMG studies. A muscle biopsy should not be taken from a muscle recently examined with needle EMG, and creatine phosphokinase levels should be drawn before the EMG examination.

## Myelopathy

Electrodiagnostic tests have been used to evaluate patients suspected of having injuries to the spinal cord or a disease process affecting the central nervous system (CNS). Typically nerve conduction studies are not helpful in evaluating the CNS with the exception of F-wave and H reflex studies, which may reveal prolonged latencies at the involved level. Needle EMG usually displays decreased recruitment but is otherwise unremarkable. SSEPs allow complete evaluation of the dorsal column sensory pathway within the CNS, including the spinal cord.

Spinal stenosis at any level within the spine can lead to myelopathy. SSEPs can determine the effect of stenosis on spinal cord function within the posterior column sensory pathways. Spinal stenosis commonly involves multiple roots. Therefore, stimulation of peripheral nerves representing multiple nerve roots, such as the peroneal or tibial nerves, are more sensitive in detecting spinal cord compression from cervical spinal stenosis. SSEPs have several shortcomings in evaluating stenosis. The SSEPs are generally nonspecific for spinal cord lesions and do not differentiate stenosis from other possible disorders. The SSEPs also do not necessarily correlate with the clinical presentation of a patient with cervical stenosis.[31]

Motor-evoked potentials with magnetic stimulation of the motor cortex have been investigated over the past 10 years as a means of evaluating the motor pathways of the spinal cord. Electrical stimulation of the motor cortex has been used in the past. The advantages of magnetic over electrical stimulation include deeper penetration of brain structures and little to no discomfort to the patient. Full approval of cortical stimulation by the Food and Drug Administration is currently lacking. Evaluation of the motor pathways by motor-evoked potentials would complement SSEPs by providing a more complete electrophysiologic assessment of spinal cord function.

SSEPs have been used in several different clinical settings to evaluate the spinal cord, including spine surgery, aorta bypass/resection surgery, and spinal stenosis.

Scoliosis surgery is the most common surgical procedure that uses SSEPs to monitor spinal cord function; it involves a 1% chance of spinal cord injury due to vascular insufficiency.[27] The "wake-up" test has been used to monitor neurologic function during surgery; the patient is intermittently awakened and asked to move the extremities. This method of spinal cord monitoring is limited by the intermittent nature of the observations and the lack of sensory testing. SSEPs allow continuous monitoring of the sensory pathways during surgery under general anesthesia. Only halogenated agents used for anesthesia have a profound effect on the recordability of the SSEPs. The one limitation of SSEPs is that they do not evaluate the motor function of the spinal cord. Despite this shortcoming, the presence of intraoperative SSEPs without decrement has a high correlation with the absence of motor and sensory neurologic function after scoliosis surgery. The success of SSEP monitoring during scoliosis surgery has encouraged surgeons to apply this method of monitoring to other types of spinal surgery, including fusion procedures and spinal cord tumor resections. SSEP monitoring also has been used during aortic aneurysm or bypass surgery to evaluate spinal cord function, which may be compromised by ischemia during surgery.

## CONTRAINDICATIONS AND COMPLICATIONS

Patients with bleeding disorders or patients receiving antiplatelet or anticoagulant therapy may be referred for electrodiagnostic testing. There has been one report of a bleeding complication from needle EMG in a patient with prolonged prothrombin time (PT) and partial thromboplastin time (PTT).[3] The risk of bleeding is increased with platelet counts that are less than 50,000 and a PT or PTT greater than 1.5–2 times control.[25,26] Thus electrodiagnostic testing, especially needle EMG, may be relatively contraindicated in patients who have bleeding disorders or receive anticoagulation. Such patients need to be evaluated on a case-by-case basis.

The advent of disposable needles has allowed safe evaluation of patients with transmissible disorders such as hepatitis, HIV infection, and Jakob-Creutzfeldt disease. Strict universal precautions should be used with all patients undergoing electrodiagnostic testing. Precautions should include the use of gloves and proper protocol for limiting inadvertent skin puncture during handling of EMG needle electrodes.

In general, electrodiagnostic studies involve little risk for patients with implanted pacemakers. The patient should be properly grounded before the nerve conduction studies are begun. The risk of inhibiting the pacemaker is greater with percutaneous nerve stimulation close to the pacemaker than distally in the extremities. Stimulation of the brachial plexus ipsilateral to the pacemaker should be performed with caution. Nerve conduction studies are *not* recommended in patients with external pacemakers with external conducting leads that terminate in or near the heart.

Special attention to proper grounding is advised in performing nerve conduction studies of critically ill patients with multiple catheters and electrical monitoring equipment. If possible, all nonessential equipment should be disconnected and catheter sites dried and covered in an attempt to prevent leakage current, which may pass through the patient with serious complications.

Needle EMG of the intercostal, scapular, cervicothoracic paraspinal, and abdominal muscles risks the development of pneumothorax; peritonitis is also a risk in needle EMG of abdominal muscles. The use of small-diameter EMG needles and sterile technique helps to reduce the risk of complication during the needle EMG of these regions. The risk of developing soft tissue infection during needle EMG of the extremities is remote; nonetheless, the study should be performed with fully sterilized electrodes that are not allowed to become contaminated during the study.

## CONCLUSION

The electrodiagnostic evaluation is an adjunct to a complete history and physical evaluation of a patient with a suspected soft tissue, musculoskeletal injury. Electro-diagnostic studies are helpful in the evaluation of soft tissue pain complicated by muscular weakness or other sensory disturbances suggesting impairment of the peripheral nervous system. They are also helpful in the evaluation of patients thought to have compression mononeuropathy, radiculopathy, or peripheral neuropathy. Electrodiagnostic tests assist with the differential diagnosis of soft tissue injuries by determining their presence or absence. They also provide prognostic information by measuring the extent and nature of neuromuscular compromise as well as determining the degree of recovery.

## REFERENCES

1. Baer RD, Johnson EW: Motor nerve conduction velocities in normal children. Arch Phys Med Rehabil 46:698–704, 1965.
2. Bolton CF, Sawa GM, Carter K: The effects of temperature on human compound action potentials. J Neurol Neurosurg Psychiatry 44:407–414, 1981.
3. Braddom RL, Johnson EW: Standardization of H reflex and diagnostic use in S1 radiculopathy. Arch Phys Med Rehabil 55:161–166, 1974.
4. Buchthal F, Rosenfalck P: Spontaneous electrical activity of human muscle. Electroenceph Clin Neurophysiol 20:321–336, 1966.
5. Campbell WW, Ward LC, Swift TR: Nerve conduction velocity varies inversely with height. Muscle Nerve 4:520–523, 1981.
6. Chu-Andrews J, Johnson RJ: Electrodiagnosis: An Anatomical and Clinical Approach. Philadelphia, J.B. Lippincott, 1986, pp 232–235.
7. deGroot J, Chusid JG: Signaling in the nervous system. In deGroot J, Chusid JG (eds): Correlative Neuroanatomy, 2nd ed. East Norwalk, CT, Appleton & Lange, 1988, pp 22–31.
8. DeJesus PV, Huasmanowa-Petrusewicz I, Brachi RL: The effect of cold on nerve conduction of human slow and fast nerve fibers. Neurology 23:1182–1189, 1973.
9. Denys EH: The influence of temperature in clinical neurophysiology. Muscle Nerve 14:795–811, 1991.
10. Deschuytere J, Rosselle N: Identification of certain EMG patterns of spinal cord reflexive activity in man. Electrophysiological study of discharges from spinal origin in anterolateral muscles of leg in normal adults. Electromyogr Clin Neurophysiol 11:331–363, 1971.
11. Deschuytere J, Rosselle N: Identification of certain EMG patterns of spinal cord reflexive activity in man. Electrophysiological study of discharges from spinal origin in forearm flexors in normal adults. Electromyogr Clin Neurophysiol 14:497–511, 1974.
12. El-Nagamy E, Sedgwick EM: Delayed cervical somatosensory potentials in cervical spondylosis. J Neurol Neurosurg Psychiatry 42:238–241, 1979.
13. Falco FJE, Hennessey WJ, Braddom RL, Goldberg G: Standardized nerve conduction studies in the upper limb of the healthy elderly. Am J Phys Med Rehabil 71:263–271, 1992.
14. Falco FJE, Hennessey WJ, Goldberg G, Braddom RL: H reflex latency in the healthy elderly. Muscle Nerve 17:161–167, 1994.
15. Falco FJE, Hennessey WJ, Goldberg G, Braddom RL: Standardized nerve conduction studies in the lower limb of the healthy elderly. Am J Phys Med Rehabil 73:168–174, 1994.
16. Ganeriwal SK, Reddy BV, Surdi AD, et al: Influence of age on motor nerve conduction. Indian J Physiol Pharmacol 27:337–341, 1983.
17. Gilliatt RW, Taylor JC: Electrical changes following section of the facial nerve. Proc R Soc Med 52:1080–1083, 1959.
18. Halar EM, DeLisa JA, Soine TL: Nerve conduction studies in the upper extremities: Skin temperature corrections. Arch Phys Med Rehabil 66:605–609, 1985.
19. Hennessey WJ, Falco FJE, Goldberg G, Braddom RL: Gender and arm length: Influence on nerve conduction parameters in the upper limb. Arch Phys Med Rehabil 75:265–269, 1994.
20. Jabre JF: Surface recording of the H-reflex of the flexor carpi radialis. Muscle Nerve 4:435–438, 1981.
21. Jasper H: The ten-twenty electrode system of the international federation. Report of a committee on clinical examination in EEG. Electroencephalogr Clin Neurophysiol 10:371–375, 1958.
22. LaFratta CW, Canestrari RE: A comparison of sensory and motor nerve conduction velocities as related to age. Arch Phys Med Rehabil 47:286–290, 1966.
23. LaFratta CW, Smith OH: A study of the relationship of motor conduction velocity in the adult to age, sex, and handedness. Arch Phys Med Rehabil 45:407–412, 1964.

24. Magladery JW, McDougal DB: Electrophysiological studies of nerve and reflex activity in normal man. I: Identification of certain reflexes in the electromyogram and the conduction velocity of peripheral nerve fibres. Bull Johns Hopkins Hosp 86:265–290, 1950.

25. Marcus AJ: Hemorrhagic disorders: Abnormalities of platelet and vascular function. In Wyngaarden JB, Smith LH (eds): Cecil Textbook of Medicine, 17th ed. Philadelphia, W.B. Saunders, 1985, pp 1028–1040.

26. McKee PA: Disorders of blood coagulation. In Wyngaarden JB, Smith LH (eds): Cecil Textbook of Medicine, 17th ed. Philadelphia, W.B. Saunders, 1985, pp 1040–1058.

27. Nash CL, Brown RH: The intraoperative monitoring of spinal cord function: Its growth and current status. Orthop Clin North Am 1:919–926, 1979.

28. Siivola J, Sulg I, Heiskari M: SSEPs in diagnostics of cervical spondylosis and herniated disc. Electroenceph Clin Neurophysiol 52:276–282, 1981.

29. Taylor PK: Non-linear effects of age on nerve conduction in adults. J Neurol Sci 66:223–234, 1984.

30. Trojaborg W: Early electrophysiologic changes in conduction block. Muscle Nerve 1:400–403, 1978.

31. Yu YL, Jones SJ: Somatosensory evoked potentials in cervical spondylosis. Brain 108:273–300, 1985.

## 17

# General Principles of Rehabilitation of Musculoskeletal Disorders

### STEVE OPERSTENY, M.D., P.T.

This chapter covers the general principles of rehabilitation for disorders commonly seen in the practice of musculoskeletal medicine. The overview of conservative treatments includes a discussion of modalities commonly used by physical therapists or chiropractors, such as exercise and mobilization and manipulation techniques.

The physician or other health care provider who serves as the case manager should treat all musculoskeletal injuries, whether they are work-related, personal injury (e.g., cervical whiplash from a motor vehicle accident), or sports-related, from a sports medicine approach. Many practitioners believe that a personal injury will not improve until after litigation has been settled. However, prospective studies show improvement despite litigation status.[27] Another study reports that patients involved in litigation tend to report higher levels of subjective pain but that pain-related disability was not affected.[30] Proponents of the sports medicine approach recommend conceptualizing rehabilitation in three phases:[13] acute phase, recovery, and maintenance. The goals to be achieved in each phase are outlined in Table 1.

The sports medicine approach requires close follow-up and good communication among the members of the rehabilitation team so that the case manager can move the patient through the three phases as quickly as the patient's progress allows. In addition, follow-up and communication allow timely adjustment of the rehabilitation program if the patient does not respond appropriately. The case manager must realize that, as managed care proliferates, treatment options and decisions become increasingly subject to critical pathways or treatment guidelines.[21] Critical pathways and treatment guidelines clarify which services are deemed reasonable and medically necessary. Among such guidelines are time recommendations for diagnostic interventions and referrals. For example, a request for a magnetic resonance (MR) scan of the spine for an injury that is less than 6 weeks old most likely will be denied by the third party payor unless special circumstances can be demonstrated. If a patient cannot be graduated into the next phase of rehabilitation within 6–8 weeks, secondary level intervention needs to be considered. After an additional 8 weeks have elapsed, the case manager should should begin tertiary level interventions, which have been recommended to span 6 weeks (Table 2). The Texas Treatment Guidelines[21] for nonoperative care of the spine allocate 0–8 weeks for primary level intervention, 8 weeks for secondary level intervention, and 6 weeks for tertiary level intervention, for a total of 5½ months. In other words, by the end of 5½–6

**TABLE 1.**
Sports Medicine Phase of Rehabilitation

| Phase | Goals |
|---|---|
| Acute | Diagnosis: to formulate a treatment plan<br>Relative rest of injured segment, pain relief, initial rehabilitation efforts<br>Patient counseling for reassurance and education about injury and rehabilitation process |
| Recovery | Restoration of strength and flexibility of injured segment<br>Development of task-specific exercises for return to activity |
| Maintenance | Return to work or sports activity<br>Independence in a self-paced exercise program to maintain or increase strength and flexibility<br>Patient education about prevention of reinjury and management of recurrent injuries |

From Herring S: Sports medicine early care. In Mayer T (ed): Contemporary Conservative Care for Painful Spinal Disorders. Philadelphia, Lea & Febiger, 1991, with permission.

months the case manager should have completed all appropriate diagnostic studies and referrals. If the patient's progress through the three phases of rehabilitation is arrested or plateaus and no progress is seen within a reasonable time, the patient should be placed at maximal medical improvement (MMI) at the end of 5½–6 months, according to both the Texas and the American Medical Association guidelines.[1] The time frame for nonoperative care of the spine also applies to nonoperative care of most other musculoskeletal problems. Other states have different time frames.

**TABLE 2.**
Levels of Intervention

| | |
|---|---|
| **Primary level of intervention** (duration: 0–8 weeks) | |
| Clinical interventions | Initial evaluation, including history and physical examination<br>Rule out surgical lesion, if suspected<br>Refer for rehabilitation if symptomatic after reevaluation in 1 week |
| Diagnostic interventions | Plain radiographs<br>Laboratory tests |
| **Secondary level of intervention** (duration: 0–8 weeks or 8–16 weeks after injury) | |
| Clinical interventions | Reevaluation: history and physical examination<br>Review of rehabilitation course<br>Consider psychologic assessment to rule out psychologic and/or psychosocial barriers to progress |
| Diagnostic interventions (only those that apply to patient's symptoms) | Computed tomographic (CT) myelograms or MR scan; MR with gadolinium only if suggested by history or previous surgery<br>Electromyography/nerve conduction studies, bone scan, epidural steroid injection |
| **Tertiary level of intervention** (duration: 0–6 weeks or 16–22 weeks after injury) | |
| Clinical interventions | Document history of failure to respond to rehabilitation<br>Document all negative studies and determine whether any other studies may help with diagnosis<br>If no operative lesion is found and patient cannot show progress with rehabilitation, consider referral for participation in chronic pain program |
| Diagnostic interventions | CT discography of lumbar spine<br>Diagnostic facet joint injections<br>Neuropsychologic assessment to determine whether patient is a candidate for chronic pain program |
| The tertiary level of care is the last remaining medical option before declaring the patient at maximal medical improvement. | |

From Meyer et al: Texas Treatment Guidelines. Public Law, 1995.

## ACUTE PHASE

One of the goals in the acute phase of rehabilitation is accurate diagnosis. To achieve this goal, an adequate history and physical examination are mandatory. Description of a detailed musculoskeletal examination is beyond the scope of this chapter, but several good references are available.[19,20,33] If the history determines that the injury is traumatic, one should order radiographs of the affected part, which help to ensure that a patient with an acute fracture is not referred for rehabilitation and also provide medicolegal documentation. If the history determines that the injury is due to repetitive overuse, radiographs probably are not indicated until later, after the patient fails to respond to rehabilitation.[29] Other paraclinical examinations, such as serum laboratory studies, bone scan, computed tomographic (CT) myelogram, and MR scans, should be reserved for patients suspected of having serious trauma or neoplasm and patients with fever and an inflammatory process or significant neurologic deficit.[29] What constitutes a significant neurologic deficit is often a clinical judgment call. The author recommends an urgent MR scan or CT myelogram for patients who present with intolerable pain and positive findings in two of the three basic neurologic categories (sensory, motor, or deep tendon reflex changes that correlate with a specific nerve root level). Other obvious reasons to proceed with an MR scan or CT myelogram in the acute phase are a progressive neurologic deficit, signs and symptoms of cervical myelopathy, and cauda equina syndrome.[7,28]

Pain relief is also a significant goal in the acute phase. Pain relief is often achieved through a combination of medications, physical modalities, manual therapy, and exercise. Medications used in musculoskeletal medicine fall into one of three categories: (1) antiinflammatory medications (steroidal or nonsteroidal); (2) antispasmodics (e.g., muscle relaxers), and (3) narcotics.

Antiinflammatory steroids include the commonly used tapering dose of cortisone (Medrol Dosepak). The side effects of steroids include gastritis, fluid retention, and bone demineralization; avascular necrosis also has been reported.[3] Side effects are minimized, however, when steroids are taken for a brief period (1–2 weeks). Steroids produce their analgesic effect by attenuating the inflammatory response to acute injury. If oral steroids are used, one must taper the dose to avoid iatrogenic Cushing's syndrome.

Nonsteroidal antiinflammatory drugs (NSAIDs) also have both antiinflammatory and analgesic properties. There are at least seven different chemical classes of NSAIDs,[4] and numerous choices are commercially available. Cost varies widely and should be kept in mind during the selection process. Patients with prescriptions for NSAIDs should be warned about gastritis as a potential side effect so that they can stop the medication before developing a more serious gastric ulcer. Another side effect of NSAIDs is hepatotoxicity. Contraindications to NSAIDs include anticoagulation with intravenous heparin or Coumadin, recent gastric ulcer, previous allergic reactions to a particular class of NSAIDs, or previous episode of hepatotoxicity induced by a particular class of NSAIDs. Patients with a history of gastritis may be managed with the combination of an NSAID and Cytotec. According to manufacturer recommendations, however, Cytotec should not be used by women of childbearing age.

Muscle relaxants are commonly prescribed. Many exert their antispasmodic action by depressing the central nervous system. Benzodiazepines are useful for treating spasticity in patients with spinal cord lesions as well as acute spasms, but they have sedating effects and are potentially addictive. Some also have the potential for development of dependence.[16,25] For these reasons, muscle relaxers should be reserved for patients in whom pain is not adequately relieved by antiinflammatory agents and/or acetaminophen. If muscle relaxers are used, they should be limited to bedtime doses to avoid sedation during the day.

Narcotics may be used on a short-term basis for relief of acute pain; however, there is no justification for their long-term use in musculoskeletal disorders. Every effort should be made to wean the patient from narcotics as soon as possible. Physicians who treat musculoskeletal disorders are likely to encounter patients with chronic conditions such as failed back syndrome.[6] Patients with chronic conditions may be difficult if not impossible to wean from narcotics. In such difficult cases, a neuropsychologic evaluation to determine whether the patient is a candidate for a structured pain management program is the most appropriate course of action. The author does not prescribe any narcotic stronger than class III. If a class II agent is required, the patient should be hospitalized for diagnostic studies and/or pain management. A more detailed discussion of the use of narcotics to treat chronic pain is beyond the scope of this chapter.

Another goal in the acute phase is rest. Rest should be broken down into bedrest and relative rest. The most often quoted study of bedrest is that of Deyo, who concluded that bedrest beyond two days has no benefit.[8] Other studies propose up to two weeks of bedrest in patients with radicular compression.[5] For the vast majority of patients with acute musculoskeletal injuries two days of bedrest should be more than adequate. Relative rest may be defined as resting the specific injured joint while maintaining strength and endurance as best possible for the rest of the kinetic chain.[13] For example, patients with knee injury should maintain the strength of the hip flexors and extensors by exercising on a hip flexor and extensor machine that does not allow forces to be transmitted through the knee joint (Fig. 1). As the injured segment recuperates, range-of-motion exercises should be initiated and encouraged. As the injured segment becomes less painful with range-of-motion activities, a gentle strengthening program can be initiated and titrated upward as the patient tolerates. This approach limits deconditioning of the remainder of the kinetic chain while the knee is rehabilitated. Patients with lumbar spine injury should maintain lower extremity strength while stabilizing the injured spinal segment by performing wall slides with or without a corset and strengthening the knee extensors and flexors on a machine that does not transmit a loading force through the spine.

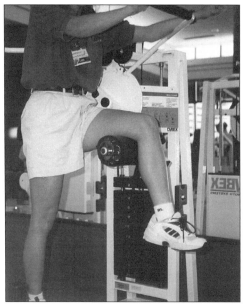

**FIGURE 1.**
Hip extensor.

Passive use of physical modalities or agents is a controversial subject in regard to both what types of modalities should be used and how long they should be used. Most authorities recommend a brief course of passive modalities for no more than 2 weeks.[21] Given that 90% of patients with low back pain recover in 6 weeks, regardless of the treatment program,[26] and that severe pain can be relieved significantly in approximately 35% of patients by double-blind placebo,[10,26] it is difficult to determine that most treatments are better than reliance on placebo and the natural history of the disease.[32] No randomized, controlled trials indicate that any particular physical agents are effective.[9,29] Therapists who believe that one specific modality works better than another are likely to communicate this belief to their patients; therefore, treatment is likely to be successful even if it gives only a placebo response.[5] Physical agents commonly used in a physical therapy practice include heat, cold, ultrasound, transcutaneous electrical nerve stimulation (TENS), iontophoresis, high-voltage pulsed galvanic stimulation, and traction. A general understanding of the physiologic effects and limitations of these modalities helps the physician to choose the appropriate modality for desired goals. Specific details are beyond the scope of this chapter; for more information about the physiologic effects of specific modalities, the reader is referred to Krusen.[15]

Spinal manipulation is another modality that may be used to help restore normal motion and joint function. However, the author is aware of no prospective, randomized study that has demonstrated its effectiveness. The Texas Treatment Guidelines limit spinal manipulation therapy to no longer than 8 weeks.[21] A clinician would find it difficult to justify to third party payors the need for spinal manipulation beyond that period. The Quebec Task Force reported that a few studies have shown temporary relief of pain, but long-term benefits have not been demonstrated.[29] Spinal manipulation as a cause of injury is a controversial topic, especially in terms of whether it can cause or aggravate disc herniations. According to one study, spinal manipulation does not transfer a greater load through the spine than normal manual handling of materials.[31] The complications of spinal manipulation are probably equivalent to the potential complications of other treatment modalities. Estimates of vertebral artery aneurysms range from 1/20,000 to 1/1,000,000, and the incidence of cauda equina syndrome is estimated at less than 1/1,000,000 treatments.[2]

## RECOVERY PHASE

Once range of motion is relatively pain-free and swelling of the injured part is minimal, rehabilitation can begin. The goals of rehabilitation exercises are restoration of normal range of motion and strength, followed by return to sport- or task-specific activities (Table 3). Normal range of motion and soft tissue mobility are important in preventing injury or reinjury. A recent study demonstrated a correlation between tight ligaments and muscles and injury in collegiate male athletes.[14] During the recovery phase the physical therapist should instruct each patient in an individualized stretching and warm-up routine before work-outs and games. Exercise to restore strength is an integral part of the recovery phase. The therapist or trainer must assess carefully which muscles need training to restore the normal muscle balance of the affected joints.

**TABLE 3.**
Steps of the Rehabilitation Exercise Program

| |
| --- |
| Step 1: Restore range of motion to normal or equal to that of the uninvolved limb. |
| Step 2: Strengthen the muscles of the affected joint to 80% or greater of the unaffected joint. |
| Step 3: Plyometric exercises or sport-specific activities |

**TABLE 4.**
Types of Exercises for the Recovery Phase

| Type and Definition | Advantages | Disadvantages |
|---|---|---|
| **Isometric:** static contraction held for length of time with no change in the angle of the joint and little or no change in the length of the contracted muscle | Simple and inexpensive Safe in that patient is less likely to overload the muscle | May cause elevations in blood pressure during static contraction, may be contraindicated in cardiac patients Does not train muscle throughout its full range, lacks exercise specificity Lack of feedback |
| **Isotonic:** contractions in which muscle fibers shorten throughout a range against resistance | Strengthens muscle throughout range Feedback and progress easily seen Relatively inexpensive | May cause injury if exercise and lifts are performed incorrectly |
| **Isokinetic:** contraction throughout a range at a constant velocity | Strengthens muscle throughout its range Feedback can be monitored Little danger of injury from handling too much weight | Costly Equipment not readily available Resistance can be moved easily and patients sometimes fail to work at maximal intensity |
| **Plyometric:** explosive movements | Inexpensive Similar to movements of actual performance | High-impact nature of exercise may cause joint and ligament injury |

Available options are isometric, isotonic, isokinetic, and plyometric exercises (Table 4). Isometric strengthening is useful if the affected joint is too painful to exercise through a protected arc. For example, quadriceps sets may be used to begin strengthening the vastus medialis muscle or isometric external rotation for early strengthening of an injured rotator cuff. Isometrics also may be used to strengthen a muscle at a particular length that has a strength lag (Fig. 2). For example, while an athlete is performing bench presses during the rehabilitation phase of a shoulder injury, the trainer notices a

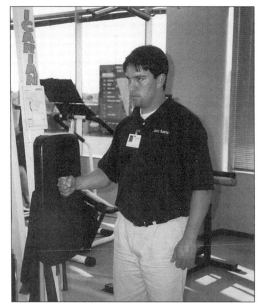

**FIGURE 2.**
Isometric shoulder external rotation.

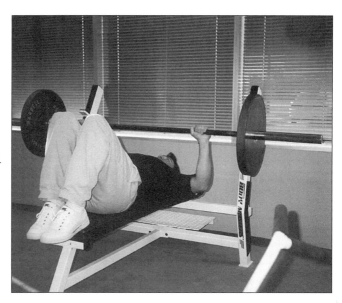

**FIGURE 3.**
Bench press sticking point.

"sticking point" at approximately midway (Fig. 3). The trainer may place the barbell in the portion of the sticking point at mid-range of the bench press maneuver on a power rack and instruct the athlete to perform isometric bench presses at the weak range for preferential strengthening (Fig. 4).

Isotonic exercises allow strengthening of the muscle throughout the affected range. To the author's knowledge, no studies have compared isotonic and isokinetic exercises in terms of muscle performance. Isotonic exercises have the advantage in that progress can be seen by performing more repetitions or adding more weights. Isotonic exercise equipment is more readily accessible and less costly than isokinetic equipment. An example of isotonic exercise is the traditional barbell curl.

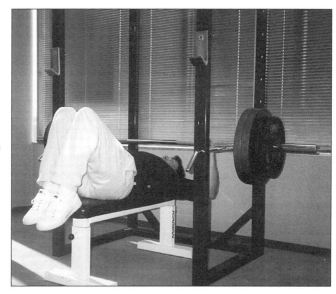

**FIGURE 4.**
Isometric bench press on power rack.

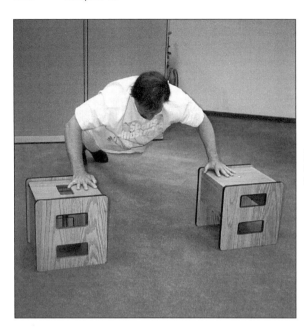

**FIGURE 5.**
Starting position on upper extremity plyometric exercise.

Isokinetic equipment can control speed of movement, thereby minimizing the potential for injury, and be adjusted to block out a particular arc of motion that is not desired (e.g., terminal phase of knee extension). Strength can be developed at different velocities that more closely resemble the speeds at which an athlete performs. Isokinetic equipment also can be used for testing. Periodic testing during rehabilitation can be used to monitor progress and to determine whether the patient is making a valid effort.[18] However, the use of isokinetic testing devices to determine validity (submaximal effort) remains controversial.[22,24] One study demonstrated that clinical observation during testing was even more accurate than curve variability on isokinetic testing.[12]

Plyometric training involves explosive movements; for example, jump training. Plyometric motions facilitate explosive power by recruiting the maximal number of large, powerful, type II muscle fibers through the stretch reflex. The energy developed in landing is stored in the elastic structures of the muscles and tendons and then converted back to kinetic energy.[11,35] Plyometrics also can be used for the upper extremities (Figs. 5–7).[34] Plyometric training can be dangerous and result in injury if warm-up is inadequate or if one trains past the fatigue point. Plyometric exercises are as close to sport- or task-specific activities as one can achieve.

## MAINTENANCE PHASE

The goal of the maintenance phase is to maintain proper ligament, muscle, and joint mobility to prevent reinjury.[14] The ingenuity and resourcefulness of the health care practitioner will help the athlete or injured worker to develop plyometric or sport- or task-specific drills to enhance power and performance.

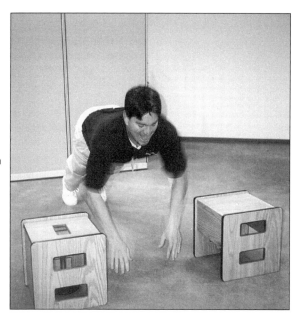

**FIGURE 6.**
Plyometric exercise in
progress.

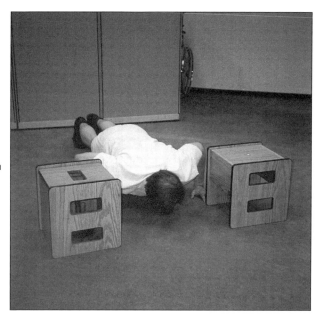

**FIGURE 7.**
Upper extremity
plyometric finish
point.

## REFERENCES

1. American Medical Association: Guides to the Evaluation of Permanent Impairment, 3rd ed. Chicago, American Medical Association, 1989.
2. Assendelft WJ: Complications of spinal manipulation. A comprehensive review of the literature. J Fam Pract 42:474–480, 1996.
3. Bradbury G: Avascular necrosis of bone after cardiac transplantation: Prevalence and relationship of administration and dosages of steroids. J Bone Joint Surg 76A:1385–1388, 1994.
4. Brooks P: Nonsteroidal anti-inflammatory drugs—Differences and similarities. N Engl J Med 234: 1716–1725, 1991.

5. Bruxelle J: Placebo effect in the treatment of pain: Review. Rev Pract 44:1919–1923, 1994.
6. Colemont J, Zielle K: Surgical treatment of failed back syndrome. In Textbook of Spinal Surgery, vol 2. Philadelphia, J.B. Lippincott, 1991, pp 739–745.
7. Coscia M: Acute cauda equina syndrome: Diagnostic advantage of MRI. Spine 19:475–478, 1994.
8. Deyo R: How many days of bed rest for acute low back pain? A randomized clinical trial. N Engl J Med 315:1064, 1986.
9. Deyo R: Historic perspective on conservative treatments for acute back problems. In Mayer T (ed): Contemporary Conservative Care for Painful Spinal Disorders. Philadelphia, Lea & Febiger, 1991.
10. Evans FJ: The placebo response in pain reduction. Adv Neurol 9l 4:289–296, 1974.
11. Fisher AG: Scientific Basis of Athletic Conditioning, 3rd ed. Philadelphia, Lea & Febiger, 1984.
12. Hazard RG, et al: Isokinetic trunk and lifting strength measurements: Variability as an indicator of effort. Spine:54–57, 1988.
13. Herring S: Sports medicine early care. In Mayer T (ed): Contemporary Conservative Care for Painful Spinal Disorders. Philadelphia, Lea & Febiger, 1991, pp 235–242.
14. Kirvickas L, Feinberg H: Lower extremity injuries in college athletes: Relation between ligamentous laxity and lower extremity muscle tightness. Arch Phys Med Rehabil 77:1139–1143, 1996.
15. Kruger F, Kottke F, et al (eds): Krusens Handbook of Physical Medicine and Rehabilitation, 3rd ed. Philadelphia, W.B. Saunders, 1982.
16. Liltrell RA: Carisoprodol (Soma): A new and cautious perspective on an old agent. South Med J 86:753–756, 1993.
17. Maitland GP: Vertebral Manipulation, 5th ed. London, Butterworths, 1986.
18. Mayer TG, Smith SS, et al: Quantification of lumbar function. II: Sagittal plane trunk strength in chronic low back pain patients. Spine 10:765–722, 1985.
19. McKenzie RA: The Lumbar Spine: Mechanical Diagnosis and Therapy. Waikanae, NZ, Spinal Publications, 1981.
20. McVemyre RA: The Cervical and Thoracic Spine: Mechanical Diagnosis and Therapy. Waikanae, NZ, Spinal Publications, 1989.
21. Meyer et al: Texas Workers Compensation Commission Rule No. 134.1001: Spine Treatment Guidelines. Public Law, 1995.
22. Nicholas JJ, et al: Isokinetic testing in young nonathletic able-bodied subjects. Arch Phys Med Rehabil 70:210–213, 1989.
23. Norton A: Cushing's syndrome/disease. In Rovel R (ed): Saunders Manual of Medical Practice. Philadelphia, W.B. Saunders, 1996, pp 651–652.
24. Rothstein JM, Lamb RL, Mayhew TP: Clinical uses of isokinetic measurements. Crit Issues Phys Ther 67:1840–1844, 1987.
25. Rust GS: Carisoprodol as a drug of abuse. Arch Fam Med 2:429–432, 1993.
26. Scheer S, et al: Randomized controlled trials in industrial low back pain relating to return to work. Int Arch Phys Med Rehabil 76:966–973, 1995.
27. Schofferman J, Wasserman S: Successful treatment of low back pain and neck pain after a motor vehicle accident despite litigations. Spine 19:1007, 1994.
28. Shapiro S: Cauda equina syndrome secondary to disc herniation. Neurosurgery 32:743–747, 1993.
29. Spitzer WO: Quebec Task Force Study. Spine 12(Suppl):8–59, 1987.
30. Swartzman L, et al: The effect of litigation status on adjustment to whiplash injury. Spine 21:53–58, 1996.
31. Triano JDC: Assessment of biomechanical risks from lumbosacral manipulation. Presented at the 11th Annual Conference of the North American Spine Society, Vancouver, October 1996.
32. Waddell G: A new clinical model for the treatment of low back pain. Spine 12:632–644, 1987.
33. Weber H: Lumbar disc herniation: A prospective study of prognostic factors, including a controlled trial. J Oslo City Hosp 28:33–64, 1978.
34. Wilk UE, et al: Stretch shortening drills for the upper extremities: Theory and clinical application. J Orthop Sports Phys Ther 17:225–239, 1993.
35. Yessis M: Plyometrics. Muscle Fitness 57(4):81–84, 1996.

# 18

# Psychologic Factors Affecting Soft Tissue Injury: Psychodynamics, Psychopathology, and Impact on Recovery

DAVID B. ADAMS, PhD
LORI B. WASSERBURGER, MD

The rehabilitation of patients with soft tissue injury requires identification of pre-existing psychologic factors that (1) increase vulnerability to injury, (2) result in decreased mobilization after injury, and (3) create pathologic adaptation to the disability role and lifestyle. The relationship between soft tissue injuries and psychologic factors influencing subjective complaints due to such injuries has been addressed most frequently in research on chronic low back pain.[75] Back injury is the primary cause of disability in people under the age of 45 years in industrialized countries.[32] It is the single most expensive medical condition, costing more than 16 billion dollars annually and contributing to the annual expenditure of 27 billion dollars for all muscular trauma. Low back complaints have grown more than 14 times more rapidly than the population.[40]

Ten percent of the cases account for 80% of the cost.[101] Ninety percent of back pain episodes are self-limited, often resolving independently of which method of intervention is chosen.[29] Fifty percent of patients with back pain have resolution of symptoms within 2 weeks and are not disabled by their injury. Almost three-fourths recover within the first month, and 90% recover in less than 6 months. Of the remaining 10%, most remain out of work at the end of 1 year, with the majority not returning to work after 2 years.

Resistance to recovery, failure to improve, and progression to a role of chronic, dependent incapacity in the remaining 10% account for the majority of frustrations, costs, and patient management problems that arise from all back injuries.[72] Thirty percent of all disabling work injuries and 19% of all workers' compensation costs arise from work-related upper extremity disorders.[66] The cost of the average cumulative trauma disorder is 50% greater than the cost of the average single-event traumatic injury, and the time lost from work is far longer. Recent studies have examined the efficacy of psychodynamic assessment to determine which acutely injured patients are most likely to evolve into a role of chronic disability.[31]

## PHYSICAL COMPLAINTS: CULTURAL BIASES

Early psychodiagnosis and appropriate time-limited psychologic care, when indicated, have been demonstrated not only to improve the quality of overall physical health but also to facilitate recovery from injury and surgery.[60,63] Such care may reduce nonproductive or overutilized medical care by as much as 75%.[62] Studies indicate that more than 50% of office visits to primary care physicians are for psychologic, somatoform, and psychophysiologic disorders regardless of the subjective complaints with which the patient presents.[75] Sociocultural factors in industrialized nations cause most patients to assume that all somatic symptoms arise from pathophysiologic origins. In American society, the taboo against psychologic disorders has not lessened significantly. Despite research and media attention in both stress-related illnesses and injury-related stress, the continued perception is that somatic pain and psychopathology are disparate entities and that control of the latter is not a viable means of addressing the former.[16] In effect, patients suffering from psychologic disorders before or after soft tissue injury most often seek a purely physiologic basis for their lingering complaints. They typically are apprehensive that an identified psychologic component will minimize the nature of the complaint or indicate constitutional weakness in dealing with life's demands.

## THE INJURED INDUSTRIAL WORKER AS AN ANALOG

Any loss or limitation of ability to work and provide for a family is one of the most psychologically devastating problems that a person must face. It can occur with any type of injury or illness. Injuries within a work setting possess a unique subset of problems for rehabilitation and recovery.[55] These problems are observed most readily in workers in labor-intensive employment. Such workers must struggle harder for recognition and status than their often more educated counterparts in other job markets. They constitute the largest segment of the working population; educational requirements are often less, and credentialing may be limited. Their investment in physical labor may serve as a means of justifying either premature termination of education or the avoidance of contained office work.

Although work may be repetitive and inconsistently available, with the potential to terminate suddenly, workers focus on obtaining higher income levels through overtime, high-risk work settings, or perceptions of themselves as independent contractors. Injured workers frequently have little capacity to tolerate a temporary loss of income because they typically do not have significant savings accounts, disability policies, or other liquid assets.

Any reduction in productivity in this fragile, labor-intensive job market, therefore, results in immediate change in status with rapid loss of financial position and assets and immediate decrease in financial backing by lending agencies. The power base for such workers is brittle at best. Even a return to employment generally does not restore their preinjury financial and social status.[67] The psychologic impact of decreased work capacity can be lessened if the lack of gainful employment arises as a result of "unavoidable" industrial injury. The cause of injury can then be attributed to factors outside the patient's control.

The patient who cannot or does not return to the premorbid form of employment has three options. The first is retraining. For a person with inadequate academic background and limited intellectual capacity, a return to school is not only costly but also runs appreciable risk of potentially humiliating failure through exposure of limitations.

The second option is alternate employment, which may fail to produce the same income, seniority, mobility, or prestige as the preinjury position. Typically the patient perceives this option as demeaning, because chances for advancement are minimal and perceptions of self-direction are absent. The patient's insight into the differences between the psychologic threat inherent in reeducation and the threat from potentially demeaning alternate employment may be minimal. In reality, few if any alternate positions may be available to the patient with complaints of chronic pain, regardless of verbalized willingness to return to work with limitations.

The third and often least psychologically threatening option is the disability role. The patient may be forgiven earlier life decisions that led to incomplete education and high-risk, low-stability employment. This option allows injured workers to perceive social acceptance of their inability to generate the same levels of income. They can maintain the illusion that they would return to work, prior life roles, and prior income levels if only such an option were physically viable.

## THE MYTH OF DIAGNOSIS BY EXCLUSION

Each person tends to find a unique course of adaptation to individual problems based on predisposing psychologic factors and socioemotional resources. Attempts to measure psychologic reaction to injury cannot predict the path to recovery. Certain at-risk workers have limited plans for improving health and general musculoskeletal conditioning and hold the belief that few or no options exist other than seeking workers' compensation.

Psychologic consultation should be considered when subjective complaints exceed objective findings or when complaints persist despite resolution of objective findings. Rarely, however, is such a psychologic consultation made during this time frame. In industrial injuries, referral should be made with the earliest indices of discord between employee and employer or family. It also may be appropriate before discussions of disability and impairment rating, if it seems to be a focus of care. In practice, the psychologic referral is usually made only after exclusion of all potential pathophysiologic causes.

Regardless of the objective physical findings, in every patient psychologic factors are involved in (1) the etiology of the complaint; (2) sequelae of injury or illness; or (3) determinants of how the patient copes with and responds to health care. Rarely are patients consciously aware of these factors.[91] When clinicians fail to detect psychologic factors affecting the medical condition and symptoms do not resolve or become amplified, a conditioning process ensues. The patient learns that each new complaint elicits additional diagnostic studies and attempts at therapeutic intervention. This open-ended health care format may create an excessive vigilance within the patient. In the quest to be seen for follow-up, the patient scans every minute symptom, frequently recording each to offer the treating clinician documentation of ongoing pain or lack of pain resolution.[105] Subjective complaints become a blend of unresolved injury residuals and anxiety-evoked somatizing components. The context of the industrial injury and injury-related care creates an environment conducive to excessive preoccupation with bodily function.

Although many injured employees simply cannot be restored to premorbid levels of functioning, the expectancy is restoration of comfort and preinjury activity levels. This expectation entangles the patient in a web of desire to be better and psychologic need not to be better. The conflict is often unresolvable. In the workers' compensation system, the concept of compensability often governs the direction of care. When psychologic intervention occurs only after all possible physiologic determinants are ruled out (diagnosis by exclusion), the patient's resistance to considering psychologic determinants or consequences has been maximized.[87] A psychologic referral near the end of the physical diagnostic and treatment process implies to the patient that the complaints are now being minimized and relegated to a position of lesser importance.[74] It is a rare patient who expresses the possibility that symptoms may be the result of emotional factors triggered or exacerbated by the work-related injury. It is certainly even rarer at the endpoint of diagnostic work-up and treatment.

## PREDISPOSING PSYCHOLOGIC FACTORS

Five factors may be considered in the management of a patient with residual soft tissue complaints. Each suggests the interplay of psychodynamic features in the establishment and maintenance of a pattern of physical symptoms:

1. Was injury the result of trauma, such as physical assault? If so, the emotional complications are likely to affect the speed of physical recovery and return to work.[19]

2. Were the patient's subjective physical complaints from the onset in excess of physical findings, improbable based on the mechanism of injury, migratory, or contradictory? Have reasonable diagnostic studies failed to reveal a cause for the complaints or their degree?

3. Does the patient fail to show positive indications of willingness to accept residual discomfort or limitations?

4. Do people involved in rehabilitating the patient consistently report concern for the patient's mood, attitude, or behavior?

5. Does the patient lack a viable occupational option to which to return?

If the answer to one or more of these questions is yes, psychological factors related to both injury and care have a high probability of influencing rate of recovery, perceptions of disability, concerns for the future, and compliance with care.


## CONTEXTUAL CONCERNS IN COMPENSABLE INJURIES

Patients expect continuity of care whether they sustain a soft tissue injury away from work with full responsibility for wage loss and return to work or in the workplace with provision of benefits and compensation. The outcome of care becomes clouded by the correlation between pain and financial restitution or liability. The patient becomes more reluctant to relinquish complaints of pain when such complaints are directly related to the amount of remuneration. Similarly, clinicians treating such complaints are vulnerable to seeing them as due to malingering for financial betterment or neurotic need for social and emotional gains. The multiple factors involved in the physical and emotional trauma, when taken as a whole, frequently govern the direction of recovery more than the specific injury or care.[13,15,43]

When financial compensation and quality of care are central concerns for the injured patient, the complexities of treatment become apparent. Without continuing physical complaints, financial compensation does not continue. Associated psychologic complaints, if acknowledged by the patient, are often conceptualized in the common phrase "pain and suffering." Pain is open to subjective interpretation, and suffering diffusely describes most states of dysphoria.

Ideally, when injuries occur in a financially compensable context, insurers and employers are concerned and supportive and facilitate recovery. Because this is not uniformly the case, the adversarial context of compensable injuries gives rise to resistance to recovery as well as escalating expectations of remuneration, distrust of clinicians, failure in compliance, and equivocal efforts.[79] Therefore, both the context in which the injury occurred and the conditions under which treatment is delivered need to be addressed.[41] Within the framework of work-related injuries, some employers initially complicate recovery by failing to assist the patient in securing care, discouraging the reporting of injuries, or isolating the patient from coworkers after injury.

In addition, employers frequently indicate to patients that they cannot return to work until they are "100%" well or can perform all of their duties without problems. This attitude sets up unrealistic expectations. Limiting patients' abilities to return to work in a light-duty capacity continues to isolate them from their coworkers and sets up an adversarial relationship because the patient is not working (and getting paid for "not working"). Insurers may restrict diagnostic and therapeutic interventions. They also may create an antagonistic relationship in which the injured worker is made to feel that the insurer does not believe that the injury is real. This antagonism may compound behaviors of symptom magnification. Such behaviors, consciously or unconsciously, ensure that the physician, insurance company, supervisors, and coworkers know that the patient is injured.

Providers who are contractually accountable to the employer may be perceived by the patient as providing inadequate diagnostic studies in an attempt to contain costs. Although this concern may have a partial basis in reality, the motivation of some injured workers does not lie in recovery but in extension of the compensation process in the form of primary or secondary gain.[53] The context of the conditions of injury, work environment, and treatment often creates a complex constellation of factors that encourages patients to exaggerate suffering and limitations.

## PRIMARY GAIN, SECONDARY GAIN, AND MALINGERING

Primary gain refers to the patient's unconscious need for the pain complaints to resolve a central underlying and often long-standing problem.[21] The patient may have no awareness of the underlying problem. The symptoms that the patient projects shield the patient from the threat arising from psychosocial problems that predated the soft tissue injury.[23] The patient seeks protection from a memory, emotion, or behavior that the patient finds unacceptable. The behaviors are often of a conflicting aggressive or sexual nature. The symptoms effectively protect the patient from awareness of unacceptable information.[53] This phenomenon operates entirely on an unconscious level. The primary gain is the relief obtained from avoidance.

Patients who were sexually abused during their developmental period may find that an injury later in life avoids responsibility for being sexually active and affords sexual protection (the primary gain) while ensuring attention, affection, and monetary (secondary) gains for the physical pain.

Secondary gain is the most frequently cited functional component in the presentation of injured patients. The concept describes a complex series of factors that influence not only the outcome of treatment but also compliance with care. Many clinicians believe that secondary gain and malingering are functional equivalents; they are not. Secondary gain is often viewed merely as an indirect reference to conscious embellishment or symptom magnification;[39] it is more effectively conceptualized, however, as a series of definable incentives. These incentives are largely unconscious and intangible factors that motivate the patient to continue to be symptomatic. The patient may not have voluntary control over the production of symptoms that result from the secondary gain aspect of injury. The psychologic needs met by the production of symptoms—in the form of support, affection, attention, and relief from responsibility—may have been otherwise unattainable. The symptoms may be associated with a temporary or permanent resolution of relationship issues or avoidance of aversive work conditions. The symptoms may serve as a covert means of passive aggression against the employer or family or may simply relieve the patient of responsibility for deciding on a future life course.[2]

In contrast to secondary gain, malingering is conscious deception for the purpose of tangible gain. Symptoms may hold the promise of settlement awards or establish a financial base otherwise unobtainable by the patient. The malingering patient recognizes the potential value of an injury and begins a long and often skilled manipulation of others by varying symptoms to ensure that expectations of tangible gain are realized.[80] The actions of the malingering patient are governed by external and conscious incentives. The most common is a definite financial goal.[18,81]

Malingering patients may simulate the symptoms of serious sequelae from injury while concealing other problems such as substance abuse, past injuries, or pending criminal charges. They also may falsely assert that the complaints arose from a compensable injury rather than an injury or problem that occurred in an unreported and noncompensable (non–work-related) context.[109] Malingering patients may have demonstrable diagnostic findings but still engage in conscious amplifying of complaints for definable and tangible rewards. In patients with positive diagnostic findings, clinicians may inaccurately discount the potential for partial malingering. The patient may use the positive findings as a means of justifying claims of disabling discomfort, inability to work, and "pain and suffering." The rate of detection by clinicians of malingering patients with a paucity of findings is poor at best. Detection is even more improbable in the patient with demonstrable orthopedic findings. Health care providers typically expect that a malingering patient will be detected by the absence of diagnostic findings.[57] In the case of pure malingering, this expectation is accurate. In the case of partial malingering, the patient embellishes subjective complaints, feeling that objective pathology will support the bid for financial or other goals.[83]

A practical conceptual model is that secondary gain influences the emotionally vulnerable patient, whereas the malingering patient influences the vulnerable clinician. Regardless of the nature of the injury or the extent of presenting symptoms, when a patient consciously exaggerates or distorts complaints for the purposes of manifest gain, the patient is malingering.[37]

## FACTITIOUS DISORDER

Factitious disorder also involves involuntary amplification or production of physical and psychologic symptoms. The symptoms, in contrast to malingering, are not generated for monetary or personal reward. Instead, patients with factitious disorder consciously mimic and exaggerate complaints because of an internal need to prolong their role as patients.[95] Patients with factitious disorder willfully submit to painful, potentially dehumanizing, and dangerous diagnostic and therapeutic procedures to meet the unconscious need to be ill. In medical clinics, it is not unusual to find patients who have undergone multiple invasive procedures designed to treat conditions or disease processes. Despite such interventions, the problem is not found or the condition is not "cured."[63]

Factitious disorder is a diagnostic entity. Patients may exhibit signs and symptoms of physical disorders, psychologic disorders, or both to ensure that the patient role is not relinquished.[106] The process is conscious and deliberate but not under voluntary control; it is a compulsive and relentless impulse. Patients cannot willingly yield their striving to maintain the role. Settlement awards do not resolve the symptoms, as they typically do for malingering patients.

Return to productivity occurs only when factors that the patient associates with the disability are identified by the practitioner.[3] Recognition and gauging of the amount of patient anger, helplessness, resentment, fear, or even relief from responsibility as a result of injury is central to full understanding of factors affecting patient recovery. In effect, it must be determined whether more needs of a conscious or unconscious nature are met by persistence than by resolution of physical complaints.[17]

## RECOVERY AND PATIENT EXPECTANCY:
## PSYCHODYNAMICS OF THE RECOVERY PROCESS

The differences in patient expectancy with regard to parameters of health care management and compensation lead to (1) variances in time of recovery; (2) differences in compliance with care; and (3) discrepancies between what is and what is not subjectively perceived as a permanent and partial disability.[94] A patient who is compensated for lost time often displays a lesser degree of urgency for recovery and return to productivity than a patient for whom nonproductivity means lost wages and significant financial risk. Rate of recovery and expectancy of compensation are not separable concepts.[103] Many people continue to be productive, even with chronic pain and musculoskeletal or medical disorders. This suggests that the time frame in which a patient recovers and progresses is not determined solely by physical findings.[107] Multiple factors determine disability and recovery intervals, including (1) a patient's acceptance vs. fear of residual physical complaints; (2) assessment of the timeliness, quality, and adequacy of health care to date; (3) the patient's concept of self and the change in that concept accrued from the disability role; and (4) the patient's perception of the expectancies of others in regard to recovery.

Determination of factors that complicate the recovery process is integral to appropriate patient care.[106] Identification of operative factors does not determine degree or time frame of the recovery process. It may explain the persistence of complaints despite what should have been effective therapies.[70,102] Simple diagnosis of a somatoform, mood, or anxiety disorder or identification of a developmental personality disorder does not determine psychologic functional capacity. Certainly, some patients who are depressed, anxious, and preoccupied with pain can and often do work. Others with clinically less significant psychologic pathology may fail to progress. Psychologic diagnosis and disability are correlated but not synonymous with determination of the patient's responsiveness to care.[85]

The difference between psychologic disorder and psychologic functional capacity has created appreciable confusion. Patients may show significant weight loss, sleep disturbance, anhedonia, feelings of worthlessness, and preoccupation with guilt or thoughts of death. Despite such symptoms, depression may remain undetected by friends, family, or the health care system.[12] Approximately 5–9% of women and 2–3% of men have a point prevalence for symptoms of major depressive disorder.[50] Many attempt to continue to be productive in the work force and within a family structure, despite significant neurovegetative symptoms of depression. Many will do so without treatment.[42]

As with physical limitations, the emotional conviction that productivity is mandatory and the belief that the disability lifestyle is aversive can be more powerful determinants of psychologic capacity than any specific diagnosis of mood disorder.[22] Endogenous and exogenous motivators may well override the limitations otherwise implied by a psychologic or physical diagnosis. Conversely, antidepressants and anxiolytics may provide appropriate symptomatic relief, but control of symptoms does not ensure that recovery will occur. Mood disorder after soft tissue injury also may resolve without return to productivity.[26]

## MOOD DISORDERS BEFORE AND AFTER SOFT TISSUE INJURY

Major depressive disorder is not only a common mood disorder but also a complex neurochemical process.[30,99] It has a point prevalence of 5–9% for women and 2–3% for men, with a lifetime risk as low as 25% in women and 5% in men. Major depressive disorder is quite different from situational disappointment. Patients with major depressive disorder often reject depression as a label. In contrast, situationally aggrieved individuals often embrace this temporary designation. The sociocultural difference between depression and anger, as conceptualized by most patients, is synonymous with the differences between weakness and strength. The physically injured patient may be consciously aware that depression is a major factor in the clinical presentation of pain after soft tissue injury.[95] They also find, however, that seeking care for the physical complaint is much more acceptable to self, family, and providers. Depression is erroneously perceived by the patient, and often by others, as something that should be under personal control.

The diagnosis of major depressive disorder is made after clinically significant alterations in mood, appetite, weight, or sleep; psychomotor changes; cognitive decline; and diminished self-worth have been present for at least 2 weeks and represent a documentable change from premorbid functioning. Additional symptoms may include complaints of chronic fatigue; increased irritability; problems with attention, concentration, and decision-making; anhedonia; and decreased libido. Symptoms often show diurnal variation ; the patient is often more symptomatic in the early hours of the day. In the characteristic sleep pattern the patient may fall asleep rapidly with a particular sleep architecture in which rapid-eye-movement sleep occurs too precipitously, causing the patient to awaken in the early hours. This pattern results in morning exhaustion. Feelings of worthlessness and guilt, sullen and withdrawn presentation, and preoccupation with thoughts of death and suicide are also common.

Patients often perceive that clinicians treating the pain complaint expect and are motivated to address only physiologic pathology—not psychopathologic complaints.[77] This perception is often warranted because clinicians are trained or attuned to recognizing only physical pathologic processes.

Patients often attribute sleep maintenance problems to pain alone. Careful clinical examination and questioning may reveal that even if the patient awakened in pain, the thoughts that occur upon awakening cause the insomnia to persist. The intrusive thoughts are often of a foreboding future, financial destitution, emotional abandonment, and relentless discomfort.[86] The sleep maintenance disorder is attributed to pain complaints, which the clinician will address, rather than the underlying mood disorder, which is feared to warrant less attention.

Clinicians, in turn, may misdiagnose mood disorder as situational anxiety. This misdiagnosis is common when the presenting symptoms of depression are agitation, irritability, impatience or overreactivity, and low frustration tolerance.[5] In the attempt to identify concurrent, preexisting, or injury-related psychopathology, the treating physician is misdirected by the similarity in presentation among the various psychopathologic entities.[45] Both clinically depressed patients and patients with anxiety disorder ruminate obsessively and are indecisive. The use of habituating anxiolytics with a clinically depressed patient is ineffective. In addition, if the patient begins to self-titrate medication or to entertain suicidal ideation, the misdiagnosis may become life-threatening. In elderly injured patients, depression is often confused with dementia. In adolescents, it may be confused with a personality disorder, especially when the adolescent expresses depressed mood primarily as petulance, impatience, and anger.[44]

## DYSTHYMIC DISORDER VS. MAJOR DEPRESSION

In contrast to major depression, the symptoms of dysthymic disorder are milder but last continuously for at least 2 years. They are associated with appetite changes but not with clinically significant weight gain or loss. Interest in formerly pleasurable events is decreased but without the marked anhedonia of major depression. These symptoms affect but usually do not preclude social and occupational functioning. The lifetime prevalence rate is approximately 3%.

Some patients with dysthymic disorder experience periods of major depressive disorder. Some clinicians refer to this concurrent expression of disorders as "double depression"—the superimposition of the significant neurovegetative symptoms of major depression on the chronic depressive pattern of dysthymic disorder. At least 75% of patients suffering from dysthymic disorder have another concurrently diagnosed disorder such as panic or anxiety attacks, drug or alcohol dependence, and eating disorders. Dysthymic disorder, therefore, is considered a secondary diagnosis and in fact may be reactive to the primary disorder. A patient with a pain disorder or generalized anxiety disorder, especially when symptoms are not resolved, may develop symptoms of dysthymic disorder in response to the persistent symptoms of the primary disorder.[51]

The most effective intervention for depression occurs only with early detection through appropriate diagnostic work-up.[56] With each succeeding month, the depressed patient in pain will increasingly somatize the mood disorder, expressing frustrations and concerns with reproduction and amplification of pain complaints. Often patients are depressed for long periods, believing themselves to be physically ill, aging, or victimized by situational events. Recognizing the early signs of the insidious progression of depression is the first step toward effective intervention and resolution.

Ideally, the symptoms of depression should be noted by a patient's self-assessment. More often the initial detection is left to the clinician to whom the patient reports the physical sequelae of the mood disorder.[88] Although some patients may accept the presence of a mood disorder when subjective complaints are interpreted for them, patients in pain are rarely offered depression as a diagnostic possibility. Even patients with some insight into their situation fear that agreeing to a diagnosis of depression will jeopardize care for the physical or pain complaint.[64]

Depressed patients presenting with pain complaints feel that they are unable to earn a living and no longer enjoy the pleasurable parts of life, such as social interactions, sexual activity, and physical or avocational activities, because of physical limitations. The concept of "learning to live with the pain" seems implausible and unfair and is often conceptualized by the patient as a sign of resignation.

The patient with chronic pain perceives life as out of control with consequent feelings of helplessness and hopelessness. Activities are avoided in an attempt to prevent the experience of pain.[93] Patients develop an almost superstitious pattern of gauging the risk involved with activities on future days on the basis of pain experienced on past days. If subjective pain is increased, patients assert that they must have engaged in some activity that precipitated the increase. As a result, even simple activities are increasingly avoided and the days become more empty. The patient increases caloric intake and may seek other forms of oral gratification, such as increased smoking, in an attempt to fill empty days. The sedentary lifestyle denies the physical activity that tends to promote a feeling of well-being and to facilitate restful sleep. The ensuing weight gain, deconditioning, and abnormal sleep cycles of the sedentary lifestyle may not only exacerbate pain but also lead to potential vulnerability to additional injury, pain, and loss of self-esteem. The maladaptive cycle, therefore, is established.

An estimated 70–80% of patients with chronic pain can be expected to develop secondary depression. Pain complaints, such as headache, backache, and diffuse musculoskeletal pain, may be symptoms of depression. It has been suggested that depression is the third stage of chronic pain and arises between 6 months and 1 year after onset of the pain complaints. In effect, a clinician examining a patient for the origins of chronic pain must also consider the possibility that depression is either causing or amplifying the patient's experience of painful symptoms.[59]

## SOMATIZATION AND SOMATOFORM DISORDERS

The process of somatization and somatoform disorders is *not* a defense against depression. Clarification of terms is essential in discussing these disorders.[6] *Somatization* is often used as psychologic insurance that emotional needs are met without risking the rejection inherent in acknowledging psychologic limitations.[47]

The term *psychosomatic* refers to physical responses to or consequences of psychologic problems, wherein potentially dangerous physical changes can result from stressors that the patient may be unable to resolve successfully. The term is applied to the interaction between physical symptoms and the underlying and often causative psychologic influences. Examples include (1) muscle contraction headaches; (2) some types of peptic ulcer disease; (3) frequency and duration of asthmatic attacks; (4) some forms of cardiac disease; and (5) diseases of and conditions in which the immune system is increasingly compromised by the physiologic demands of anxiety. The psychosomatic (or psychophysiologic) disorders are best conceptualized as the physical toll exacted by the demands of psychologic stressors.

The relationship between emotional symptoms and physical illness has received much attention in the field of psychoneuroimmunology. Past approaches emphasized the effect of treating the mental disorder on the process of recovery from physical injury. In instances of psychosomatic disorders, the goal is treatment of the emotional symptoms to change the context and course of the physical disease or condition.[1]

*Somatoform disorders* refer to a patient's significant unconscious needs for physical complaints to meet psychologic needs. The patient does not consciously produce or feign the physical complaints. The subjective complaints of pain, however, exceed objective findings.[6] Patients are neither malingering nor suffering from factitious disorder, because the somatoform process is not conscious. Either there is no organ pathology, or the pathology does not account for the extent of the subjective symptoms.[83] Psychologic mechanisms are either demonstrated or presumed to be causative of the symptoms.[36,46] Patients rarely understand or accept that the process is occurring. They may vehemently deny that unconscious needs have any effect on assumed physical symptoms. They vigorously protest the concept of a somatoform disorder or somatoform component to their chronic pain process. Patients perceive that psychologic factors minimize and somehow demean their physical complaints. It is important to recognize that somatization and somatoform disorder are not synonymous. The somatization process is the use of bodily complaints to communicate and conceptualize emotional states and environmental stressors in terms of medical symptoms. When the somatization process becomes fixed and consistent or disrupts social and occupational functions, it is pathognomonic of a somatoform disorder.[79] Among the somatoform disorders are hypochondriasis, somatization disorder, conversion disorder, and pain disorder.[52]

*Hypochondriasis* is diagnosed in the patient with excessive preoccupation with health and disease. The patient unrealistically interprets normal bodily functioning as indicative of disease processes and clings to these beliefs despite medical reassurance. In general medical practices, hypochondriasis is seen in 3–14% of patients and is slightly more predominant in men.[4,69] There is clinical support for the theory that hypochondriacal complaints meet not only dependency needs but aggressive needs as well. Aggressive needs are met by burdening others with relentless complaints that fail to resolve.[39]

*Somatization disorder* is a diffuse presentation in which the patient has more than a dozen physical complaints that cannot be completely explained by organic processes. Symptoms include gastrointestinal, cardiopulmonary, and sexual complaints as well as conversion and pain symptoms.[48] The disorder has a prevalence rate of 0.2–2% in women and is quite rare in men.

In *conversion disorder*, the patient reports a loss or alteration of physical functioning in the absence of physical disease. Whereas a hypochondriacal disorder involves complaints of physical symptoms without objective physical dysfunction, conversion disorder is characterized by actual loss or disorder of bodily functions.[52] This loss or alteration has a temporal relationship with an environmental event or trigger and often can be related to an unconscious psychologic conflict. Both primary and secondary gain operate in conversion disorder. Lessening of internal tension is the primary gain, and securing of psychologic support is the secondary gain of conversion disorder. In general hospital settings, the incidence rate of conversion disorder is believed to be 5–16%; it is typically 2–5 times more common in women.

Of the somatoform disorders, *pain disorder* has been the most problematic, because it may not be a diagnostic entity in itself. It is conventionally considered a form of illness behavior in which certain personality disorders respond poorly to the onset of acute pain or residuals of chronic pain.[10] The patient then engages in unconscious illness behaviors. Physical findings are inadequate to explain the degree of pain, and psychologic factors increase the patient's need to be in pain. Physician shopping, excessive drug use, requests for surgery with marginal to no surgical indications, and assuming the role of an invalid are common features. Other common findings are family members with chronic pain problems, ongoing psychologic conflict, and depression. The point prevalence of pain disorder is less easily specified, although it is twice as common in women.[104]

The association of pain complaints from early in life with subsequent support and nurturance is the probable psychodynamic cause of pain disorder. The health care system and society can condition the patient to believe that pain in itself is a valid cause for inability to participate in school, work, and domestic responsibilities. There are also interpersonal sources of pain behaviors. Pain can be an effective means for controlling the action of others or internal behaviors and emotions that the patient feels would not otherwise be manageable.

The mechanisms of pain may not have similar neurophysiologic effects on all patients. The decreased availability of serotonin and endorphins in some patients with chronic pain may explain some of the variance among patients with similar soft tissue injuries but disparate pain complaints.[82]

## PERSONALITY DISORDER AND RESIDUAL PAIN

Character pathology (i.e., personality disorders) is defined as developmental defects in psychologic growth. The defects may be in cognition, affect, interpersonal functioning, and impulse control. Maladaptive patterns contribute to disturbances in social and occupational roles. They arise in childhood and adolescence and are entrenched by adulthood; they are also pervasive, inflexible, and unalterable.[71] Personality disorders are not the result of adult trauma or experiences. Patients often carry such pathology into their early employment but may function adequately in the workplace.

Personality disorders differ from clinical disorders. Patients with clinical disorders such as major depression, posttraumatic stress disorder, or sexual disorders are made uncomfortable by their symptoms. Although they may resist seeking psychologic care, they at least seek relief from their symptoms. Patients rarely seek care for personality disorders but may seek care for the affective or anxiety disorders to which the personality disorder makes them vulnerable.[24]

Personality disorders occur in 5–15% of the population. In some studies, as many as one-half of patients with complaints of chronic low back pain had some form of personality disorder that predated the onset of chronic low back pain.

Many patients with personality disorders seek disability roles in a vain attempt to resolve long-standing internal conflict. The conflict often represents a combination of dependency and resentment toward those on whom they are dependent.[98] The attention and compensation from others as well as the potential passive aggression against others may be conscious enticements. If these maladaptive behaviors are permitted to continue or are further rewarded verbally or financially, they merely increase in scope. Patients become even more reluctant to relinquish them, knowing that the disability role is the most powerful in which they have found themselves.

Patients with personality disorders not only have a maladaptive response to stress, but also elicit dysfunctional responses by a pervasive pattern of interpersonal stress.[25] Such patients rapidly learn to use externalized events (e.g., unfaithful spouse, financial deprivation, social embarrassment, occupational disappointment, physical complaint) to justify their quest to meet long-standing pathologic needs. Feeding into maladaptive behaviors does not assist the patient. Supporting patients' beliefs that they are "disabled" is not only erroneous but harmful rather than rehabilitative. For some patients, the nourishing of the disability lifestyle is the ultimate in chronic dependency.

## Differential Presentation of Personality Disorder

*Passive-aggressive personalities* are often referred to as negativistic. They put off completion of tasks and fail to meet deadlines. When required to do what they do not want to do, they tend to become moody or irritable. Their work is characterized by inordinate slowness of completion or repeated errors, even though it could be performed more rapidly or correctly. Without justification, they complain of demands that others make of them. There is an important association between injury and passive-aggressive personality, because the individual learns by adulthood that physical symptoms, whether real or exaggerated, can be used as effective means of controlling others. Compliance can be especially difficult because of inappropriate or subversive expression of anger in such patients.

Patients with *histrionic personality disorder* are excessively emotional, attention-seeking, and melodramatic. Interpersonal relationships are characterized by egocentric, self-indulgent, and dependent behavior or at least by requirements of constant reassurance. Although they continually seek attention, they deny the presence of psychologic conflict or even anxiety in association with physical symptoms. In contrast to the emotional isolation and associated alienation created by *schizoid personality* or the withdrawing presentation of *avoidant personality*, the histrionic patient is dramatic and offers lengthy discourse that lacks specificity and detail. Emotions are hollow and shallow, and psychologic defenses are characterized by denial.

*Borderline personality disorder* is probably the most clinically challenging. Patients have unstable moods, impulsive behavior, fluctuating identity, feelings of chronic boredom, and a tendency toward alcohol and drug addiction. At the center of all behaviors, however, is a chaotic personality structure, sometimes a product of child abuse or neglect. Patients often seek to escape dysphoria by mood-altering substance abuse, promiscuous sex, gambling, and other impulsive acts. They frequently have recurrent symptoms of major depression. Suicidal attempts may follow.[33] Patients may attempt to escape emotional problems by focusing anxieties on somatic complaints such as chronic musculoskeletal pain, headaches, gastrointestinal disturbances, and other physical problems. People with borderline personality disorder tend to be highly resistant to treatment.[68] Medication must be monitored carefully because patients often self-medicate and exhibit drug-seeking behavior. Reports of overdose of prescribed medications are not uncommon because of their tendency toward suicide. Patients with borderline personality disorder may successfully draw their primary provider into complicated destructive situations.

Managing pain patients with *narcissistic personalities* may be quite complex. A central factor in dictating the response of narcissistic personalities to demands placed on them is the concept of the narcissistic insult. Patients may see the sequelae of physical injury as marring their striving for perfection and self-gratification. Delay in self-gratification is intolerable. Patients may be unable to meet educational demands but are offended that their economic problems are secondary to inadequate employment. They may purchase objects perceived to enhance social image, resulting in significant debt. Narcissistic patients are often intolerant of compromises. Injury often involves compromises with regard to medication and meeting the needs of others (including coworkers, treating physician, and family). A grandiose sense of self-importance, malicious envy of others, arrogance, and demand for both attention and admiration may characterize most interactions, even in clinical settings. The injury and limitations resulting from pain may represent an intolerable compromise in the quest for being viewed as special or unique, unless the patient perceives health care symptoms or needs as unique. Most patients are unwilling to empathize with or recognize the needs of others involved in the health care process such as providers, employers, and significant others.

The *obsessive personality* is preoccupied with details, rules, and schedules. Patients exhibit an inflexible presentation, often detailing and recording subjective complaints in a precise manner.[76]

The *dependent personality* demonstrates indecisiveness, often relying on the spouse or any perceived authority figure to make decisions. Patients also harbor feelings of helplessness and lack of control.

The *paranoid personality* presents with endless suspicious and unjustified doubts about care, creating problematic management problems. Patients present as guarded, evasive, and easily affronted; they require reassurance that never completely dissipates their distrust.

*Antisocial personality disorders* are of great concern to the general public as well as to the health care provider. Patients are characterized by disregard for the safety of others; they are consistently irresponsible, impulsive, deceitful, aggressive, and irritable. They do not benefit from past punitive experience and often are characterized as "knowing right from wrong" but not caring about the difference. Patients have a special sense of entitlement, which is often of great concern when the issue of malingering is addressed.

Although not all injured workers have personality disorders, many exhibit traits consistent with these disorders. It is important to recognize such traits in treatment of physical problems.

## DIAGNOSTIC AND THERAPEUTIC PSYCHOLOGIC CONSULTATION

When physical findings fail to account for the level of impairment or an injured worker has other risk factors, it is important to identify relevant psychosocial and personality traits. Psychologic examination is a lengthy process, often requiring several hours. The examination must clarify issues about the patient's perception of his or her condition, needs for ongoing medical care, and expectancies of degree of recovery. Psychologic consultation also indicates factors, both injury-related and exogenous to the compensable injury, that interfere with the recovery process and contribute to the persistence of pain and psychologic dysfunction.[7] Most importantly, consultation may determine whether the patient truly wishes to relinquish pain complaints and return to work at premorbid levels. This determines the degree to which a clinician will pursue treatment or defines the endpoint. Psychologic assessment is central to the clinical examination to understand not only the patient's subjective assessment of pain, both quality and quantity, but also what methods the patient uses for pain management and coping.

During the history-taking, patients tend to reveal which aspects of pain behavior are under voluntary control. Although malingering and factitious disorders should not be immediate suspicions, they are common enough to warrant diagnostic consideration. If the patient achieves direct gain from symptoms, either in the form of positive outcome or avoidance of negative events, conscious deception may be an element. A number of factors may be sufficient to set the foundation for false symptoms, including litigation, remuneration, attention, sympathy, removal from work or domestic tasks, and avoidance of unpleasant emotional, social, or sexual responsibility. Although psychologic evaluation is mandatory, psychologic treatment is not appropriate for all patients with chronic pain. Not all patients are psychologically oriented or benefit from psychologic intervention.[8,14,28] Before embarking on a path of intervention, the patient should be evaluated thoroughly for willingness to attempt to take control of life's demands rather than holding out for an elusive cure. Psychologic treatment of patients with pain complaints cannot proceed without assessment of factors such as intellectual capacity, emotional preparedness, motivation, and capacity for insight.

Patients with ongoing litigation are especially problematic. It must be determined whether the patient accepts and pursues care with the goal of productive change or seeks to entrench more deeply the disability role and potential remuneration.[27] No amount of therapy, procedures, psychologic support, or, at times, monetary investment and reward will improve a functional outcome unless the patient is willing to give up the disability role.

The Minnesota Multiphasic Personality Index (MMPI) and revised MMPI-2 are commonly used assessments. A major problem with these tools is the difficulty of determining whether elevations on clinical profiles are determinants or results of a chronic or soft tissue pain problem. A commonly described MMPI profile related to injury is *conversion V*, which refers to the V-shaped pattern of elevated scores on scale 1 (hypochondriasis) and scale 3 (hysteria) with a low score on scale 2 (depression). The elevations on scales 1 and 3 indicate that the patient endorses a large number of vague or specific physical complaints but a relatively smaller number of symptoms of depression. Although common among patients with chronic pain, it does not distinguish between organic and nonorganic pathology. Elevated scores on scales 1 and 3 have been associated with poor response to surgery but are equivocal indicators of response to epidural injections, nerve blocks, or spinal cord stimulation.[58]

Elevated conversion V profiles do not preclude successful treatment with pain management programs, although one must remain cautiously optimistic and terminate such a program when appropriate goals are not met. High scores on scale 6 (paranoia) and scale 8 (schizophrenia) with low scores on ego strength are associated with poor prognosis and treatment outcome. This association may be explained by true psychopathology that precedes injury rather than the combined pre- and postinjury psychopathology of the typical patient with a conversion V profile.[58]

Psychologic treatment that may benefit many patients with soft tissue disorders includes (1) teaching cognitive and behavioral skills; (2) training in assertiveness, stress management skills, and relaxation techniques; and (3) education of patient and family. Psychotherapy that is directive and behavioral (rather than purely insight-oriented) and geared toward assisting the patient to focus on future goals and productivity may be beneficial.[29] The cognitive-behavioral approach attempts (1) to reduce emotional distress related to pain or physical impairment; (2) to reduce attendance to pain; and (3) to increase functional capabilities.[89] Clinical biofeedback, hypnosis, and stress reduction therapies provide adaptive means of dealing with pain through visual imagery, verbal cues, appropriate exercise, muscle relaxation, and associated physiologic components of the pain experience.[35,73]

Patients seen by a psychologist soon after injury are able to address fears, doubts, and resentments related to their care, their condition, and its probable course. Psychologic evaluation should be strongly considered for patients with risk factors for protracted care for soft tissue injury. Risk factors include (1) job, supervisor, or coworkers dissatisfaction, (2) ongoing litigation, (3) predisposing psychologic factors, and (4) low education levels and language or cultural barriers.

Psychologic diagnosis and care soon after injury may offset distortion arising from erroneous and inadequate information from friends and family. Lay information may entrench misperceptions about the pain problem, which health care providers often find difficult to offset. Psychologic care offers patients an effective means to deal with subjective complaints, helping them to resolve the effect of pain complaints on lifestyle and empowering them to develop an effective plan for future productivity, even if their injuries preclude return to the preinjury status.

## CONCLUSION

For most patients, the most tragic consequence of injury-related soft tissue pain may be creation of a pattern of isolation and alienation. Soft tissue injuries affect more severely patients with less capacity to understand the physiologic process. Such patients poorly internalize data that may be rapidly and tersely provided by health care providers and are often offset by bad medical information from family and friends. Nonetheless, the patient's capacity to understand and benefit from the information yielded by diagnostic and prognostic findings is central to the psychologic aspects of the recovery process.

Physical disorders cannot be considered independently of psychologic functions. Somatoform disorders have long confounded and frustrated clinicians who seek a purely pathophysiologic cause for disease or a clear delineation between somatic and psychologic influences. Reliance on physical criteria enables the clinician to establish an endpoint to medical intervention, but if predisposing psychologic factors are present or subjective complaints continue beyond resolution of objective findings, we must assume that other factors are intervening in the recovery process. The experienced clinician continually considers the probability of concurrent physical illness, psychologic disorder, and personality disorder as well as the potential for all three to interact.

## REFERENCES

1. Achterberg J, Kenner C, Casey D: Behavioral strategies for the reduction of pain and anxiety associated with orthopedic trauma. Biofeedback Self Regul 14:101–144, 1989.
2. Bacon NMK, Bacon SF, Atkinson JH, et al: Somatization symptoms in chronic low back pain patients. Psychosom Med 56:118–127, 1994.
3. Barksy AJ: Amplification, somatization, and the somatoform disorders. Psychosomatics 33:28–34, 1992.
4. Barsky AJ: Hypochondriasis: Medical management and psychiatric treatment. Psychosomatics 37:48–56, 1996.
5. Baum A, Lorenzo C, Hall M: Control and intrusive memories as possible determinants of chronic stress. Psychosom Med 55:275–286, 1993.
6. Bayer TL, Chiang E, Coverdale JH, et al: Anxiety in experimentally induced somatoform symptoms. Psychosomatics 34:416–423, 1993.
7. Bernstein L, Garzone PD, Rudy T, et al: Pain perception and serum beta-endorphin in trauma patients. Psychosomatics 36:276–284, 1995.
8. Blanchard JJ, Neale JM: Medication effects: Conceptual and methodological issues in schizophrenia research. Clin Psychol Rev 12:345–362, 1992.
9. Budman SH, Stone J: Advances in brief psychotherapy: A review of recent literature. Hosp Commun Psychiatry 34:939–946, 1983.
10. Bradley LA: Pain-related correlates of MMPI profile subgroups among back pain patients. Health Psychol 3:157–174, 1984.
11. Carling PJ: Reasonable accomodations in the workplace for individuals with psychiatric disabilities. Consult Psychol 25:46–62, 1993.
12. Cavanaugh SV: Depression in the medically ill: Critical issues in diagnostic assessment. Psychosomatics 36:48–60, 1995.
13. Chamberlin B: Mayo seminars in psychiatry: The psychological aftermath of disaster. J Clin Psychiatry 41:238, 1980.
14. Chu JA: The rational treatment of multiple personality disorder. Psychotherapy 31:94–100, 1994.
15. Coalson B: Nightmare help: Treatment of trauma survivors with PTSD. Psychotherapy 32:381–389, 1995.
16. Cohen S, Manuck SB: Stress, reactivity and disease. Psychosomat Med 57:423–426, 1995.
17. Cohen S, Rodriquez MS: Pathways linking affective disturbances and physical disorders. Health Psychol 14:274–379, 1995.
18. Cornel DG, Hawk GL: Clinical presentation of malingerers diagnosed by experienced forensic psychologists. Law Hum Behav 13:375–384, 1989.
19. Cotler LB, Compton WM, Mager D, et al: Post-traumatic stress disorder among substance abusers from the general population. Am J Psychiatry 149:664–670, 1992.
20. Deyo R: Conservative therapy for low back pain: Distinguishing useful from useless therapy. JAMA 250:1057–1062, 1983.

21. Dush DM, Simons LE, Zimostrad SW, et al: MMPI classification of chronic pain patients: Toward a finer analysis. Am J Pain Manage 4:17–22, 1994.
22. Eimer BN: The chronic pain patient: Multimodal assessment and psychotherapy. Med Psychother 1:23–40, 1988.
23. Eliashof BA, Streltzer J: The role of "stress" in workers' compensation stress claims. J Occup Med 34:297–302, 1992.
24. Emerson J, Pankratz L, Joos S, Smith S: Personality disorders in problematic medical patients. Psychosomatics 35:469–473, 1994.
25. Eysenck HJ: The definition of personality disorders and criteria appropriate for their description. J Personality Disord 1:211–219, 1987.
26. Farmer R, Nelson-Gray RO: Personality disorders and depression: Hypothetical relations, empirical findings, and methodological considerations. Clin Psychol Rev 10:453–476, 1990.
27. Fishbain DA, Goldberg M, Rosomoff RS, Rosomoff R: Chronic pain patients and the nonorganic physical signs of nondermatomal sensory abnormalities (NDSA). Psychosomatics 32:294–303, 1991.
28. Francis JH, Pennal BE: The MMPI as a predictor of the refractory headache. Am J Pain Manage 6:21–25, 1996.
29. Frank JD: Treatment of the focal symptom: An adaptational approach. Am J Psychother 20:564–575, 1966.
30. Free ML, Oei TPS: Biological and psychological processes in the treatment and maintenance of depression. Clin Psychol Rev 9:653–688, 1989.
31. Frymoyer JW: Epidemiology of spinal disease. In Mayer TG, Mooney V, Gatchel RJ (eds): Contemporary Conservative Care for Painful Spinal Disorders. Philadelphia, Lea & Febiger, 1991, pp 10–23.
32. Frymoyer J, Rosen J, Clements J, Pope M: Psychological factors in low back pain disability. J Clin Orthop Rel Res 195:178–184, 1985.
33. Fromm MG: What does borderline mean? Psychoanal Psychol 12:233–247, 1995.
34. Gatchel RJ, Polatin PB, Kinney RK: Predicting outcome of chronic back pain using clinical predictors of psychopathology: A prospective analysis. Health Psychol 14:415–420, 1995.
35. Geisser ME, Robinson ME, Richardson C: A time series analysis of the relationship between ambulatory EMG, pain, and stress in chronic low back pain. Biofeedback Self-Regul 20:339–356, 1995.
36. Goldring JM: Sexual assault history and physical health in randomly selected Los Angeles women. Health Psychol 13:130–138, 1994.
37. Gross JJ, Munoz RF: Emotion regulation and mental health. Clin Psychol Sci Pract 2:151–164, 1995.
38. Hendler NH, Kozikowski JM: Overlooked physical diagnoses in chronic pain patients involved in litigation. Psychosomatics 34:494–501, 1993.
39. Hiller W, Rief W, Fichter MM: Further evidence for a broader concept of somatization disorder using the somatic symptom index. Psychosomatics 36:285–294, 1995.
40. Holbrook T, Grazier K, Kelsey J, Stauffer R: The Frequency of Occurrence, Impact and Cost of Selected Musculoskeletal Conditions in the United States. Park Ridge, IL, American Academy of Orthopedic Surgeons Press, 1984.
41. Homes JA, Stevenson CA: Differential effects of avoidant and attentional coping strategies on adaptation to chronic and recent-onset pain. Health Psychol 9:577–584, 1990.
42. Huszonek JJ, Montosh JD, Donnelly BA: Factors associated with antidepressant choice. Psychosomatics 36:42–47, 1995.
43. Hyder L, Summers MN, Braswell L, Boyd S: Posttraumatic stress disorder: Silent problem among older combat veterans. Psychotherapy 32:348–364, 1995.
44. Iezzi A, Garnett S, Adams H, et al: Somatothymia in chronic pain patients. Psychosomatics 35:460–468, 1994.
45. Ingram RE, Atkinson JH, Slater MA, et al: Negative and positive cognition in depressed and nondepressed chronic-pain patients. Health Psychol 9:300–314, 1990.
46. Jones JC, Barlow DH: The etiology of post-traumatic stress disorder. Clin Psychol Rev 10:299–328, 1990.
47. Karoly P, Lecci L: Hypochondria and somatization in college women: A personal projects analysis. Health Psychol 12:103–109, 1993.
48. Kashner MT, Rost K, Cohen B, et al: Enhancing the health of somatization disorder patients: Effectiveness of short-term group therapy. Psychosomatics 36:462–470, 1995.
49. Reference deleted.
50. Kathol RG, et al: Diagnosing depression in patients with medical illness. Psychosomatics 31:434–440, 1990.
51. Kelner R: Psychosomatic Syndromes and Somatic Symptoms. Washington, DC, American Psychiatric Press, 1991.
52. Kent DA, Tomasson K, Coryell W: Course and outcome of conversion and somatization disorders: A four-year follow-up. Psychosomatics 36:129–137, 1995.
53. Kirmayerm LJ, Robbins JM: Current Concepts of Somatization: Research and Clinical Perspectives. Washington, DC, American Psychiatric Press, 1991.

54. Koss MP, Tromp S, Tharan M: Traumatic memories: Empirical foundations, forensic and clinical implications. Clin Psychol Sci Pract 2:111–132, 1995.
55. Leavitt F: The role of psychological disturbance in extending disability time among compensable back injured industrial workers. J Psychosom Res 34:447–453, 1990.
56. Levenson H, Glenn N, Hirschfield ML: Duration of chronic pain and the Minnesota Multiphasic Personality Inventory: Profiles of industrially injured workers. J Occup Med 30:809–812, 1988.
57. Lillienfeld SO: The association between antisocial personality and somatization disorders: A review and integration of theoretical models. Clin Psychol Rev 12:641–643, 1992.
58. Love AW, Peck CL: The MMPI and psychologic factors in chronic low back pain: A review. Pain 28:1–12, 1987.
59. Manos NE, Vasilopoulo E, Sotiriou M: DSM-III diagnosed borderline personality disorder and depression. J Personality Disord 1:263–269, 1987.
60. Mayer TG, Gatchel RJ: Functional Restoration for Spinal Disorders: The Sports Medicine Approach. Philadelphia, Lea & Febiger, 1988.
61. Mayou R, Sharpe M: Patients whom doctors find difficult to help: An important and neglected problem. Psychosomatics 36:323–325, 1995.
62. Miller RJ, Hafner J: Medical visits and psychological disturbance in chronic low back pain: A study of a back education class. Psychosomatics 32:309–316, 1992.
63. Miranda J, Pérez-Stable E, Munoz R, et al: Somatization, psychiatric disorder, and stress in utilization of ambulatory medical services. Health Psychol 10:46–51, 1994.
64. Merriken KJ, Overcast TD, Sales BD: Workers' compensation law and the compensability of mental injuries. Health Psychol 1:373–387, 1982.
65. Nachemson AL: Newest knowledge of low back pain. Clin Orthop Rel Res 279:8–20, 1992.
66. National Safety Council: Accident Facts, 1993. Ithaca, IL, National Safety Council, 1993.
67. Nietzel MT, Harris MJ: Relationship of dependency and achievement/autonomy to depression. Clin Psychol Rev 10:279–298, 1990.
68. Noring C: Borderline personality organization and prognosis in eating disorders. Psychoanal Psychol 10:551–572, 1994.
69. Noyes R, Kathol R, Fisher M, et al: One-year follow-up of medical outpatients with hypochondriasis. Psychosomatics 25:533–545, 1994.
70. Ogden J: Effects of smoking cessation, restrained eating and motivational states on food intake in the laboratory. Health Psychol 10:114–121, 1994.
71. Oldham JM: DSM-III personality disorders: Assessment problems. J Personality Disord 1:241–247, 1987.
72. Organista PB, Miranda J: Psychosomatic symptoms in medical outpatients: An investigation of self-handicapping theory. Health Psychol 10:427–431, 1991.
73. Peebles MJ: Through a glass darkly: The psychoanalytic use of hypnosis with post-traumatic stress disorder. Int J Clin Exp Hypnosis 37:192–206, 1989.
74. Pimental PA, Lucia CM, O'Hara JV, Newton NA: Cultural issues in the psychological management of pain. Am J Pain Manage 3:60–64, 1993.
75. Polatin PB, Kinney RK, Gatchel RJ, et al: Psychiatric illness and chronic low-back pain, the mind and the spine—which goes first? Spine 18:66–71, 1993.
76. Pollak J: Obsessive-compulsive personality: Theoretical and clinical perspectives and recent research findings. J Personality Disord 1:248–262, 1987.
77. Putnam SH, Millis SR: Psychosocial factors in the development and maintenance of chronic somatic and functional symptoms following mild traumatic brain injury. Adv Med Psychother 7:1–22, 1994.
78. Reasor GL: The magnitude of the pain problem along with treatment history, pain classification and reimbursement. Am J Pain Manage 3:120–125, 1995.
79. Reief W, Hiller WD, Geissner E, Fichter MM: A two-year follow-up study of patients with somatoform disorders. Psychosomatics 36:376–386, 1995.
80. Rogers R, Sewell KW, Goldstein AM: Explanatory models of malingering: A prototypical analysis. Law Hum Behav 18:543–552, 1994.
81. Rogers R, Harrell EH, Liff CD: Feigning neuropsychological impairment: A critical review of methodologial and clinical considerations. Clin Psychol Rev 13:255–274, 1993.
82. Rogers MP, Weinshenker NJ, Warshaw MG, et al: Prevalence of somatoform disorders in a large sample of patients with anxiety disorders. Psychosomatics 37:17–22, 1996.
83. Roy A: Hysteria. New York, John Wiley & Sons, 1982, pp 21–40.
84. Russo J, Katon W, Sullivan M, et al: Severity of somatization and its relationship to psychiatric disorders and personality. Psychosomatics 35:546–556, 1994.
85. Salmon P: Psychological factors in surgical stress: Implications for management. Clin Psychol Rev 12:681–794, 1992.
86. Sandler JL, Becker GE: Addressing the relationship between back pain and distress in your patients. J Musculoskel Med Dec:28–39, 1993.

87. Scheier MF, Carver CC: Optimism, coping, and health: Assessment and implications of generalized outcome expectancies. Health Psychol 4:219–247, 1995.

88. Schumaker RG: Orienting the physician-referred patient to psychological intervention. Med Psychother 3:141–146, 1990.

89. Slater MA, Hall HF, Atkinson JH, Garfin SR: Pain and impairment beliefs in chronic low back pain: Validation of the pain and impairment relationship scale (PAIRS). Pain 44–51, 1991.

90. Smith GR: Somatization Disorder in the Medical Setting. Washington, DC, American Psychiatric Press, 1991, pp 2–25.

91. Smith GR: The course of somatization and its effects on utilization of health care resources. Psychosomatics 35:263–267, 1994.

92. Smith TW, Christensen AJ, Peck JR, Ward JR: Cognitive distortion and depressed mood in rheumatoid arthritis: A four-year longitudinal analysis. Health Psychol 13:213–217, 1994.

93. Stone AA, Kennedy-Moore E, Neale JM: Association between daily coping and end-of-day mood. Health Psychol 14:341–349, 1995.

94. Supernaw RB: The chronic pain-depression complex. Am J Pain Manage 2:4–7, 1992.

95. Spivak H, Rodin G, Sutherland A: The psychology of factitious disorders: A reconsideration. Psychosomatics 35:25–34, 1994.

96. Stein RA, Murray EJ, Gorelick DA: Impairment of memory by fluoxetine in smokers. Exp Clin Psychopharmacol 1:188–193, 1993.

97. Stewart DE: The changing faces of somatization. Psychosomatics 31:153–158, 1990.

98. Tracey TJ, Ray RB: Stages of successful time-limited counseling: An interactional examination. J Counsel Psychol 31:13–27, 1984.

99. Tsuang M, Simpson J: Schizoaffective disorder: Concept and reality. Schizophren Bull 10:14, 1984.

100. Ukestad LK, Wittrock DA: Pain perception and coping in female tension headache sufferers and headache-free controls. Health Psychol 15:65–68, 1996.

101. U.S. Department of Labor, Bureau of Labor Statistics; Occupational injuries and illnesses in the United States by Industry, 1991. Washington, DC, U.S. Government Printing Office, 1993.

102. Weiss WU: Psychophysiologic aspects of reflex sympathetic dystrophy syndrome. Am J Pain Manage 4:67–72, 1994.

103. Wheeler AH: Evolutionary mechanisms in chronic low back pain and rationale for treatment. Am J Pain Manage 5:62–66, 1995.

104. Whitehead WE: Assessing the effects of stress on physical symptoms. Health Psychol 13:99–102, 1994.

105. Whitehead WE, Crowell MD, Heller BR, et al: Modeling and reinforcement of the sick role during childhood predicts adult illness behavior. Psychosomatics 56:541–550, 1994.

106. Wood CA, Barsky AJ: Do women somatize more than men? Gender differences in somatization. Psychosomatics 35:445–452, 1994.

107. Zautra AJ, Burleson MH, Matt KS, et al: Interpersonal stress, depression, and disease activity in rhematoid arthritis and osteoarthritis patients. Health Psychol 13:139–148, 1994.

108. Zautra AJ, Burleson MH, Smith CA, et al: Arthritis and perceptions of quality of life: An examination of positive and negative affect in rheumatoid arthritis patients. Health Psychol 16:399–408, 1995.

109. Zelinski JL: Malingering and defensiveness in the neuropsychological assessment of mild traumatic brain injury. Clin Psychol Sci Pract 1:169–184, 1994.

# 19

# Psychopharmacologic Considerations in Management of Acute and Chronic Pain

DAVID B. ADAMS, PhD
ROBERT E. WINDSOR, MD

## FACTORS INFLUENCING THE EXPRESSION OF PAIN

Although patients differ in their threshold, interpretation, and endurance of painful stimuli, there is an innate drive to avoid the experience of pain. The management of acute and chronic pain[3] has been problematic for clinicians of many health care disciplines. Because most analgesia was derived from narcotic and dependency-producing agents, the complaint of pain and the unwillingness to tolerate the experience of pain became an area of increasing concern. In health care management, pain is among the most common complaints, but its definition has been imprecise. The existence of pain is inferred by the patient's verbal and motor behavior and has defied objective measurement. The term pain is used metaphorically to refer to the most negative human experience, physical or emotional, and the experience of pain has become associated with concepts of loss, damage, upset, onslaught, and physical discipline.

Social, psychological, and biochemical influences of pain determine the patient's clinical presentation. The social aspect is marked by the patient's reaching into the interpersonal environment for support, nurturance, explanation, and reassurance during the experience of pain and even in anticipation of activities or procedures that precipitate pain. Consequently, there are social and cultural differences to the experience and expression of pain. The role of the patient's support system can determine whether the patient complies with care and takes appropriate action in response to the complaint or retreats into a disability role,[19] permitting others to assume the patient's responsibilities. The socially reinforcing aspects of litigation, contradictory and continuous diagnostic processes, and vagaries among the treating staff in response to patient complaints modify the expression of pain.

Both short-lived and enduring psychologic components influence the experience and expression of pain. To some patients, pain may represent aggression against others and an effective means of controlling behavior. For other patients, the experience of pain represents an extension and expression of self-repudiation, guilt, and remorse, an effective means of atoning for actions for which the patient feels culpable. The alexithymic patient, unable to express distress verbally and tending to somatize emotional

349

concerns, uses pain as a means of communicating emotions that do not emerge from an otherwise constricted lexicon. For many patients, the experience of pain is a conditioned response evoked by unmanageable psychological conflict—a learned means of resolving interpersonal conflict that was not managed verbally.

The biochemical mechanisms[4] of pain have been described in terms of increased analgesia due to elevated serotonin[14] levels in the periaqueductal gray areas and increased inhibition at the spinal cord level. T-cells in the substantia gelatinosa of the dorsal horn are believed to be influenced by both small facilitory and large inhibitory fibers from the peripheral nervous system and by descending brain input. Individual differences in central nervous system structures[26] account for the variability in response latency and degree after exposure to painful stimuli. An increase in available serotonin may be associated with inhibition of pain. The increase of norepinephrine or the blockage of dopamine in the lateral aspect of the reticular formation, on the other hand, may increase the experience of pain. Psychoactive agents based on these bioamine actions may modulate pain but less markedly than analgesics that act on opiate receptors.

## MEDICATION AND THE EXPERIENCE OF PAIN

Regardless of the appraisal of the variable pain experience among patients or even within the same patient, at some point in the therapeutic process most treating clinicians become increasingly uncomfortable with the patient's reliance on habituating analgesics for pain management. Clinician discomfort is associated with duration, frequency, and dose of analgesic consumption. Concern escalates when the patient makes no demonstrable attempt to reduce intake or when the amount of intake has increased despite temporal distance from the acute phase of injury.

The concern for dependency on analgesics leads many clinicians to early consideration of surgery, sensory or physical therapies, biofeedback, hypnosis, psychotherapies, and alternate pharmacologic approaches.[16] Patients frequently resist movement to nonnarcotic pharmacologic intervention. The patient in chronic pain often feels that the goal in medication management is amelioration of all pain experience, not merely the management of residual discomfort. Concurrently, past experiences with narcotic analgesia create within many patients the perception that it is something for which to bargain, demand, plead, or manipulate, further confounding clinically effective intervention.

## DEPRESSION, INSOMNIA, AND PAIN AS FUNCTIONAL ANALOGS

Anxiolytics, neuroleptics, and antidepressants (Tables 1 and 2) have been used in various combinations as adjuncts or alternatives to narcotic analgesia. Both tricyclic antidepressants (TCAs) and phenothiazines demonstrate opiate-sparing in patients with pain. This effect is believed to be associated with their interaction with enkephalins and their binding[1] to opiate receptors. By contrast, many of the benzodiazepines[18] are not only habituating but may lower pain threshold.

The history of TCAs in the management of patients with chronic pain spans several decades. Concern about the use of TCAs began to emerge when it was documented that both sedating and appetite-stimulating effects of some TCAs were associated with increased sedentary lifestyle, hypersomnia, and hyperphagia. The patient with a lumbar injury may become increasingly inactive, gain weight, and potentiate sleep problems[5] by sleeping during the day.

Concern about the use of antidepressants for patients in pain is threefold: (1) comorbid clinical depression,[12] (2) sleep disturbance due to depression or pain, and (3) the effect of antidepressants on the pain experience. Antidepressants[7] that selectively inhibit serotonin reuptake[6] (SSRIs) have not consistently been shown to be more effective in

**TABLE 1.**
Sample Overview of Antidepressants, Mood Stabilizers, and Psychostimulants

| Generic Name (Brand Name) | Range (mg) | Sedation | Anticholinergic Side Effects | Impact on Norepinephrine | Impact on Serotonin | Other Qualities |
|---|---|---|---|---|---|---|
| **Monoamine oxidase inhibitors (antidepressants)** | | | | | | |
| Phenelzine (Nardil) | 30–90 | Low | 0 | Increase norepinephrine | | |
| Tranylcypromine (Parnate) | 20–60 | Low | 0 | serotonin, and dopamine | | |
| **Heterocyclic antidepressants** | | | | | | |
| Imipramine (Tofranil) | 150–300 | Moderate | Moderate | ++ | +++ | |
| Desipramine (Norpramin) | 150–300 | Low | Low | +++++ | 0 | |
| Amitriptyline (Elavil) | 150–300 | High | High | + | ++++ | |
| Nortriptyline (Aventyl, Pamelor) | 75–125 | Moderate | Moderate | +++ | ++ | |
| Protriptyline (Vivactil) | 15–40 | Moderate | Moderate | ++++ | + | |
| Trimipramine (Surmontil) | 100–300 | High | Moderate | ++ | ++ | |
| Doxepin (Sinequan, Adapin) | 150–300 | High | Moderate | +++ | ++ | |
| Maprotiline (Ludiomil) | 150–225 | High | Moderate | +++++ | 0 | |
| Amoxapine (Asendin) | 150–400 | Moderate | Low | ++++ | + | |
| Trazodone (Desyrel) | 150–400 | Moderate | 0 | 0 | +++++ | |
| Fluoxetine (Prozac) | 20–80 | Low | 0 | 0 | +++++ | Anti-obsessional |
| Bupropion (Wellbutrin) | 200–450 | Low | 0 | + | 0 | |
| Sertraline (Zoloft) | 50–200 | Low | 0 | 0 | +++++ | Anti-obsessional |
| Paroxetine (Paxil) | 20–50 | Low | Low | 0 | +++++ | Anti-obsessional |
| Venlafaxine (Effexor) | 75–375 | Low | 0 | ++ | +++ | |
| Nefazodone (Serzone) | 100–500 | Moderate | 0 | 0 | +++++ | |
| Clomipramine (Anafranil) | 150–250 | High | High | | | Anti-obsessional |
| Fluvoxamine (Luvox) | 50–300 | Low | Low | 0 | +++++ | Anti-obsessional |
| **Mood stabilizers** | | | | | | |
| Lithium carbonate (Eskalith, Lithonate) | 600–2400 | Serum level: 0.6–1.5 mEq/L | | | | |
| Carbamazepine (Tegretol) | 600–1600 | Serum level: 4–10+ µg/ml | | | | |
| Valproic acid (Depakene) | 750–1500 | Serum level: 50–100 µg/ml | | | | |
| **Psychostimulants** | | | | | | |
| Methylphenidate (Ritalin) | Adult daily dosage: 5–50 mg | | | | | |
| Dextroamphetamine (Dexadrine) | Adult daily dosage: 5–40 mg | | | | | |
| Pemoline (Cylert) | Adult daily dosage: 37.5–112.5 mg | | | | | |

Adapted from Preston J: Quick Reference to Psychotropic Medication. Cameron Park, CA, P. A. Distributors, 1995.

the management of pain than lower-than-customary dosages of TCAs. Nonetheless, co-morbid depression in patients with chronic pain can be substantial, and the SSRIs have a lower side-effect profile and thus a higher rate of patient compliance than TCAs.

The use of TCAs for the management of pain complaints has three primary goals: (1) the neurovegetative symptoms of depression must be addressed; (2) the patient must have sufficient restful sleep to deal with diurnal variations in agitation and psychomotor retardation; and (3) if the patient can be managed effectively with monitored psychoactive agents, reliance on narcotics can be lessened or eliminated.

Depression may be a natural response to pain both neurochemically and psychosocially. If unaddressed, it merely complicates the efficacy of other attempted interventions. The patient with both pain and depression exhibits cognitive changes with attendant problems in attention, concentration, and decision making. The depressed patient's increased irritability, low tolerance of frustration, and overreactivity creates problems with compliance and management for the clinician and problems with tolerance for the family. Anhedonia, guilt, and decreased libido further erode the patient's self-esteem.

The proper antidepressant in conjunction with a decrease in narcotics facilitates sleep, enhances the patient's inherent ability to manage pain, ensures that pain does not

**TABLE 2.**
Sample Overview of Antipsychotic and Anxiolytic Agents

**Antipsychotics**

| Generic Name (Brand Name) | Range (mg) | Sedation | Anticholinergic Side Effects | Extrapyramidal Side Effects | Equivalence to Thorazine (mg) |
|---|---|---|---|---|---|
| Chlorpromazine (Thorazine) | 50–1500 | High | ++ | ++++ | 100 |
| Thioridazine (Mellaril) | 150–800 | High | + | +++++ | 100 |
| Clozapine (Clorazil) | 300–900 | High | 0 | +++++ | 50 |
| Mesoridazine (Serentil) | 50–500 | High | + | +++++ | 50 |
| Molindone (Moban) | 20–225 | Low | +++ | +++ | 10 |
| Perphenazine (Trilafon) | 8–60 | Moderate | ++++ | ++ | 10 |
| Loxapine (Loxitane) | 50–250 | Low | +++ | ++ | 10 |
| Trifluoperazine (Stelazine) | 10–40 | Low | ++++ | ++ | 5 |
| Fluphenazine (Prolixin) | 3–45 | Low | +++++ | ++ | 2 |
| Thiothixene (Navane) | 10–60 | Low | ++++ | ++ | 5 |
| Haloperidol (Haldol) | 2–40 | Low | +++++ | + | 2 |
| Pimozide (Orap) | 1–10 | Low | +++++ | + | 2 |
| Risperidone (Risperdal) | 4–16 | Low | + | + | 2 |

**Anxiolytics (benzodiazepines and others)**

| Generic Name (Brand Name) | Single Dose (mg) | Equivalence (mg) | Other Comment | Examples of Psychotropic Side Effects |
|---|---|---|---|---|
| Diazepam (Valium) | 2–10 | 5 | | *Anticholinergic effects* |
| Chlordiazepoxide (Librium) | 10–50 | 25 | | • Dry mouth |
| Flurazepam (Dalmane) | 15–60 | 15 | Insomnia | • Constipation |
| Prazepam (Centrax) | 5–30 | 10 | | • Urinary retention |
| Clorazepate (Tranxene) | 3.75–15 | 10 | | • Blurred vision |
| Temazepam (Restoril) | 25–30 | 10 | Insomnia | • Memory impairment |
| Clonazepam (Klonopin) | 0.5–2 | 0.25 | | • Confusion |
| Lorazepam (Ativan) | 0.5–2 | 1 | | *Extrapyramidal effects* |
| Alprazolam (Xanax) | 0.25–2 | 0.5 | | • Parkinsonian symptoms |
| Pazepam (Serax) | 10–30 | 15 | | • Dystonias |
| Triazolam (Halcion) | 0.25–0.5 | 0.25 | Insomnia | • Akathisia |
| Estazolam (ProSom) | 1–2 | 1 | Insomnia | • Tardive dyskinesia |
| Quazepam (Doral) | 7.5–30 | 7.5 | Insomnia | |
| Zolpidem (Ambien) | 5–10 | 5 | Insomnia | *Autonomic effects* |
| Buspirone (BuSpar) | 5–20 | | | • Orthostatic hypotension |
| Hydroxyzine (Atarax, Vistaril) | 10–50 | | | *Sedation* |
| Diphenhydramine (Benadryl) | 25–100 | | Antihistamine | • Drowsiness |
| Propranolol (Inderal) | 10–80 | | Antihypertensive | • Impaired reaction time |
| Atenolol (Tenormin) | 25–100 | | Antihypertensive | |
| Clonidine (Catapres) | 0.1–3 | | Antihypertensive | |

Adapted from Preston J: Quick Reference to Psychotropic Medication. Cameron Park, CA, P. A. Distributors, 1995.

stimulate excessive appetitive drive counterproductive to recovery, and ideally energizes a lethargic mind and body.

The indication that 60–80% of patients benefit from the use of TCAs and monoamine oxidase inhibitors (MAOIs) must be tempered with concern for dosage levels and appropriate patient education about their sedating and anticholinergic side effects. The sedating properties can be used to benefit if medication is taken two hours before bedtime with the goal of restful, productive sleep.[8] The sleep disturbance among patients in pain can be inordinately problematic. Clinicians must be concerned not only about the sedating effects of antidepressants but also about their effects on sleep quality or architecture. Some clinicians concurrently prescribe anxiolytics[8] with the antidepressant in an attempt to ensure adequate sleep onset and maintenance. However, the disadvantages of potential dependence and daytime sedation provide further complications rather than resolution.

A central concern is not only that sleep disorders[22] arise in the patient with chronic pain but also that the patient with chronic pain who does not sleep is more vulnerable to the development of a sleep disturbance. Depression worsens as sleep disturbance

**TABLE 3.**
Potential Effects of Antidepressants on Sleep Architecture

| Tricyclic Antidepressants | Monoamine Oxidase Inhibitors | Selective Serotonin Reuptake Inhibitors |
|---|---|---|
| Affect latency and continuity Suppress REM and/or REM latency May increase awakenings and sleep stages 1 and 2 | Prolong sleep latency and reduce continuity Suppress REM and increase REM latency Produce REM rebound when discontinued | Increase latency, REM latency, and stage 1 Decrease REM time and sleep efficiency Increase wakefulness and arousals |

REM = rapid eye movement.

continues. Attempts to treat the mood disorder as a primary sleep disorder by prescribing anxiolytics run the risk of anxiolytic dependence without addressing the true primary disorder. Concurrently, patients who do not sleep begin a cycle of anticipatory anxiety at bedtime that further disrupts sleep, potentiates pain, and ensures poor coping skills during the following day. Poor coping may include not only an increase in caloric intake with consequent weight gain but also increased irritability toward support systems, failure to comply with care related to the cause of pain, and increased seeking of other analgesia. A concern not often addressed is the higher incidence of mortality from cerebrovascular accident and myocardial infarction in patients with abnormal sleep patterns.

For the pain patient with complaints of sleep disturbance, TCAs, MAOIs, and SSRIs have an appreciable effect on sleep architecture and continuity (Table 3). Bupropion and nefazodone[2] prolong rapid-eye-movement (REM) sleep. Trazodone and nefazodone[23] increase sleep continuity. Trazodone is associated with appreciable daytime sedation. Amitriptyline and doxepin are sedating and increase sleep continuity; both, however, decrease REM sleep and may promote daytime somnolence and lethargy. Imipramine, nortriptyline, desipramine, and clomipramine are less sedating than doxepin and amitriptyline, but all four—most notably clomipramine—decrease REM sleep,[24] as do the MAOIs, phenelzine and tranylcypromine. The SSRIs—fluoxetine,[17] paroxetine, and sertraline—have less sedating effects but may decrease sleep continuity and REM sleep. Both fluoxetine and paroxetine, for example, increase sleep latency. Fluoxetine also increases stage I sleep and REM latency while decreasing REM time, whereas paroxetine increases sleep phase shifts, arousal, and wakefulness while decreasing sleep efficiency.

In addressing the combination of depression and sleep disturbance in patients with chronic pain complaints, some clinicians prefer a combination of a morning SSRI to address clinical signs of depression, especially lack of mobilization during daytime hours, and an agent such as trazodone to promote sleep onset and continuity.

## ANXIETY, ANXIOLYTICS, AND PATIENT COMPLIANCE

Concern about the use of anxiolytics[15] in the management of anxiety symptoms arising from pain complaints has not lessened. The patient may learn to fear the lack of adequate sleep[28] and become obsessively anxious about the effect on future family, social, and occupational functioning. The rapid effect of anxiolytics[29] in contrast to antidepressants leads not only to their more ready acceptance by patients but also to the risk of dependency.

In addition, an agitated, depressed patient with signs of psychomotor retardation may be misdiagnosed as suffering from situational anxiety[9] (i.e., adjustment disorder) or anxiety disorder rather than clinical depression. Anxiolytics should be considered powerful adjuncts for anxious patients as long as the clinician has distinguished appropriately between anxiety and clinical depression.[20] When the patient suffers from situational anxiety (e.g., before surgery) or when a preexisting or injury-consequent anxiety disorder threatens the efficacy of care for injury-related pain, the use of anxiolytics may be indicated. Realistic concerns about dependency on diazepam or alprazolam have too often discouraged an appropriate contract with the patient for a specific anxiolytic regimen with preestablished duration and discontinuance of use. During the time of acute management with anxiolytics, the patient may be treated concurrently with nonpharmacologic methods of anxiety management such as psychotherapy, cognitive therapies, biobehavioral procedures, or interpersonal skill training.

## COROLLARY CONSIDERATIONS

The prescribing clinician needs an adequate understanding of differential therapeutic levels, including blood levels of agents used for the treatment of affective vs. pain disorders in the absence of a treatable mood disorder.[13] The schedule of medication administration, whether divided daily dosages of SSRIs, evening administration of TCAs, or fixed daily schedules of anxiolytics, needs to be established and clearly communicated to the patient and the patient's support system.

Major considerations include the schedule of medication increase, targeting of specific neurovegetative symptoms to determine when asymptotic levels have been reached, and prophylactic use of antidepressants in patients with a prior major depressive disorder. Patient education about the inadvisibility of abrupt discontinuation of antidepressant medication as well as clarification about the nonhabituating nature of antidepressants may be central to compliance and therapeutic response. Education about the dependency risks of anxiolytics is a consideration, along with differences in schedules and effects of agents with a long half-life (e.g., diazepam) vs. agents with a short half-life (e.g., lorazepam) and the relative merits and goals of each. Although some patients readily incorporate an as-needed schedule in the brief use of anxiolytics to manage situational anxiety, the same patients may fail to understand readily that antidepressants[27] cannot be taken as subjectively needed merely because they may produce sedation. This attitude suggests that antidepressants are needed only on evenings when sleep is problematic. Patients need information about the differences between anticipated and benign side effects that subside vs. valid adverse reactions that imply increased health risk.

Finally, education of the patient about the intent, action, and nature of the prescribed medications may be the most efficacious means of ensuring compliance. Patients receiving antidepressants need to be educated to ensure that there are no gaps in the refill pattern. Many clinicians discontinue an effective TCA when the patient reports self-termination of treatment with the first anticholinergic signs of dry mouth and sedation. Similarly, other clinicians persist in the use of a specific antidepressant despite sufficient documentation that the patient is hypersomniac, hyperphagic, and gaining weight. Such symptoms are not only deleterious to health but also adversely affect the chief complaint of pain. The latter practice is generally ill advised except when other reasonable medications have failed.

## CONCLUSION

The appropriateness and efficacy of psychopharmacologic agents for adjunctive or primary management of patients with pain complaints can be determined only by differential psychodiagnostic approaches. Both pain and depression may present with appreciable sleep disruption. The use of antidepressants for the management of sleep, although now commonplace, demands appropriate understanding of their effect on sleep architecture.[25] Simply prescribing a sedating agent does not ensure that the patient's sleep disturbance has been adequately or appropriately addressed. The coexistence of affective[21] and anxiety disorders in some patients who present with pain as a chief complaint requires differentiation of the role of the psychologic disorder in the etiology and maintenance of pain complaints. Many patients in pain are depressed as a result of attempts to manage painful residuals. Similarly, major depression may present initially with pain as a primary complaint. The preexistence or coexistence of depression is a major differential diagnostic factor in such situations.

In addition, consideration of the use of anxiolytics to address sleep disturbance or symptoms of agitation also requires differentiation among anxiety, agitated depression, insomnia related to analgesia,[11] and a myriad of interpersonal and intrapsychic upheavals that confront the patient in chronic pain.

## REFERENCES

1. Anton RF: New directions in the psychopharmacology of alcoholism. Psychiatr Ann 25:353–362, 1995.
2. Armitage R, Rush AJ, Trivedi M, et al: The effects of nefazodone on sleep architecture in depression. Neuropsychopharmacology 10:123–127, 1994.
3. Blackwell B: Chronic pain. In Kaplan HI, Sadock BJ (eds): Comprehensive Textbook of Psychiatry, vol. V. Baltimore, Williams & Wilkins, 1989, pp 1264–1271.
4. Carpenter MB, Sutton J: Human Neuroanatomy, 8th ed. Baltimore, Williams & Wilkins, 1983.
5. Dement WC, Milter MM: It's time to wake up to the importane of sleep disorders. JAMA 269:1548–1550, 1993.
6. Dubovsky SL: Beyond the serotonin reuptake inhibitors: Rationales for the development of new serotonergic agents. J Clin Psychiatry 55:33–44, 1994.
7. Eison AS, Eison MS, Torrente JR: Nefazodone: Pre-clinical pharmacology of a new antidepressant. Psychopharmacol Bull 26:311–315, 1990.
8. Ford DE, Kamerow DB: Epidemiologic study of sleep disturbance and psychiatric disorders: An opportunity for prevention? JAMA 262:1479–1484, 1989.
9. Fordyce WF: Pain and suffering: A reappraisal. Am Psychol 43:276, 1988.
10. Gelenberg AJ: Buspirone: Seven-year update (academic highlights). J Clin Psychiatry 55:222–229, 1994.
11. Gillin JC, Byerley WF: The diagnosis and management of insomnia. N Engl J Med 322:239–248, 1990.
12. Kupfer DJ, Spiker DG, Coble PA, et al: Sleep and treatment prediction in endogenous depression. Am J Pyschiatry 138:429–433, 1981.
13. Kupfer DJ, Reynolds CF: Sleep and affective disorders. In Paykel ES (ed): Handbook of Affective Disorders, 2nd ed. Edinburgh, Churchill Livingstone, 1992, pp 311–323.
14. Leonard BE: Pharmacological differences of serotonin reuptake inhibitors and possible clinical relevance. Drugs 43(Suppl 2):3–10, 1990.
15. Mellinger GD, Balter MB, Uhlenhuth EH: Prevalence and correlates of the long-term regular use of anxiolytics. JAMA 251:375–379, 1984.
16. Merskey H: Psychological approaches to the treatment of chronic pain. Postgrad Med 60:886, 1994.
17. Nicholson AN, Pascoe PA: Studies on the modulation of the sleep wakefulness continuum in man by fluoxetine, a 5-HT uptake inhibitor. Neuropharmacology 27:597–602, 1988.
18. Olajide D, Lader M: Depression following withdrawal from long-term benzodiazepine use: A report of four cases. Psychol Med 14:937–940, 1984.
19. Pilowsky I, Spence ND: Patterns of illness behavior in patients with intractable pain. J Psychosom Res 19:297, 1975.
20. Reich J, Tubin JP, Abramowitz SI: Psychiatric diagnosis of chronic pain patients. Am J Psychiatry 140:495, 1983.
21. Reynolds CF, Kupfer DJ: Sleep research in affective illness: State of the art circa 1987. Sleep 10:199–215, 1987.
22. Reynolds CF, Dew MA, Monk TH, Hoch CC: Sleep disorders in late life: A biopsychosocial model for understanding pathogenesis and intervention. In Cummings J, Coffey CE (eds): Textbook of Geriatric Neuropsychiatry. Washington, DC, American Psychiatric Press, 1994.
23. Sharpley AL, Walsh AES, Cowen PJ: Nefazodone—a novel antidpressant—may increase REM sleep. Biol Psychiatry 31:1070–1073, 1993.
24. Shenck CH, Mahowald MW, Kim SW, et al: Prominent eye movements during NREM and REM sleep behavior disorder associated with fluoxetine treatment of depression and obsessive-compulsive disorder. Sleep 15:226–235, 1992.

25. Thompson TL, Moran MG, Nies AS: Psychotropic drug use in the elderly. N Engl J Med 308:134–138, 1983.

26. Wall PD: The gate control theory of pain mechanisms: A reexamination and restatement. Brain 101:1, 1978.

27. Walsh TD: Antidepressants in chronic pain. Clin Neuropharmacol 6:271, 1983.

28. Wingard DL, Berkman LF: Mortality risk associated with sleeping patterns among adults. Sleep 6:102–107, 1983.

29. Woods JH, Katz JL, Winger G: Use and abuse of benzodiazepines: Issues relevant to prescribing. JAMA 260:3476–3480, 1988.

# 20

# Disability and Impairment

## DAVID C. CRADDOCK, JD, LLM

The concepts of disability and impairment necessarily start with definitions; however, it is important to understand how these concepts relate to real-life situations. This chapter focuses on the interaction between the medical and legal communities in determining disability and impairment and its impact on the patient. The definitions of disability vary with the purposes and intellectual disciplines of the definers.[1]

*Impairment* is a medical term defined as "the loss, loss of use or derangement of any body part, system or function."[2] *Permanent impairment* has become static or will stabilize with or without medical treatment and is not likely to remit despite medical treatment.[2] To understand the interaction between the determination of impairment and the determination of disability, one must understand the historical development of these concepts. Early writers used the term *handicapped*, and until recently it was used in most federal legislation. The term was used to indicate that a person who was either impaired or disabled was in some way handicapped in the ability to function in the everyday world, either by actual impairment, barriers, or prejudicial attitudes.[3] Handicapped has been defined as "an imputation of difference from others; more particularly, imputation of an undesirable difference."[4] The term is thought to imply that a person is seeking charity, as in "hand in a cap." The more appropriate term is *disabled* or *physically challenged.*

Currently about 43 million Americans fall in the broad category of disabled persons.[3,4] It is important to distinguish when a disability actually prevents adequate functioning in a particular life activity and when the inability to engage in the activity results from external sources such as prejudice and architectural barriers. When the disability is related to a physical or mental impairment and the disabled person is seeking compensation, definitions are generally related to the loss of earning capacity. When the disability is related to discrimination, terms are broadly defined to protect all persons who may benefit from the legislation. The problem is that a physical impairment may be a disability to one person and not to another. The existence of a disability is related to age, race, education level, income, and other socioeconomic factors.[5] Clearly the loss of a finger would be greater disability to a surgeon than a lawyer.

## HISTORICAL OVERVIEW

The first major federal legislation providing protection for people with disabilities was the Social Security Act of 1935.[6] The Social Security Act initially provided medical and therapeutic services for children who were "crippled." The LaFollette-Barden Act of 1943, which was amended by the Vocational Rehabilitation Amendment in 1954, made vocational training and rehabilitation services available for persons older than 15 years.[7] In 1968 the Architectural Barriers Act (ABA) was passed and required certain buildings to be accessible to people with disabilities.[8] In 1973 one of the most significant federal statutes was enacted—the Rehabilitation Act of 1973.[9] This act mandated nondiscrimination and affirmative action by federal employers and recipients of federal funds. Currently the most important statute related to disability rights is the Americans with Disabilities Act (ADA) of 1990. The ADA extended protection for people with disabilities to areas outside federal employers and recipients of federal funds. The ADA contains the most comprehensive definition of a disability:

A. A physical or mental impairment that substantially limits one or more of the major life activities of an individual;

B. A record of such an impairment; or

C. Being regarded as having such an impairment.[10]

Physicians are frequently asked to evaluate people with impairments and to give opinions about their disabilities. This request may occur in various legal settings, including federal laws such as the Social Security Act, the ADA, and the Family and Medical Leave Act. More commonly such questions arise in workers' compensation claims and personal injury actions. An understanding of these laws and actions helps the physician to evaluate a patient's impairment and resulting disability.

## WORKERS' COMPENSATION

Claims under workers' compensation laws are governed by the individual states. Although these laws differ, they share a common purpose—to compensate an employee injured on the job. The separate states adopted these laws in the early 1900s in response to the industrial revolution and the special needs of injured employees. Before the enactment of workers' compensation statutes, an injured employee had to prove negligence or fault on the part of the employer. Conversely, the employee had to be free from fault to recover damages. A further obstacle was the theory that if a worker's injury was caused by a fellow employee, the employer was not liable.[1] These concepts created an almost insurmountable barrier for the injured employee, often resulting in financial ruin. Countries in Europe adopted so-called no-fault rules in the late 1800s, and the American system of compensation closely follows these laws. In general, an employee may be compensated for an accident and injury that occurred during the course of employment without regard to fault or negligence. The swap-out is a system of compensation that often limits the recovery in amount and time.

All workers' compensation laws define disability in a similar manner. The usual definition is the inability, as a result of a work-connected injury, to perform or obtain work suitable to the claimant's qualifications and training. The degree of disability depends on the impairment of earning capacity.[11] Confusion sometimes occurs because workers' compensation laws speak of impairment of earning capacity. This type of impairment is obviously different from the medical concept of physical impairment. As in other disability statutes, workers' compensation laws recognize that people with different physical impairments will have different disabilities. The distinctive feature of the compensation system is that its awards are not usually made for physical injury as such, but for disability produced by physical injury. However, some states have so-called scheduled injuries, which compensate injured employees on the basis of physical impairment, such as loss of a hand or eye, with no requirement that the impairment actually results in loss of earning capacity. Scheduled injuries usually result in an insignificant amount of compensation and today are of little practical significance. Most such claims are converted to claims based on loss of earning capacity, which historically render larger sums for the employee and his or her attorney. Because attorneys for injured employees are usually compensated with a percentage of the recovery, there is often a built-in conflict for the attorney representing the injured worker. Many employees would fare better over the course of their employment if they did not have a record of a permanent disability claim. There is real or perceived discrimination against injured employees in the work force. Recognizing this problem, states have created second injury funds to assist employers in compensating workers who have subsequent injuries. The purpose of these funds is to promote the hiring of injured employees by insuring the risk of a second injury that results in disability. Such laws have little impact on the problem because of their narrow application and because their availability is limited by administrative agencies.

Should a physician render an opinion about the degree of disability suffered by a patient? The American Medical Association's (AMA) *Guides to the Evaluation of Permanent Impairment*[2,11] states that the evaluation or rating of a disability is a nonmedical assessment of the degree to which a person does or does not have the capacity to meet social, occupational, or other demands or to meet statutory or regulatory requirements. The AMA *Guides* further states:

> The Physician's tasks are to (1) identify impairments that could affect performance and determine whether or not the impairments are permanent; and (2) identify impairments that could lead to sudden or gradual incapacitation, further impairment, injury, transmission of a communicable disease, or other adverse occurrence.

In a legal claim for workers' compensation benefits, the claimant's attorney usually employs a vocational expert to testify about the degree of disability associated with a specific impairment. The physician should render such opinions only when there is sufficient information about the patient's necessary job skills and transferable skills.

## SOCIAL SECURITY DISABILITY

Social Security disability has a fact-specific set of rules, regulations, tables, and agency policies to determine whether a claimant meets the definition and criteria of disabilities under the Social Security Act. To be found disabled and therefore entitled to Social Security disability benefits, a person must be unable to perform any substantial gainful employment due to an impairment (physical or mental) that can be expected to last at least 12 months.[12] Substantial gainful employment is generally based on whether the claimant is capable of earning $500.00 per month.[13] The issue is not whether the person can do the same work as before he or she became disabled, but whether the person can perform any type of work that will earn $500.00 per month.

In determining whether a person is capable of substantial gainful employment, the Social Security Administration considers criteria set out in "listings" and "grid tables." The listings are a set of the most commonly encountered disabling conditions that lead to an impairment severe enough to qualify as disability. The listings not only identify the impairment (e.g., spinal disorders, psychologic disorders) but also set out the criteria that must be met by a person whose claim is based on a particular listing. Each listing contains the functional limitations that specify what a claimant must be unable or limited in doing to meet the standards of the listing. Each listing also has what is called the *theory of the case*. The theory is simply the logical reason that allows a claim to be approved when the claimant meets the required criteria of the listing. The claimant's impairment must meet the medical requirements of the listing and result in the specified functional limitations, and the claimant must not have transferable skills or education.[13] The existence of a disabling condition must be supported by a medical report, signed by a duly licensed physician. Social Security will not accept the subjective opinions of physicians unless supported by objective evidence such as radiographs and laboratory tests. Because pain is a subjective finding according to Social Security, a complaint of pain unsupported by objective evidence is not adequate to sustain a finding of disability.[14] The physician for a patient who is applying for Social Security disability should be aware of the specific criteria used in determining disability. The physician and attorney for the patient should communicate to determine whether the patient's impairment meets the criteria and, if so, the proper manner in which to state the limitation.

## PERSONAL INJURY

Physicians also treat patients who have been injured in accidents, typically motor vehicle accidents. Such patients may have pending or prospective litigation to recover monetary damages against a third-party tortfeasor. A claimant may recover for pain and suffering, disfigurement, temporary and permanent disability, lost wages, and medical expenses. Proof of these damages can be obtained from several different sources. Typically the claimant describes his or her injuries and pain to a jury, medical records may be introduced as evidence, and the medical testimony of physicians is submitted, usually by way of depositions. When the injury is not obvious and no objective proof of injury is available, juries are usually reluctant to grant large awards. Medical proof obviously plays a lesser role in such personal injury cases, and judgments depend more on the skill of the attorneys than the medical condition of the claimant. It is usually difficult for a person to describe pain in a formal atmosphere such as a jury trial. Attorneys now use more sophisticated techniques, such as a video deposition, to prove damages in personal injury cases. In some cases the jury is shown a "day-in-the-life" film of the claimant attempting to perform day-to-day activities.

The role of the physician in a personal injury case obviously varies with the circumstances. It is important to remember that the complete medical record may be introduced at trial and read by the jury. Cases are sometimes won or lost based solely on such records. If a claimant testifies that he or she had intense pain on a certain date but the medical record indicates otherwise, the claimant's credibility is irreversibly damaged. Physicians must review their records and be prepared to answer hostile questions in a medical deposition. The defense attorney may question the need for treatment and the veracity of the treating physician. There are usually questions about physical impairment or disability. Attorneys sometimes either intentionally or unintentionally confuse the two terms, and it is important for the physician to clarify the question and to respond only to the extent of his or her knowledge and expertise.

## AMERICANS WITH DISABILITIES ACT

An increasingly fertile ground for litigation and medical proof is the ADA. Physicians should keep in mind the ADA definition of a disability as (1) a physical or mental impairment that substantially limits one or more of the major life activities of an individual; (1) a record of such an impairment; or (3) being regarded as having such an impairment.[15] A review of the regulations and case law gives a clearer indication of the scope of the ADA. Existing impairments are to be determined without regard to mitigating measures such as medicines or prosthetics. Physical characteristics that are within "normal" range and do not result from a physiologic disorder are not disabilities.[16] Obesity is an impairment if the person is 100% over normal weight.[17] Stress and depression may or may not be considered impairments, depending on whether they result from a documented physiologic or mental disorder.[18] A person with a contagious disease has an impairment.[19] Major life activities under the ADA are the basic activities that the average person can perform with little or no difficulty, such as caring for one's self,

performing manual tasks, walking, seeing, hearing, and speaking.[20] If a person is incapable of performing one or more of these major life activities, he or she may be disabled.

Of particular interest to the physician is what constitutes "a record of a disability."
The physician's medical record, if it documents an impairment or disability, may qualify
as a record under the ADA. The medical history, however, must be related to the impairment that substantially limits a major activity.[21] An employer who relies on educational,
medical, or employment records containing information about a previous disability to
make an adverse employment decision is subject to challenge under the ADA.[1,21]

## FAMILY AND MEDICAL LEAVE ACT

To a limited degree patients may seek benefits or protection under various other
federal legislation, such as the Family and Medical Leave Act of 1993 (FMLA). The
FMLA entitles eligible employees to take up to 12 weeks of unpaid, job-protected leave
in a 12-month period for specified family and medical reasons. The FMLA applies to
public agencies and private sector employers with more than 50 employees.[22] Under the
FMLA a "serious health condition" means an illness, injury, impairment, or physical or
mental condition that involves (1) inpatient care and any corresponding period of incapacity or subsequent treatment or (2) continuing treatment by a health care provider.[2,22]

## ROLE OF PAIN IN DETERMINING DISABILITY AND IMPAIRMENT

Pain is considered subjective and cannot by measured by objective testing. The
AMA *Guides* states that the impairment percentage applicable to permanent impairment of the various organ systems should include allowances for the pain that may
occur with such impairments.[2,22] The *Guides* further states that in estimating the extent
of pain-related impairment, the following criteria should be observed:

1. Acute pain is not a "permanent impairment."
2. Psychogenic pain is a mental disorder that should be evaluated according to the
criteria for mental and behavior disorders.
3. Recurrent acute pain is likely to be classified as primary and nociceptive or
neurogenic. Such pain relates clearly to well-defined diseases or pathologic entities.
4. Chronic pain (chronic pain syndrome) is likely to be classified as secondary
pain. Chronic pain in the absence of objective validated diseases or impairments should
be evaluated on a multidisciplinary basis by physicians with a special interest and background in pain medicine and with consideration of the effects of the pain on the patient's ability to carry out daily activities.[3,22]

Given the medical difficulties in assessing pain, it is understandable that govern-
mental agencies also struggle with the concept. As discussed in the section on Social
Security, generally pain is not a factor in determining disability unless supported by objective evidence. The Social Security listings are based on four levels of ability to work:

1. *Sedentary* refers to work that requires mainly sitting and no physical labor.
2. *Light* refers to work that requires slightly more effort than sedentary.
3. *Medium* refers to work that requires average physical ability.
4. *Heavy to very heavy* refers to work that requires extensive physical ability.[23]

Arguably, pain that prevents a person from performing the level of work for which he
or she is qualified by age, education, and experience should qualify for disability benefits. However, the Social Security Administration determines whether there is any type
of work a person may perform, regardless of whether such jobs are actually available.

Pain may be a factor in determining whether a person is disabled under the ADA.
The definition of disability under the ADA includes a physical impairment that substantially limits one or more of the major life activities.[2,23] Major life activities include

caring for one's self, performing manual tasks, and basic abilities such as walking, seeing, hearing, and speaking. The AMA *Guides* provides for the rating of pain intensity as slight, moderate, or marked, depending on diminution of the ability to carry out daily activities. One may conclude, therefore, that pain that limits one or more of the major life activities will qualify as a disability under the ADA.

The role of pain in workers' compensation depends to a large extent on the evaluation of physical impairment by the physician. If the pain is severe enough to interfere with the ability to work, it is relevant to determining disability under workers' compensation. As a practical matter, the administrative law judge evaluates the credibility of a claim based on pain by taking into account the medical testimony and the claimant's ability to describe the pain. Because the decisions in workers' compensation cases are rarely reviewed or reversed, the judge may consider any factors in determining the degree of disability and loss of ability to earn money. In a personal injury action, pain is definitely a factor in determining the amount of the award. Any and all factors may be considered by the judge or jury in rendering a monetary judgment for "pain and suffering." Generally the court instructs the jury that pain and suffering are incapable of being measured in an exact manner; the amount of compensation is left to the discretion of the jury.

## CONCLUSION

A review of this chapter should give one some understanding of the various and confusing usages of the terms impairment and disability. A physician should be cognizant of any current or proposed legal action by the patient before rendering an opinion about impairment or corresponding disability. At least a passing familiarity with the various statutes and types of claims will assist the physician in these tasks. Perhaps the most important point to understand is when *not* to render an opinion that may be based on incomplete information and result in permanent harm to the patient's claim.

## REFERENCES

1. Liachowitz C: Disability as a Social Constraint. Philadelphia, University of Pennsylvania Press, 1988.
2. American Medical Association, Guides to the Evaluation of Permanent Impairment, 4th ed. Chicago, American Medical Association, 1993.
3. Rothenstein LF: Disabilities and the Law. New York, McGraw-Hill, 1992.
4. Reference deleted.
5. Bickenbach JE: Physical Disability and Public Policy. Toronto, Canada, University of Toronto Press, 1993.
6. 42 USC secs. 301-399.
7. Pub. L. No. 78-113 and 83-565.
8. 42 USC secs. 4151-4157.
9. 29 USC secs. 790-796.
10. 42 USC 12102(2).
11. Larson A: The Law of Workmen's Compensation. New York, Matthew Bender & Co., 1972.
12. 42 USC sec. 423 (d)(l)(a).
13. Reference deleted.
14. 42 USC 12102(2); 29 C.F.R. sec. 1630.2(g).
15. 29 C.F.R. sec. 1630.2(h).
16. Comp. Man. sec. 902.2(c)(4).
17. A Technical Assistance Manual on the Employment Provisions of the ADA, EEOC Jan 1992 sec. 2.1(a).
18. School Board of Nassau County v. Arline, 480 U.S. 273 (1987).
19. Appendix to 29 C.F.R. sec 1630.2(i).
20. 29 C.F.R. sec. 1630.2(l).
21. 29 C.F.R. sec. 1630.2(k).
22. FMLA sec. 825.113.
23. Tucker B, Goldstein B: Legal Rights of Persons with Disabilities: An Analysis of Federal Law. Horsham, PA, LRP Publications, 1996.

# Index

Page numbers in **boldface type** indicate complete chapters.

ABC syndrome, 189
Abductor pollicis longus, 132–133
Abductor pollicis longus tendon, in intersection
  syndrome, 135, 136
Acceleration/deceleration injury. *See also* Whiplash
  injury
  as headache cause, 214–215
  as temporomandibular dysfunction cause,
    234–237
Achilles tendon, injuries to, 124
Acromioclavicular joint
  anatomy of, 162, 164, 165
  arthritis of, 162
  injuries to, 162, 168, 169
  sprains of, trigger point injection treatment of, 95,
    96
Action potentials, generation of, 296–297
Acupressure, as trigger point inactivation technique,
  89
Acupuncture, as posttraumatic headache treatment,
  220
Adductor muscles, strains of, 108
Adhesions, as anterior elbow pain cause, 161
Adolescents, depression diagnosis in, 338
Airbags, as facial trauma cause, 232, 233
Alar ligament, function of, 17
Alcohol, as headache cause, 218
Alexithymia, 349–350
Algometry, pressure, 85, 86, 87–88
Algoneurodystrophy, 189
Allodynia, experimental models of, 193
Alpha blockers, as reflex sympathetic dystrophy
  treatment, 202
Alprazolam, dependency on, 354
AMBRI mnemonic, for shoulder instability, 166
American College of Rheumatology, 101, 102, 103
American Medical Association
  *Guides to the Evaluation of Permanent
    Impairment* of, 359, 361–362
  treatment intervention guidelines of, 322
Americans with Disabilities Act, 358, 360–361
Amino acids deficiency, 218
Amnesia, posttraumatic, 207
Amputation
  as complex regional painful syndrome treatment,
    190
  as refractory reflex sympathetic dystrophy
    treatment, 199

Amyotropathy, diabetic, 257
Analgesics, as zygapophyseal joint pain treatment,
  55–56
Aneurysm, of vertebral artery, spinal manipulation-
  related, 325
Aneurysm clips, cerebral, as magnetic resonance
  imaging contraindication, 281
Anger, differentiated from depression, 337
Angiogenesis, in soft tissue injury, 3
Angiospasm, traumatic, 189
Ankle
  instability of, 124
  inversion sprains of, 122–123
  ligament sprains of, 2
Ankylosing spondylitis
  as sacroiliac joint inflammation cause, 71–72
  zygapophyseal joints in, 52
Annular ligament
  anatomy of, 148
  disruption of, 161
Annulus fibrosus
  anatomy of, 36
  fissures of, imaging of, 285–286, 287
  imaging of, 283, 285–286, 287, 288, 290
  nerve fibers of, 38
  tears of
    in degenerative discs, 37, 285–286
    imaging of, 283, 288, 290
    thermographic evaluation of, 200
Anterior capsule, strains and tears of, 161
Anterior interosseous syndrome, 250–251
Antidepressants
  appetite-stimulating effects of, 350, 351–352,
    354
  as symptomatic treatment, 337
  as zygapophyseal joint pain treatment, 56
Anti-inflammatory drugs. *See also* Nonsteroidal
  anti-inflammatory drugs
  as pain treatment, 323
  as reflex sympathetic dystrophy treatment, 202
  as soft tissue injury treatment, 1
Antisocial personality disorders, 343
Anxiety
  head injury-related, 209
  effect on immune system, 340
  pain-related, 353–354, 355
  posttraumatic headache-related, 216
  reflex sympathetic dystrophy-related, 195, 196